P9-EFH-376

100, 184, 226, 233, 291,
293, 307

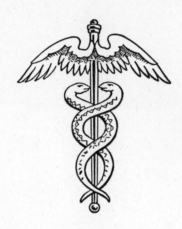

A SKETCH OF MEDICINE
AND PHARMACY

Cover Design

AESCULAPIUS, HYGEIA, AND WORSHIPPERS
A votive tablet from the Athenian Asclepion
(National Museum at Athens)

A

Sketch of Medicine

and

Pharmacy

*and a view of its progress by the
Massengill family from the fifteenth
to the twentieth century.*

By

SAMUEL EVANS MASSENGILL, M. D.

COPYRIGHT, 1942
BY
THE S. E. MASSENGILL COMPANY

SECOND EDITION

PRINTED AT THE S. E. MASSENGILL COMPANY, BRISTOL, TENNESSEE
IN THE UNITED STATES OF AMERICA

TO INA, MY WIFE, AND TO

JOSEPHINE, MY MOTHER,

THIS BOOK IS DEDICATED

❧

610.9
M384s

51023

THERE is no pretense to any original investigation in the history of medicine, nor to any consultation of original documents. I have selected what seemed to be fitting from well-known biographies, monographs, and from standard histories.

"And if so be any man object unto me that this discourse is only compilede together of certayne rapsodyes of the antique Chyrurgians, I willingly heere confes and acknowledge that in this Treatise there is verye little, or nothing at all, of myne own Invention."

—Jacques Guillemeau
A. D. 1594.

Contents

Illustrations

Introduction

ANTIQUITY means ancient or obsolete, and when it is applied to physicians it refers to those who practiced in a misty, distant age. The term usually refers back to the doctors of Egypt, or even Babylon, or early Asiatic countries. But it is a wrong assumption to look upon the physicians of those countries as obsolete.

When history dawned, we find therapeutics well advanced as a science. The Assyrians, Babylonians, and Egyptians had well-established drug stores, which were used as clinics by the leading doctors of the various cities and villages. They had well-written books on materia medica which gave valuable descriptions of several hundred drugs, their preparation and uses.

The history of medicine may be divided into three periods or ages, to be denominated respectively:

    I.   The Mythological;

    II. The Dogmatic or Empirical; and,

    III. The Rational

The Mythological age extends from the infancy of the human race to about the year 400 B. C., and includes what is known from tradition of the early evolution of medicine, together with the meager facts gained from history during this interesting epoch.

The history of medicine really begins with the Dogmatic or Empirical age, and includes that portion of the time between the Hippocratic period (400 B. C.) and the close of the eighteenth century, A. D., or the death of the last Dogmatic system, the Brunonian.

The Rational age in medicine begins where dogmatism leaves off; viz., about the close of the eighteenth century and the beginning of the nineteenth. It is founded upon the ruins of the ancient dogmatic schools, together with the new facts discovered about this time by the rapid evolution of anatomy, physiology, pathology, chemistry and the collateral sciences. The latter two ages are necessarily more or less blended, and seem to overlap each other.

S. E. M.

CHAPTER ONE

Medicine in the Stone Age

THE HISTORY of the physician begins with the dawn of humanity, as disclosed by the fossil records. The great lesson yielded by examinations of the earlist bones of fossil men is that they were subjected to the same accidents and diseases as we are.

The practice of medicine is the oldest and most esteemed of the professions. Primitive man, hundreds of thousands of years ago, was attended in his sickness by men who were expert in medicine.

Before the priest, politician, and lawyer began their practices, the doctor pursued his noble calling and exercised the principal power in his community.

Man learned the practice of medicine at an early age in his development by watching the curative powers of nature, and the practices of animals and birds.

Finger, arm, and other amputations were performed with crude flint instruments. The early Stone Age surgeon was particularly skilled in setting fractures. LeBaron studied the skeletons of eighteen men who had fractured limbs, and found only three had healed badly.

Looking backward, the life of primitive man appears simple to us, but he was probably sufficiently occupied in keeping himself alive. At any rate, he was either not fastidious, or his women had not learned the art of housekeeping, for the floors of his caves were never swept. With the passing generations, layers of debris were covered with accumulating layers, but what was rubbish then is archeology now.

Primitive man himself is depicted as straight and slender, but he liked his women round, and thus the pendulous breasts and overdevelopment of the buttocks were due not only to too much cave-life and too much meat, but to selection.

Rock-shelters and caves were plentiful in those days. In the hills of Ariege, France, is a cavern called The Grotto of the Three Brothers. Some twenty or thirty thousand years ago it sheltered a tribe of those primitive men called Cro-Magnon. Traces of their sojourn still remain after all of the thousands of years that have passed since the dissolution of the tribe; bones and knives, tools and weapons, left in that dry stone cave, have been preserved. There is pictured there the first known representation of a physician, the tribal medicine-man. He is shown clothed in the skin of a deer, and he bears upon his head the antlers of that animal.

The first weapon in the hands of the first surgeon was a flint, and trepanning for the release of demons is the earliest surgical operation of which any evidence remains. Skulls bear witness to what was done aeons before the dawn of civilization.

They also practiced bleeding and the kindred practices of cupping, leeching, and scarifying. All are varieties of blood-letting and are based on the theory that a demon is causing pain or swelling and an exit must be provided if the patient is to be relieved. Also, there are evidences of cauterization.

The surgery of this period began in mystery and magic. Medicine and religion have marched down the centuries hand in hand. For hundreds and thousands of years, the medical man was also a priest and magician. Medicine and chemistry are really the offspring of magic. In primitive societies today the doctor is considered to be a magician.

12

CHAPTER TWO

Medicine in Ancient Egypt

EGYPT was the medical center of the ancient world. The Biblical admission, "And Moses was learned in all the wisdom of the Egyptians," indicates the origin of Mosaic magic. The medical history of Egypt, in early times, is really the history of all the peoples having contact with the Egyptians, because the Egyptians were a people ever alert to copy all which they found admirable in other peoples. From the remains of papyri, from stone tablets and various other inscriptions on monuments and tombs, it has been definitely determined that Egyptian medicine was largely a discipline established under the authority of the gods.

By the time the Egyptians began to write about medicine, the art was so old that they either forgot or ignored its crude beginnings, and preferred to attribute its origin to the gods. They could not eliminate magic from their medicine, or divorce their sacred and secular knowledge. All diseases were regarded as caused by the displeasure of the gods, and of course, according to that view of their pathology, they could be cured in no other way than by appeasing this displeasure, and no other means could be employed by the multitude in order to approach these gods, than through the medium of the priests who administered in the temples. The sick were bewildered with imposing rites and ceremonies. They used venesection, cathartics, emetics and clysters. They claimed to have been taught venesection by the hippopotamus, which, it is said, performed this operation upon itself by striking its leg against a sharp reed and opening a vein in this way, and after the blood had flowed as long as it thought proper, filled the wound with mud. They also claim to have learned the use of clysters from their sacred bird, Ibis, which is said to have administered them to itself with its bill.

According to Herodotus there was in Egypt a special physician for every part of the body. They were thoroughly conversant with such ordinary hygienic measures as baths, massage and inunctions; they studied foods from the point of view of health, appreciated the role played by vermin in disease and practiced fumigation as a means of offsetting epidemics.

Mythology was well developed in Assyrian times, and in Babylonia and Egypt as well, the gods are often referred to in the medical literature. The gods of medicine were developed from outstanding surgeons and physicians, just as the Greeks deified Asklepios, a remarkably bold and successful surgeon, and made him supplant Jove as god of medicine.

There is a remarkable case of this character in Egypt, a country which was always famous for its medical arts and medical schools. Imhotep, or Imouthis, was elevated to be the god of medicine. He was said to be a son of Ptah, of the great triad Ptah-Seket-Osiris, the gods of heaven and earth. Imhotep means the man who comes in peace.

There are many references in the works of romance writers, to the capacity of Imhotep to send people suffering from pain to sleep. This, apparently, refers to his ability to place sick people under anesthetics, and indicates that Egyptian physicians were familiar with anesthetic agencies.

As the good physician both of gods and men, Imhotep cured their ailments while they lived, and in the cases of men, he cared for the preservation and embalming of their bodies at death.

14

Egyptologists who have studied the history of the god Imhotep believe that he was originally a very eminent and skilled physician, whose memory after his death was so wisely and favorably kept, that he eventually was elected to be a god. He appears, also, to have had something of importance to do with the embalming processes and with drugs. This indicates that he was a broadly-learned man—a surgeon, physician, and druggist. His knowledge, too, was great, and there is no doubt that the doctor possessed an unusually broad knowledge of drugs, spices, chemicals, and bandaging materials. He is depicted as bald, but the Egyptians did not like baldness and treated the condition vigorously. Heru-tata was one of the most learned scholars of the earlier settlers in Egypt, and the coupling of his name with that of Imhotep suggests that the god of medicine practiced on the Nile at the time of the earliest Egyptian settlements.

The early Egyptian physicians made considerable use of drugs. Their drugs were of the kind usually found in early civilizations; a few effective remedies lost in a mass of substances of purely superstitious origin. They used opium, squill, and other vegetable substances, but also excrement and urine. It is said that the urine of a faithful wife was with them effective in the treatment of sore eyes. The tale concerning the difficulty in obtaining this remedy (or the ineffectiveness of its cures) has come down with variations through folk tales.

PAPYRI

The Veterinary and Gynecological Papyri from Kahun are the oldest yet discovered, dating back 2160-1788 B. C.

The Surgical Papyrus, written about 1600 B. C., is over fifteen feet in length, and originally was longer.

The Book on Surgery and External Medicine, while copied 3500 years ago, actually reveals Egyptian medicine as it was practised 4500 years ago.

Among the papyri preserved in various museums a number of medical and pharmaceutical records have been found. Some medical prescriptions inscribed on a papyrus in the British Museum (No. 10,059) are said to be as old as the time of Khufu (Cheops), reckoned to have been about 3700 years B. C.

The most complete information of the medicine and pharmacy of ancient Egypt is contained in the famous Papyrus Ebers, which was discovered by Georg Ebers, Egyptologist, in 1872-3. The date is about the year 1552 B. C.

Among the drugs named in the papyrus and identified are oil, wine, beer (sweet and bitter), beer froth, yeast, vinegar, turpentine, various gums and resins, figs, sebestens, myrrh, mastic, frankincense, opium, wormwood, aloe, cumin, peppermint, cassia, carraway, coriander, anise fennel, saffron, sycamore and cyprus woods, lotus flowers, linseed, juniper berries, henbane, and mandragora.

Iron, lead, magnesia, lime, soda, nitre and vermilion are among the mineral products which were then used in medicine.

To prevent the immoderate crying of children a mixture of the seeds of the plant Sheben with some fly-dirt is recommended. It is supposed that Sheben may have been the poppy. Incidentally, it is remarked that if a new-born baby cries "ny" that is a good sign; but it is a bad sign if it cries "mbe."

To prevent the hair turning grey anoint it with the blood of a black calf which has been boiled in oil; or with the fat of a rattlesnake. When it falls out one remedy is to apply a mixture of six fats, namely those of the horse, the hippopotamus, the crocodile, the cat, the snake, and the ibex. To strengthen it anoint with the tooth of a donkey crushed in honey.

Medicines against worms are numerous.

The animal drugs included lizards' blood, swine's teeth, putrid meat, stinking fat, moisture from pigs' ears, milk, goose grease, asses' hoofs, animal fats from various sources, excreta of various animals, including human beings, donkeys, antelopes, dogs, cats, and even flies.

Seven hundred remedies are mentioned in this papyrus, and some of these drugs are serving mankind today: opium, castor oil, acacia, squill, calamus, coriander, hyoscyamus, saffron, colchicum, gentian, pomegranate and olive oil, and the salts of various metals.

Some of the prescriptions of the Ebers Papyrus are very simple. In those for purges they used a mixture of milk, yeast, and honey, or pills compounded of honey, wormwood, and onion. For headache there was used a prescription calling for frankincense, cumin, u'an berries (unidentifiable), and goose grease, which were to be boiled together and used as an external application.

There is one headache remedy attributed to divine origin (Isis having prescribed it for Ra's headache), which contains coriander, wormwood, juniper, honey, and opium.

As a prescription for a tonic there is recommended a preparation made by compounding figs, Assyrian plums, grapes, frankincense, cumin, wine, beer, yeast, and goose grease.

A prescription, annotated as having been prepared for Schesch (a queen of the third dynasty), consisted of equal parts of the heel of an Abyssinian greyhound, of date blossoms, and of asses' hoofs, boiled in oil. This was for the purpose of making the hair grow.

They were also called upon to supply infusions, decoctions, macerations, fumigations, inhalations, gargles, injections, pills, powders, triturations, salves, plasters, confections, cataplasms, and poultices. One ancient remedy, comparatively little used at present, has come down to us through the centuries almost unchanged. This is a mixture of aloe and canella known by the Latin name of "*hiera picra*," literally "sacred bitters."

A perfume called "kyphi," made in the times of the Pharaohs from juniper berries, myrrh, frankincense, cypress wood,

17

aloe wood, calamus, mastic, and styrax, came down through the writings of Dioscorides, the father of materia medica, to later times and was used in religious observances, even in comparatively recent times in Europe.

MUMMIFICATION

The Egyptians astonish us with the lost art of mummification. Mummification failed in its principal object, but it exerted a powerful influence on medicine and surgery, and laid the foundation of anatomy and biology. It has been shown on Egyptian mummies that these ancient people suffered and died from modern diseases such as arteriosclerosis and nephritis.

Egyptian medicine was non-progressive; therefore, it went backward with the centuries. The earlier papyri contain less magic and more medicine, while in the later scrolls the incantations are predominant. The Egyptians did not fully take advantage of the opportunities to leave a scientific legacy to posterity, for during the many centuries they eviscerated millions of their dead, they learned no pathology, and their mummies are evidence of badly united bones and abscessed teeth.

Sekhetananch, the first physician mentioned in history, is but a name, Imhotep is a semi-myth, and we know nothing of their thoughts or methods. However, Egyptian surgeons have rather significant accomplishments to their credit. They bandaged well, cupped and venesected, practiced circumcision and castration, developed men particularly skillful in cutting for bladder stones (lithotomists) and in performing amputations. There were among them ophthalmic surgeons and dentists and clever artificers of surgical instruments.

CHAPTER THREE

Medicine in Ancient Greece

THE OUTSTANDING eminence of Greece in medicine and surgery has led many to believe that modern medicine was founded in Greece. That, however, is a pure fallacy. Medicine and surgery were both inherited in a high state of development. They came to Greece through a long line of other civilized peoples from a remote antiquity. The early history of Greek medicine, like that of political developments, is lost in mythology.

In the early days it must have been primitive, as at the beginning of every civilization—a mixture of religion, magic, and empirically acquired ideas and practises.

The Persians, Indians, Chinese, and other Asiatic peoples were just as much advanced in surgery, medicine, chemistry, and therapeutics as the Assyrians, Babylonians, and Egyptians. All these peoples united their medical knowledge and placed it in the hands of the Greeks to be polished and presented to us.

Ancient Greece was largely colonized by the Egyptians. These colonists brought their deities and their worship along with them, and consequently the mythology of the Greeks was largely borrowed from the Egyptians; and especially was this the case with medical divinities. The Greeks were a restless, warlike people, and soon developed a propensity for manufacturing gods that fairly eclipsed all previous efforts in that line.

19

AESCULAPIUS

Aesculapius was likely a skillful physician, but just as the Egyptian Imhotep, who was originally an historical personage, in time evolved into a deity, so Aesculapius developed into the Grecian god of medicine.

So great, as the Greeks believed, was the power of Aesculapius over disease, so wonderful were the cures which he accomplished, and so noble and pure his character, that they not only made him a god, but erected temples in his honor.

Instruction in medicine was given in the Temple of Aesculapius. This instruction was oral, since there were no written medical works among the Greeks before the fifth century before Christ.

According to legends, Aesculapius suffered many vicissitudes in his early life. By one tale he was said to be the son of Coronis and Apollo, and was saved at birth only by taking him from his mother's womb as she was brought to her funeral pyre. According to another tale his mother was Ascinoe and, while there were no difficulties in the matter of his birth, he was abandoned as an infant, but was saved from starvation by a goat. Aesculapius survived his stormy childhood and lived to marry twice. He was the father of the damsels Hygeia and Panacea, often described as allegorical figures, Hygeia representing health, and Panacea, medicine. The mother of Hygeia was a daughter of his first wife. Hygeia is present in its various forms, such as hygiene, hygienic, and hygienist. His second wife was Lampetia, a daughter of the sun-god.

He was a student of Chiron the centaur, who is said to have established the first medical college mentioned in history, in a cave or grotto at the foot of Mount Pelion, where he taught medicine, music, botany and chirurgery.

Aesculapius grew to manhood in Thessaly, learning from his wise tutor (half man, half horse) which plants had healing

20

virtues, and that many a charm could cure illness. Thus he became a physician, greatly sought after.

The votive tablets on which the god's miraculous healings were recorded, say that Ambrosia, a woman from Athens, was blind of one eye, that Aesculapius slit the eye open, rubbed in balsam, and that thereafter the patient could see perfectly with both eyes. Also, how Agestratus was cured of headaches which had been so severe that he was never able to sleep, and how Gorgias, having a suppurating wound made by an arrow that had pierced his chest, slept beside the altar and awakened with a sound skin holding the arrow point in his hand.

Aesculapius distinguished himself above all others as surgeon-in-chief of the expedition of Argonauts in search of the golden fleece, and his fame has been celebrated in poetry, more as a surgeon than as a physician. One of his principal medicines appears to have been a mixture of wine, meal and scraped cheese made from goat's milk.

Aesculapius' death has been attributed to two different causes. First, after he had restored Hippolytus to life, instead of a reward, incurred destruction by fire at the hands of Zeus because his professional skill excited the wrath of that jealous god. Second, Pluto complained to Zeus that the prolongation of life on the earth, due to the ministrations of Aesculapius, was keeping down the population of Hades. Zeus, to restore the balance of population, slew Aesculapius with a thunderbolt.

HIPPOCRATES

Hippocrates was born on the Island of Cos about 460 B. C., and graduated from the school of Cos and received his medical training in the hospital where his father, Heraclides, was a surgeon. It is claimed that his father, Heraclides, was a direct descendant of Aesculapius, and that his mother, Phenarita, was of the family of Hercules. He also studied under a prominent doctor named Herodicos of Cnidos.

The history of Dogmatic or Empirical medicine, as transmitted to us in a direct line, begins with Hippocrates and his followers. All our information prior to this date partakes largely of the prehistoric or mythological.

Medicine existed for centuries before him, and Hippocrates himself wrote a treatise entitled ON ANCIENT MEDICINE, but we properly call him the Father of Medicine. Everything that has been learned before Hippocrates has perished; and, curiously, there exists a great gap after him as well as before him, so that the writings of Hippocrates remain isolated amongst the ruins of ancient medical literature. His knowledge of medicine was so great that it is suggested that his writings represent the remains of the medical library of Cos.

The great contribution of Hippocrates was medical diagnosis. It was he who established firmly the principle that the knowledge of disease rests primarily upon the careful observation and notation of symptoms. It is questionable whether, all things considered, a more subtly critical clinical mind than his has ever graced the art of medicine.

He separated medicine from religion and philosophy, and made it an independent subject.

Hippocrates flourished when nothing or next to nothing was known of anatomy, physiology, or pathology. Chemistry was as yet an unborn science. Not a single trace of chemistry as applied to pharmacy can be found previous to or during the time in which Hippocrates lived. Little was known of botany; especially of the medicinal properties of plants.

Some of Hippocrates' divisions of diseases have scarcely been modified, and words spoken by physicians daily, in the present age, are found in his writings, with the same meanings as at present; such as acute and chronic; epidemic, endemic and sporadic; malignant and benign, crisis, and so on.

Dislocations of the hip, shoulder, and jaw are described exactly in the Hippocratic works and treated almost as we would treat them today, except that an anesthetic was not used.

Among the diseases treated are pneumonia, pleurisy, malaria, tuberculosis, wounds, bites of serpents, and occasional epidemics. Catarrhs, gout, dysentery, and lung diseases only came with luxury.

In writing of the consumptives, he says, "Many, and in fact, the most of them, died; and of those confined to bed, I do not know if a single individual survived for any considerable time." Of the forty-two case-histories detailed, twenty-five end in death.

In his writings he refers to nearly four hundred remedies. For quinsy, he burned sulphur and asphalte with hyssop. He gave narcotics, including, it is supposed, the juice of the poppy and henbane seeds, and mandragora; purgatives, sudorifics, emetics, and enemas. His purgative drugs were generally drastic ones: the hellebores, elaterium, colocynth, scammony, thapsia, and a species of rhamnus. He also used milder remedies such as, barley gruel, hydromel, oxymel, and wine, and placed his faith in the healing power of nature.

Hippocrates describes methods for what he calls purging the head and the lungs, that is, by means of sneezing and coughing.

Of Hippocrates as an individual it may be said that he was the embodiment of all that a physician should be. He was a close observer, a humane scholar, and a man filled with the desire to help his patients and to ensure that by his teaching and experience others should benefit. High ideals are set forth simply in the Hippocratic oath. This oath has been respected by physicians and surgeons of every race and creed for two thousand years.

The treatise ON THE PROGNOSTICS will always be famous for the Hippocratic description of the signs of approaching death which we still call *facies Hippocratica*: nose sharp, eyes

23

hollow, temples sunken, ears cold and contracted with their lobes turned outward, skin tense and parched, face discolored, eyelids livid, mouth open, lips loose and blanched.

There are many fables and anecdotes designed to show how great a physician was Hippocrates, for example:

Wandering from place to place, he traversed the whole of Greece, and his cures aroused general astonishment. The king of Macedon fell sick, and his doctors believed him to be consumptive. Hippocrates was called in consultation with Euryphon, the court physician, and recognized that the king's illness was not consumption but was what we should now call psychogenic—of mental causation. The philosopher Democritus had become insane, and the people of Abdera sent for Hippocrates to cure him, and also to free their city of the plague. In Athens, too, pestilence was raging. Hippocrates appeared upon the scene and noticed that the smiths were immune. Fire, then, must be a remedy, and Hippocrates had huge bonfires kept burning until the epidemic abated.

A swarm of bees is said to have settled near his tomb; the honey from this hive was reputed to possess remedial virtues for centuries thereafter. This was an example of reversion to type, for Hippocrates himself would not have countenanced such a superstitious belief.

GALEN

Claudius Galen was born in Pergamos, Greece, in 130 or 131 A. D., and is said to have died in the same city between 200 and 210 A. D.

He received instruction from distinguished teachers in both the Dogmatic and Empiric schools and undertook the task of reforming medicine. He claimed in the beginning of his career to be an Eclectic, but soon proved himself to be the most bigoted and intolerant of Dogmatics.

From the body of medical writings then available, he took whatever seemed good to him. If he recognized any master,

24

it was the founder of the healing art, Hippocrates. The Galenic system of medicine, thus established by the practical skill of its founder upon the most accessible materials which intelligent zeal could use, was servilely followed throughout the Middle Ages.

Galen was a genius, a born physiologist, a brilliant exponent of experimental methods, and a first-class anatomist. His system of anatomy was accepted by the entire civilized world, until the time of Vesalius.

Galen, the best-educated and most gifted physician of the second century—and of the centuries to come—could not be content in the provinces or in fallen Alexandria; therefore, as a stranger he entered Rome, 162 A. D.

Galen was always conscious of his own abilities and his own superiority in learning; he was always burning with ambition and hopeful for grander fields for his activities, and there was a weakness in his character which he appears to have been quite unaware of and which always handicapped him. It was his irascibility. This narrowed his vision, and, as all his writings show, constantly kept him in a combative mood. Pugnacity, and a strong desire to criticize other medical writers, are plainly featured in all his writings. Speaking of his parents, Galen wrote:

"I was blest with a calm, just, gallant, and sympathetic father, whereas my mother was of so irritable a temper that she would at times bite her maids, and was forever screaming and quarreling with my father, worse than Xanthippe with Socrates."

Galen was not only a strongly critical writer, but a boastful and conceited doctor, as his recital of his conversation with Marcus Aurelius, his patient, bears witness:

"This diagnosis called forth his praise, and he thrice repeated: 'Yes, that is it; it is exactly as you say; I feel that cold food is disagreeing with me.'

"He then asked me what was to be done. I answered him frankly that if another than he had been the patient, I should have, following my custom, given him wine with pepper.

" 'With Sovereigns like yourself, however, doctors are in the habit of employing the least drastic remedies, therefore it must suffice to apply upon the abdomen wool with warm spikenard.'

"The Emperor replied that warm ointment on purple wool was his usual remedy for pain in the stomach, and called Dr. Peitholaos to apply it and let me go. This being done, and his feet warmed by rubbing with heated hands, he demanded Sabine wine, threw pepper into it and drank, after which he said to Dr. Peitholaos that now, at last, he had a physician and a courageous one, repeating that I was the first of physicians and the only philosopher."

"I have done as much to medicine," wrote Galen, "as Trojan did to the Roman Empire, in making bridges and roads throughout Italy. It is I alone that have pointed out the true method of treating diseases: it must be confessed that Hippocrates had already chalked out the same road, but as the first discoverer, he has not gone so far as we could wish; his writings are defective in order, in the necessary distinctions; his knowledge in some subjects is not sufficiently extensive; he is often obscure after the manner of the ancients, in order to be concise; he opened the road, but I have rendered it passable."

The following quotations illustrate the varying opinions of Galen:

"They called him Paradoxologos, and Logiatros, which meant that he was a boaster and a master of phrases. It appears that he was able to hold his own in this wordy warfare."

"Galen was himself a large-sized bundle of conceit, prone both to dilate upon his own wisdom and skill and very fond of reciting his own remarkable cures and emphasizing the impossibility of less wise individuals accomplishing similar results."

26

No other physician has ever occupied the commanding position of Claudius Galen. For fifteen centuries he dominated medical thought as powerfully as did Aristotle in the schools of the day. Not until the Renaissance did daring spirits begin to question the infallibility of this medical Pope.

The more we know of Galen, however, the less surprised are we at his hold over the minds of men. Only those who are ignorant of Galen's immense knowledge, his practical common sense, and the frequent marvellous anticipations of what we think most modern, affect to despise him.

No writer of either ancient or modern times can compare with Claudius Galenus probably in the abundance of his output, but certainly in the influence he exercised over the generations that followed him. For fifteen hundred years the doctrines he formulated, the compound medicines he either introduced or endorsed, and the treatments he recommended commanded almost universal submission among medical practitioners.

Some of the diseases treated by Galen are as follows: Fevers, and everything connected with febrile affections, callosities, corns, burns, blisters, sneezing, coughing, bruised nail, headache, toothache, baldness, bleeding of the nose, loss of eyelashes, freckles, wrinkles, colic, dropsy, jaundice, coryza, asthma, dysentery, diseases of the teeth, wounds of nerves, erysipelas and emphysema.

Ancient scientific medicine reached the summit of its development when Galen's last great volume was printed. His system of medicine comprised all that was known in his time.

"Galen was the last of the Greeks and when he spoke no more, the voice of the ancient world was hushed. Galen was the final star that shone in the twilight of antiquity, and when his effulgence was extinguished, there settled over Europe a darkness that was not lifted for many centuries."

HEROPHILUS AND ERASISTRATUS

There were many great physicians during the golden age of medicine in Greece. Two of these were connected with the University of Alexandria, established in the fourth century B. C., and drew its sustenance not from Egypt but from Greece—Herophilus (about 300 B. C.), who is called the Father of Anatomy, and Erasistratus (about 360 B. C.), who is called the Father of Physiology. These two physicians are the first who publicly dissected the human body—and it has been whispered down the ages that condemned criminals were furnished to these investigators who were thus enabled to contrast dissection with vivisection. The first who made this statement was Celsus: "They procured criminals out of prison by royal permission, and dissecting them alive, contemplated, while they were yet breathing, the parts which nature had before concealed."

Because Herophilus was the first who regularly dissected the body of man and studied it systematically, he is known as the Father of Anatomy.

Examples of the sayings of Herophilus include: "He is the best physician who knows how to distinguish the possible from the impossible." "Medicines are nothing in themselves, if not properly used, but the very hands of the gods, if employed with reason and prudence." "To lose one's health renders science null, art inglorious, strength effortless, wealth useless and eloquence powerless." They deserve a place beside Sophocles' "Sleep is the physician of pain," and "Death is the supreme healer of maladies."

There are many interesting anecdotes concerning Herophilus. One of the best of these relates to the keenness of his medical insight. While he was examining the patient, Stratonice, a young woman, one of the elderly king's wives, entered the room. From the quickening of the sick man's pulse and from the flush which spread over his cheeks, the doctor recognized that the illness was mental rather than bodily—that a

28

passion for his inaccessible stepmother was at the root of the trouble.

According to another ancient tradition, Erasistratus presented the temple of the Pythian Apollo at Delphi with a pair of dental forceps made out of lead—as a hint that doctors would do well to extract only such teeth as were loose in their sockets.

AULUS CORNELIUS CELSUS

Aulus Cornelius Celsus, the most distinguished Roman writer on medicine, lived in the age of Tiberius between 14 A. D. and 37 A. D. Celsus took up the study of medicine with such good effect that he has made an immortal name for himself by his great series of books on the practice of medicine—books that have been of immense service to the medical profession and mankind. He has been called the Father of Plastic Surgery, and was admiringly known as the Roman Hippocrates.

Celsus is notable for the description of inflammation, familiar to every medical student: redness, swelling, heat and pain *(rubor et tumor, cum calore et dolore)*.

The only remaining works of Celsus, De Re Medicina, contained, among the other data, authentic principles of plastic surgery. Published 1300 years after his death, this volume was one of the first medical books to be printed (1478), passed through more editions than any other scientific treatise of that era.

Among the many accomplishments of Celsus was his description of forty skin diseases.

One of Celsus' prescriptions for preventing the decay of the teeth was called "sory." It consisted of poppy seed, pepper, and copper sulphate, made into a paste with galbanum. He also employed enemas of sea-water, and poultices of flaxseed or of foenugreek.

Celsus describes the ideal surgeon as follows:

"A surgeon ought to be young, or at any rate, not very old; his hand should be firm and steady, and never shake; he should be able to use his left hand with as much dexterity as his right; his eye-sight should be acute and clear; his mind intrepid, and so far subject to pity as to make him desirous of the recovery of his patient, but not so far as to suffer himself to be moved by his cries; he should neither hurry the operation more than the case requires, nor cut less than is necessary, but do everything just as if the other's screams made no impression upon him."

DIOCLES

In the second half of the fourth century B. C. there arose a great doctor in Athens. Diocles by name, he was born in Carystus, on the island of Euboea. He wrote a great work on hygiene.

We owe our thanks to Diocles and his Greek congeners for having formulated a regimen based upon the conception of the human being as a unity of body and mind, and at the same time one which, with few modifications, remains the hygienist's ideal for all time.

He was a dissector of animals and occasionally of human material, and wrote the first Greek herbal and the first book entitled ON ANATOMY, and was acclaimed the greatest physician after Hippocrates. He is to be grouped therefore with Alcmaeon of Croton, the discoverer of the optic nerves, and with Diogenes of Apollonia, the investigator of the blood vessels, as among the forerunners of Herophilus.

EMPEDOCLES

Empedocles, in the fifth century, B. C., was the first comparative anatomist. Empedocles must have had a crude idea of the circulation of the blood, for he says: "The heart lies in seas of blood which dart in opposite directions."

ANCIENT MEDICAL SCHOOLS

The professors in the luxurious medical colleges in Nineveh, Babylon, Thebes, Memphis, Sais, Heliopolis, Silsilis, and other cities, gave daily lectures on therapeutics and pharmacology to students from all parts of the civilized world. Their extensive knowledge of drugs was handed down to them from a remote antiquity.

The first modern university was the University of Alexandria, established in the fourth century B. C. Among the learned men who answered the summons to Alexandria were two physicians, Herophilus and Erasistratus, whose writings were of considerable note. Anatomy and physiology, the first of the basic and experimental sciences born of medicine, were cradled in Alexandria—but drew their sustenance not from Egypt, but from Greece. During the centuries that this medical school flourished, it was unrivaled. Several of these pupils acquired practice and fame, though none of the Alexandrians approached in importance the founders of the school —Herophilus and Erasistratus.

CHAPTER FOUR

Medicine in Rome

TO BEGIN with, Roman medicine had been primitive medicine. As everywhere else, so there, it had been a mixture of religious and magical ideas with empirical knowledge. One who was stricken with fever, prayed to the goddess of fever. A pregnant woman offered up sacrifices to Lucina or Carmenta. Even during the era of the republic, the art of medicine remained extremely primitive. There were domestic remedies for pains and coughs and diarrhea. Cabbage was regarded as an extremely valuable drug. A certain amount of knowledge had been acquired concerning the treatment of wounds, and splints were applied to a broken bone. But in addition to such means, or when they proved ineffective, recourse was had to spells and charms. Common, too, was the practice of wearing amulets to protect against the evil eye and other sinister powers. One who owned numerous slaves was certain to have among them a person regarded as skilled in medical matters. Such a slave was extremely valuable in the household, and commanded a high price.

Cato, the dominant Roman for three generations, stood in the path of Greek learning. Cabbage was his panacea. He wrote: "Cabbage is good for everything." And this further: "keep the urine of one who is wont to eat cabbage. Warm it. Immerse the patient in it. You will soon cure him by this

33

treatment. It has been tried. Also if you wash small children with this urine, they will never become weakly. And if there is any bruise it will break it up and heal it if you apply mashed cabbage. And if any ulcer and cancer arise in the breasts apply mashed cabbage, it will heal it."

"Averse to sexual passion, he supervised the coition of his dependents. Preaching purity, he was detected in his own home in the act of corrupting a slave-girl. The apostle of continence, in his old age he took a young bride. Such was the man without a vice, who made virtue loathsome."

While the Greeks were developing their rational system of medicine, the Romans were without any systematized medicine. They had, instead, systematized superstitions. They looked for aid from their deities, of which there was one for every disease and indeed for every stage of every disease. Their medical practice is summed up in the statement that "even the itch was not without its goddess."

The Romans at first had no laws to punish malpractice, poisoning, and the manipulation of wills by hired physicians.

Pliny, the lawyer, who lived in the first century after Christ, says of physicians: "It is at the expense of our perils that they learn, and they experimentalize by putting us to death, a physician being the only person that can kill another with sovereign impunity. Nay, even more than this, all the blame is thrown upon the sick man only; he is accused of disobedience forthwith, and it is the person who is dead and gone that is put upon trial."

When Corinth was destroyed in 146 B. C., Greece lost her dominating influence. Weakened by barbarian immigration which destroyed the vigor of the race, the better class of Greeks, and particularly the merchants and professional men, including the doctors, were among the first to migrate to and settle in Rome, where they labored and taught for several centuries.

The Greek doctors found a fertile field for their services in Rome. Ever-increasing luxurious living had a sequence of weaknesses and diseases, which were unknown before and which the herbalists, quacks, and family medicines could not cope with.

ARCHAGATHUS

The first Greek physician who settled in Rome was appropriately named Archagathus, which means a good beginning.

ASCLEPIADES

On the whole the newcomers were regarded with distrust, but finally one of them succeeded in establishing Greek medicine upon a firm footing in Rome. This was Asclepiades, who has been called the father of Fashionable Physicians.

He was born in Bithynia about 96 B. C. He began his career by teaching rhetoric. He found he could not make much money as a rhetorician, but it helped him enormously in medicine.

The Dogmatic school flourished without serious opposition until about the year 287 B. C., when there arose a formidable rival, which is known by the name of the Empiric School. They assailed the doctrines of the Dogmatic school with great fury, and abused Hippocrates, although they continued to use his medicines. But in the meantime another sect had arisen, which was known by the name of the Methodic School. The platform of principles upon which this school was founded was furnished by Asclepiades.

He knew how to blow his own trumpet. He promised *"curare tuto, celeriter, et jucunde"*—to cure safely, swiftly, and pleasantly. (This phrase originated with him). A man, he said, would be a poor physician who had not two or three remedies ready for use in every case of illness; well-tried remedies. He himself had such remedies. Nor were these remedies the violent purgatives and vomitories of his colleagues. He cured by prescribing fasts, abstinence, massage, active and passive movements.

One day a funeral procession was winding its way through the streets of Rome. Suddenly a loud voice startled all: "I am Asclepiades, and I say take this funeral feast from the pyre to the table." Asclepiades brought the body to his house, applied restoratives which reestablished respiration, and the supposed corpse participated in his own funeral festivities.

Did Hippocrates say, "Nature is the healer of disease?" Then Asclepiades said, "Not only is nature useless, it may even be harmful. A natural healing power, curing diseases by design, is a delusion. The physician must actively interfere with nature. It is the physician's duty to cure safely, quickly, pleasantly."

Pliny criticized Asclepiades in the following language: "There is, however, one thing, and one thing only, at which we have any ground for indignation—the fact, that a single individual, and he belonging to the most frivolous nation in the world, a man born in utter indigence, should all on a sudden, and that, too, for the sole purpose of increasing his income, give a new code of medical laws to mankind."

Though Asclepiades was a charlatan he had much to his credit. He was the first who definitely divided disease into acute and chronic, he described malaria, catalepsy, frenzy and lethargy, and treated the insane with gentleness, sunlight, music and song.

This ex-rhetorician was a foreigner, but he knew his Romans. His treatment consisted in massage, wine, exercise, such as walking, riding or dancing, bathing, etc. He often permitted luxurious meals, in some cases he prescribed plenty of sleep, and in others sexual intercourse.

If a doctor fell sick, laymen were wont to make fun of him, saying sarcastically *"Merice cura te ipsum"* (Physician, heal thyself). It is said that Asclepiades proclaimed that he would no longer call himself a physician if he ever fell sick. When well advanced in years, he did not die of illness but of an accident, through falling down a flight of stairs.

In medicine the Romans did little or nothing. All their medicine they borrowed from the Greeks, adding nothing of their own, except their great contribution in the field of public sanitation. The practical Romans were better plumbers than the Greeks—their aqueducts are still working; otherwise, the legacy of Rome is largely evil.

In Rome, Greek medicine reached its second climax before its ultimate fall, which was ascribed to the prohibition of human dissection.

"So bloodthirsty were the Romans of this period, that neither the populace nor the fashionables could enjoy a holiday unless contending ranks of gladiators were butchered for their sport, but they recoiled with horror at the notion of permitting a scientist to examine the murdered corpse."

"Rome, which would not attend a circus unless human blood was spilled, blunted the scalpel. Those ages which destroyed life for amusement, or took it at the least provocation, were the most stringent in protecting the cadaver."

When in 330 A. D., the capital of the Roman Empire was removed from Rome to Constantinople, the leading professional men went with Constantine to his new home.

GREEK PHYSICIANS IN ROME

There were many famous Greek physicians and surgeons who settled in Rome. A few of them will be mentioned:

CLAUDIUS GALEN entered Rome in the year 162 A. D. and practiced there for four years.

ANTYLLUS was the creator of arterial surgery, and was the first to distinguish aneurysm caused by pathological dilatation and aneurysm forming after trauma of the artery.

ARCHIGENES was one of the great surgeons of his era, operating in cancer of the breast and womb, and amputating limbs, with employment of the ligature, in a manner that we consider modern. He wrote the best contemporary account of leprosy, distinguished between primary and secondary symptoms in disease "and found time—in the intervals of using the vaginal speculum and prescribing hair-dyes for the fashionable ladies—to become the author of the most elaborate of the ancient treatises on the pulse."

ARETAEUS described asthma, tetanus, epilespy, diphtheria, hysteria, satyriasis, warned against excess of bloodletting, seems to have understood the direction of the blood-flow in the veins, and was the author of the first systematic account of diabetes.

Aretaeus made the following remarks on the treatment of epilepsy: "It is told, that the brain of a vulture, and the heart of a raw cormorant, and the domestic weasel, when eaten, remove the disease; but I have never tried these things. However, I have seen persons holding a cup below the wound of a man recently slaughtered, and drinking a draught of the blood! O the present, the mighty necessity, which compels one to remedy the evil by such a wicked abomination! And whether even they recovered by this means no one could tell me for certain. There is another story of the liver of a man having been eaten. However, I leave these things to be described by those who would bear to try such means."

Aretaeus' advice for procuring sleep was as follows: "Gentle rubbing of the feet with oil, patting of the head, and particularly stroking of the temples and ears is an effectual means; for by the stroking of their ears and temples wild beasts are overcome, so as to cease from their anger and fury. But whatever is familiar to any one is to him provocative of sleep. Thus, to the sailor, repose in a boat, and being carried about on the sea, the sound of the beach, the murmur of the waves, the boom of the winds, and the scent of the sea and the ship. But to the musician the accustomed notes of his flute in stillness; or playing on the harp or lyre, or the exercise of musical children with song. To a teacher, intercourse with the tattle of

38

children. Different persons are soothed to sleep by different means."

The following are quotations from Aretaeus' writings: "This is a mighty wonder, that in hemorrhage from the lungs, which is particularly dangerous, patients do not despair, even when near their end. The insensibility of the lungs to pain appears to me to be the cause of this; for pain even when slight makes one fear death. In most cases pain is more dreadful than pernicious, whereas the absence of it, even in serious illness, is unaccompanied by fear of death and is more dangerous than dreadful."

Aretaeus continued as follows: "For it is the semen, when possessed of vitality, which makes us to be men, hot, well braced in limbs, hairy, well voiced, spirited, strong to think and to act, as the characteristics of men prove. For when the semen is not possessed of its vitality, persons become shriveled, have a sharp tone of voice, lose their hair and their beard, and become effeminate, as the characteristics of eunuchs prove."

"If you give a medicine at the height of the dyspnea, or when death is at hand, you may be blamed for the patient's death by the vulgar."

"When he can render no further aid, the physician alone can still mourn as a man with his incurable patient: this is the physician's sad lot."

HELIODORUS' writings have been mostly lost, but the few fragments saved reveal him as a great surgeon. He says: "Amputation above the elbow or knee is very dangerous owing to the size of the vessels divided. Some operators in their foolish haste cut through all the soft parts at one stroke, but it seems to me better to first divide the flesh on the side away from the vessels, and then to saw the bone, so as to be ready at once to check the bleeding when the large vessels are cut. And before operating, it is my habit to tie a ligature as tightly as possible above the point of amputation." He wrote on operative treatment of hernia, stricture, resections, flap and circular amputa-

39

tions, bandaging, probing injuries to the skull and torsion of blood-vessels.

Juvenal has branded Heliodorus with infamy because he castrated robust young slaves so their lustful mistresses may use them with impunity: "Matron and maid, the sex has turned all whore; to escape abortion they love the eunuchs, but only such as have been gelded at manhood's age; all that the navel-string could give is present except the beard—and that's the barber's loss, not theirs."

THEMISON OF LAODICEA was the most conspicuous disciple of Asclepiades. Themison considered his doctrines a middle way or method between the dogmatists and empiricists, and was responsible for the formation of another medical sect —the Methodic School. He was once bitten by a mad dog, and therefore could not write on rabies without developing the symptoms.

Juvenal, the magnificent hater, who coined the expression of matrimonial halter, and greeted a rake's announcement that he had found a girl of old-fashioned virtue with the exclamation, "O physicians! open the middle vein, he is mad!" wrote of Themison:

"Besides all this, the little blood in the old man's chilly frame is warm except with fever. All kinds of diseases dance around him in a troop. If you were to ask their names, I could sooner tell you how many lovers Hippia had; how many patients Themison has killed off in a single autumn; how many partners Basilus has cheated; how many wards Hirrus has corrupted; how many embraces tall Maura has submitted to in a single day."

DIOSCORIDES, an army surgeon in the service of Nero, in which capacity he traveled extensively, everywhere on the lookout for medicines, is the greatest of medical botanists. In the sense that Hippocrates is the Father of Medicine, and Theaphrastus, the Father of Botany, Dioscorides is the Father of Materia Medica.

Opium was known long before his time, but Dioscorides was the first who distinctly praised it. He pointed out that it allays pain, induces sleep, is useful in chronic coughs, and in overdoses occasions a deep and terrible lethargy.

SORANUS of Ephesus in Asia Minor—nearly all the leading Greek physicians of the Roman empire came from Asia Minor—stands out as the first specialist in diseases of women and children. Like most of the famous physicians of the time, he studied in Alexandria, and settled in Rome.

CHAPTER FIVE

Arabian Medicine in the Middle Ages

FOR CONSIDERABLY over a thousand years we find that Arabian medicine was based upon the Greek systems, and Persia brought it to maturity. The influence of the doctors of Islam upon modern medicine was profound. They snatched the torch of Hellenistic culture before it was snuffed out at the beginning of the Dark Ages, and preserved the remains until scholarship was revived in the fifteenth and sixteenth centuries. Without their aid, the great works of the Greek and other ancient medical men would have been entirely lost, and the practice of medicine today would have suffered in consequence. Had the Greek texts been lost, and the vast teachings of antiquity been unknown, modern medicine would have been in a far less advanced condition.

The Arabs not only preserved the medical books and practices of antiquity, but they also raised the status of medicine in Europe from a menial condition to a learned profession, by establishing schools and insisting upon a system of rigid qualifying examination for doctors. Chemistry, as applied to medicine, was also their discovery.

In one respect the Persians were wiser than the Greeks, for they informed Heroditus: "We think that it is wrong to carry women off: but to be zealous to avenge the rape is foolish: wise men take no account of such things: for plainly the women never have been carried away, had not they themselves wished it. We of Asia regarded the rape of our women not at all; but the Greeks, all for the sake of a Lacadaemonian woman, mustered a great host, came to Asia, and destroyed the power of Priam. Ever since then we have regarded the Greeks as our enemies."

Much of the early Arabian medical practice was based upon amulets. The Arabic amulets of earlier times consisted of a phrase from the Koran, written by the priest on papyrus (and later on paper). This was then put up in a leather or metal case and worn constantly as near the afflicted part as it was possible to keep it. It was necessary that the amulet must have been written by the priest on a Friday, shortly before sunset, and with ink containing certain drugs, as myrrh and saffron.

The Arabians contributed many new drugs and encouraged the use of some older ones which had almost been forgotten. We are indebted to them for the use of senna, camphor, rhubarb, musk, myrrh, cassia, tamarind, nutmeg, clove, cubeb, aconite, ambergris, cannabis, and sandalwood. They were the originators of syrups, juleps, alcohol, and aromatic waters.

Some of the Arabian authorities speak of a form of anesthesia by inhalation. This was probably derived from the Chinese, for Hua To, the Hippocrates of China, is said to have taught this practice and used for the purpose a combination of aconite, datura, and henbane. It was later revived in the thirteenth century, when it was called the "soporific sponge."

The Hindus discovered the surgical use of loadstone, plastic surgery, and their surgical instruments were extensive, including knives of steel that could divide a hair, reedlike catheters, fluid-removing trocars, bone-dividing nippers, polypus-forceps, cupping-glasses, and one hundred-and-one blunt instruments.

RHAZES (865-925)

The most distinguished of the Arabian physicians, who was called the Galen of his time, was the man whose rather lengthy

Arabian name, beginning with Abu Bekr Mohammed, finished with el-Razi, and who has hence been usually referred to in the history of medicine as Rhazes. He was born at Raj, in Persia. He drew many pupils to Bagdad to benefit by his teaching.

Some of his aphorisms are said to have been:

"Truth in medicine is a goal which cannot be absolutely reached, and the art of healing, as it is described in books, is far beneath the practical experience of a skillful, thoughtful physician."

"At the beginning of a disease choose such remedies as will not lessen the patient's strength."

"Physicians ought to console their patients even if the signs of impending death seem to be present. For the bodies of men are dependent on their spirits."

"In treating a patient, let your first thought be to strengthen his natural vitality. If you strengthen that, you remove ever so many ills without more ado. If you weaken it, however, by the remedies that you use, you always work harm."

"The patient who consults a great many physicians is likely to have a very confused state of mind."

It was proposed to build a great hospital in Bagdad, and the Caliph consulted Rhazes about it. Rhazes selected the site by a simple but effective experiment. He had pieces of raw meat hung up in different parts of the city. The hospital was built at the point where the raw meat had decomposed least rapidly.

There is scarcely any feature of modern medicine and surgery that Rhazes does not touch, and oftener than not his touch is sure and rational. His treatment of the upper respiratory tract is much farther advanced than we might think possible at this time. He advises tracheotomy whenever there is great difficulty of respiration, and describes how it should be done. His treatment of fractures, luxations, and hernia was practical and his monograph on smallpox was eminently important. He was perhaps one of the first men to use sutures of animal gut for the repair of abdominal wounds.

Among the methods of treatment for which Rhazes is responsible may be mentioned that of phthisis, with milk and sugar; of high fever, with cold water; of weakness of the stomach and of the digestive organs, with cold water and buttermilk; and he advises sufferers from melancholia to play chess. He states that fever is not itself a disease, but an effort of nature to cast out a disease. He was particularly careful in the use of purgatives, which he said were apt to occasion irritation of the intestinal canal, and in dysentery he relied usually on fruits, rice, and farinaceous food, though in severe cases he ordered quicklime, arsenic, and opium.

Mercury in the form of ointment and corrosive sublimate were applied by him externally, the latter for itch; yellow and red arsenic and sulphates of iron and copper were also among his external remedies. Borax (which he called tenker), saltpetre, red coral, various precious stones, and oil of ants, are included among the internal remedies which he advises.

Rhazes would not have been ill-equipped for practice a thousand years before his time in the Isle of Cos or practice a thousand years later in a modern hospital.

ALI ABBAS

Ali Abbas, a distinguished Arabian physician who died near the end of the tenth century, was the successor in prestige to Rhazes.

He wrote the ROYAL BOOK OF MEDICINE. This became the leading textbook of medicine for the Arabs until replaced by the CANON OF AVICENNA some two centuries later.

Abbas realized that book-learning did not suffice for a physician. "It is incumbent," he wrote, "that the student of this Art should constantly attend the hospitals and sick-houses; pay unremitting attention to the conditions and circumstances of their inmates, in company with the most acute professors of Medicine; and enquire frequently as to the state of the patients and the symptoms apparent in them, bearing in mind what he

46

has read about these variations, and what they indicate of good or evil."

Ali Abbas perceived that both sexes are prone to depression at the approach of puberty, and he classified love under melancholia, and recommended the following for lovesick youths: "They should take baths," said Ali Abbas, "moderate horse exercise, and anoint themselves with oil of violets. They should look upon gardens, fields, meadows and flowers, listen to sweet and low sounds as of the lute or lyre, and their minds should be occupied by stories, or pleasant and interesting news. But they must also have some work or business so as to keep them from idleness, and from thoughts of the loved ones; and it is good to excite them to quarrels and arguments, that their minds may be yet further distracted. Let them also cultivate the acquaintance of other young women."

ALBUCASIS (or Abulcasis)

Albucasis, like many contributors to medical literature from among the Arabs, was born in Spain, but he wrote in Arabic. The exact year of his birth is not known, but he flourished in the second half of the tenth century. He is said to have lived to the age of 101. His work represents the only independent surgical book produced during the whole of the Arabian period. He is said to be the conservator of dentistry in this period.

The Arabs have been described as blood-shy and knife-shy, but it was Albucasis who made the actual cautery their national instrument. Albucasis and Avicenna established the cautery as being a cure for practically all the ills with which Allah had seen fit to afflict mankind. It was to be used for apoplexy, epilepsy, headache, toothache, piles, pleurisy, dropsy, sciatica, melancholia, and most other real or imaginary conditions.

AVICENNA (About 980-1037)

Ibn Sina, whose Arabic name was transformed into Avicenna, was born in Persia, at the height of Arabian influence, and is sometimes spoken of as the chief representative of Arabian medicine, of as much importance for it as Galen for later Greek medicine. His principal book is the so-called CANON. It replaced the compendium CONTINENS of Rhazes, and, in the East, continued until the end of the fifteenth century to be looked upon as the most complete and best system of medicine. The CANON is both the epitome and the summation of Graeco-Arabian medicine. What Galen did for the Romans, Avicenna accomplished for the Moslems. His book, the ANTIDOTARIUM, is the foundation of our knowledge of the drug-giving of his time.

For over three centuries after the foundation of medical schools in Europe, Avicenna was still in the hands of all those who had an enthusiasm for medical science.

He attended the sick without fees, and says he was rewarded by discovering new methods of treatment.

Avicenna has been sleeping since the year 1037, but he still treats all the invalids of Persia. His activity was extraordinary, for he composed a treatise on many other subjects. At eighteen he cured a king of a serious illness, and the fee enchanted him: he was permitted to use the royal archives with its manuscripts that had no duplicates. This irreplaceable library disappeared in fire, and before its ashes had cooled, the rumor was spread that Avicenna burned it to hide the sources of his knowledge.

His amazing career began in his childhood, for at the age of ten he memorized the Koran; neither arithmetic nor Arabic poetry presented any difficulties. He found medicine easy: "Medicine is no hard and thorny science, like mathematics and metaphysics, so I soon made great progress; I became an excellent doctor, and began to treat patients, using approved remedies. . . . At twelve years of age I disputed in law and logic. . . . When I found a difficulty, I referred to my notes and prayed to the Creator. At night, when weak or sleepy, I strengthened myself with a glass of wine."

"That he advised a louse to be inserted in the meatus of persons suffering from retention of urine, is simply additional evidence of the easy capacity of the Arabians to mix absurdities with their rational procedures. It is almost unbelievable how frequently Avicenna's louse, modified at times to a bug or a flea, reappears in the venereal literature." In treating gonorrhea, Avicenna was probably the first to use catheters made of the skin of various animals.

"The night was always young to Avicenna, and when manuscripts were put aside, the wine-jug was seldom empty, and he relaxed amid minstrels and dancing-girls. His sensualism was as famous as his scholarship, and all Islam asked: Which does Ibn Sina love the more—learning, or wine and women?"

AVENZOAR

Avenzoar, transformed from his family Arabic name, Ibn-Zohr, is counted among the greatest of the Spanish-Arabian physicians. He was probably born in Penaflor, not far from Seville. He died in Seville in 1162 at the age, it is said, of ninety-two years.

Avenzoar wrote the first account of the bezoar stone, a superstition which prevailed for centuries. The name, bezoar, is derived from the Persian words, Pad-Zahr, meaning "expel poison." The pebbles were first popularized by the Arabs, who had many superstitions about stones. They came into use in Europe about the twelfth century and because of the high price they commanded were usually a remedy only of the nobility. While the original use of the bezoar was as an antidote to poisons, it came to be the valued remedy for all kinds of fevers, was applied externally in many skin diseases, and had the reputation of being able to cure even leprosy.

These stones were concretions found in the bodies of certain animals, and were supposed to prevent melancholia and all kinds of poisoning. It was a very useful medicament in those bygone days when the art of poisoning was highly developed. In cases of suspected poisoning the bezoar was swallowed and recovery was assured. If the bezoar failed, the explanation was simple—the patient died of something else.

All superstitions, even medical ones, must have their picturesque background. Here is the legend of the bezoar. According to the current belief the stone was obtained from the deer. In reality the origin of the bezoar stones was much more prosaic than this poetic version would lead us to believe. They were pebbles found in the intestines of goats and other animals. They resemble gall-stones. Their medicinal value is the same as that of any ordinary piece of gravel.

Avenzoar's folly is wiped out by his wisdom, for he has many accomplishments to his credit. His belief in the bezoar stone is proof that delusion and discernment may dwell in the same brain. There were many others who were deluded, for they were included in the London Pharmacopoeias from 1618 to 1746. Three bezoar stones were sent by the Shah of Persia as a royal gift for his brother the Emperor Napoleon, only a hundred and thirty years ago.

Avenzoar is interesting as probably being the first to suggest nutrition *per rectum*.

AVERROES

Among the distinguished contributors to medicine at this time, though more a philosopher than a physician, is the famous Averroes. Like Avenzoar, of whom he was the intimate personal friend, he was born in the south of Spain.

Altogether there are some thirty-three works of Averroes on philosophy and science. Only three of these are concerned with medicine. One is the "Colliget," so-called, containing seven books, on anatomy, physiology, pathology, diagnostics, materia medica, hygiene, and therapy. Then there is a commentary on the "Cantica of Avicenna," and a tractate on the "Theriac."

Averroes was an industrious student, and it is said that the night of his father's death and the night of his wedding-day were the only nights which he did not devote to intellectual labor.

He wrote much on the healing art, but his observation that smallpox does not attack the same person twice constitutes his sole original contribution to medicine.

Averroes fell under the suspicion of free thinking and was brought to trial with a number of personal friends, who occupied high positions in the Moorish government. He escaped with his life, but only after great risks, and he was banished to a suburb of Cordova, in which only Jews were allowed to live. By personal influence he succeeded in securing the pardon of himself and friends. He died, not long after, in 1198.

Taking the general average, medicine was not much improved by its sojourn among the Arabians. Anatomy, physiology and surgery retrograded. Chemistry was considerably improved, as was also materia medica. Their observations were faulty and they lacked originality. The prohibition in the Koran was a fatal handicap.

ABDALLATIF

Abdallatif of Bagdad visited Cairo and during his sojourn in Egypt a chance remark about a mount of unburied bodies induced him to visit the spot, and Abdallatif stood on a hill in the midst of twenty thousand skeletons. He picked up a mandible, and could not believe his eyes: the infallible Galen had written it was composed of several pieces, but Abdallatif could see only one. He looked at two hundred of these lower jaws, he sent them to other physicians for examination, and all agreed it consisted of one bone. His experience was similar with the sacrum; Galen said it was multiple, but Abdallatif found it was usually single. Holding these bones in his hand, Abdallatif was the first who saw that Galen could be wrong, and his simple observations are the sole Arabian contributions to anatomy.

"The alleged differences between the three great Semitic religions stained continents with blood and strewed the earth with corpses, but all shrank with equal horror from the anatomist's knife. All united in the belief that whoever touches a cadaver is guilty of sin, and Medicine remained without a true basis for centuries. Hence Arabian medicine could not endure, and under accumulating knowledge it collapsed completely."

ARABIAN HOSPITALS

It is interesting to find that 5,000 years ago a hospital should exist associated with, and under the patronage of, the Pharaoh, and having its own staff of physicians.

Moslem hospitals constitute one of the brightest phases of Arabian medicine. Islam founded hospitals throughout its dominions, and infirmaries for the blind and for lepers were established as early as 707. Every mosque had its hospital. There were asylums for the insane and Arabian lunatics were treated much better than those in Europe. There were sixty hospitals in Bagdad, "All well provided from the king's stores with spices and other necessaries, and every patient who claims assistance is fed at the king's expense until his cure is completed."

Rhazes, the famous Arabian physician, was active in founding hospitals. The incident has already been mentioned that when Rhazes was invited to choose a hospital site, he exposed meat in various sections of Bagdad, and selected the location where there was the most resistance to putrefaction.

Sivarn ibn Thabit at Bagdad was a famous hospital administrator. The Buddhist king, Asoka, was the first great builder of hospitals for man and beast. Ephraim built the first large hospital in Edessa; and upon the ruins of pagan temples, Rabbula erected an infirmary exclusively for women. Duttha Gamani, feeling his earthly journey ending (161 B. C.), asked the records of his reign be read to him, and among the last words the dying king heard were these: "I have daily maintained at eighteen different places, hospitals provided with suitable diet, and medicines prepared by physicians for the infirm."

Khalil Daheri wrote that even the healthy feigned illness to gain admittance: "While making the pilgrimage to Mecca, I stayed at Damascus, and had with me a certain Russian, a man of wit and intelligence, who followed the rites of the four orthodox sects, performing them all at the same time. When he went over the hospital and saw the patients' diet, and all their comforts and advantages, which are without number, he pretended to be ill and stayed three days there. The physician having felt his pulse recognized his case and prescribed any diet he liked, so he was fed upon young chickens, cakes, and sherbet, and all manner of fruits. But after two days the doctor wrote a prescription implying that a guest should not stay beyond the third day. They say the fire has never been put out at this hospital since it was built."

The ancient wisdom and science of the Greek and Latin authors, which was so well preserved by the Arabs, was transferred, when their passion for study and research began to fail, to European nations.

CHAPTER SIX

European Medicine in the Middle Ages

THE MIDDLE or so-called Dark Ages cover, roughly speaking, the period beginning when the barbarians captured Rome in 476 and scattered the learned men throughout the west, to the discovery of the New World in 1492, or as some reckon the period, to the time that Gutenburg invented the art of printing by moveable letters in the fifteenth century. Learning descended to its lowest depths in the ninth century, followed by a revival of learning in the eleventh century, the great intellectual awakening in the thirteenth century, which resulted in the Renaissance or New Birth in the fifteenth and sixteenth centuries.

All that Hippocrates and his loyal disciples had so patiently and painfully dug out of impassive nature, all that Galen had added to this store of information, was shrouded from view for over a thousand years. The thousand years between Galen and the Renaissance have always been known as the Dark Ages. One must carefully note, however, that the light of Greek medicine only faded; it was not snuffed out.

With the passing of Galen at the end of the second century, the thread of rational medicine snaps. Wherever we turn, the era of magic is upon us. Greek medicine, which in its classic days had been free from superstition, has ceased to function. Experiments are not performed, but miracles are expected. It is a period of morbid fascination when meaningless incantations replaced medicine. Mysticism, spiritualism, superstitions and other varieties of magic were the order of the day. Miracles were related by everyone and the belief in them was considered commonplace. Holy men and women each specialized in the cure of a specific illness, so that the number of saints became legion.

Sextus Placitus treats fever by cutting a splinter from a door through which a eunuch has passed, and Marcellus Empiricus removes an abscess of the right eye by touching it with three fingers of the left hand, expectorating, and repeating thrice: "The mule brings into the world no young, nor does the stone produce wool; so may this disease come to no head, or if it comes to a head, may it wither away."

Diseases were generally regarded as a chastisement from God or a visitation of the devil. Severe acute diseases were generally held to be the result of poison; pestilences as the effect of poisoning of the springs. The monks frequently held the principle of *similia similibus,* and for example treated the poisoning occasioned by swallowing a toad, by directing the eating of another toad.

At all times people have looked to faith for the cure of illness. As in the days when Imhotep and Aesculapius were worshipped, so now.

During the Middle Ages faith healing was raised to a greater ascendancy than at any period other than the most primitive. It was the "age of faith." This would have been a golden age for Christian Scientists, those people who are mostly educated but sentimental, though the application of faith would not have been broad, as Christian Science makes no appeal to people who are poor. The best feature of Christian Science is the optimism it teaches to its followers; it teaches them not to brood over the ills of life.

Faith healing that is practiced today among civilized peoples differs only in form from the faith healing of the most primitive peoples. The howling medicine-man of former times and the quiet Christian Science healer of today use the same essential principles in their treatments. These essentials are to attract the patient's attention, to gain his confidence, and to inspire him with faith in his recovery even to the extent of denying the existence of his disease. The central element of faith healing is to inspire confidence in the patient; the patient must have sincere belief. No faith cure ever worked on an unconscious man, an animal, or an idiot, and only the crudest kinds work on children.

THE UNIVERSAL TENDENCY

It would merely try the patience of the reader to enumerate even a tithe of the absurd things which have been and are being used by people, civilized and savage, as charms, talismans, and amulets.

Catherine de Medici wore a piece of an infant's skin as a charm, and Lord Byron presented an amulet of this nature to Prince Metternich. Pascal died with some undecipherable inscription sewn into his clothes. Charles V always wore a sachet of dried silkworms to protect him from vertigo. The Emperor Augustus wore a piece of the skin of a sea calf to keep the lightning from injuring him, and the Emperor Tiberius wore laurel round his neck for the same reason when a thunderstorm seemed to be approaching.

As late as the seventeenth century King Charles II of Spain had his confessor and two friars sit beside his bed while he slept to keep away the devils. Until recent times it was believed that night air caused disease and bedroom windows were closed tightly at night. This belief in the harmfulness of night air was a remnant of the ancient belief in wandering devils as the cause of disease.

It was during the Middle Ages that Petrarch uttered his criticisms and epigram about doctors: "Now the young man appears, puts on an air of importance, and murmurs unintelligibly while the people stare at him with astonishment, and his friends congratulate and applaud him. The bells are rung, trumpets sounded, rings and kisses exchanged, and the round cap of the Magister is placed on his head. Whereupon he, who had mounted the ceremonial chair a blockhead, descends from it a wise man. This is a metamorphosis of which Ovid knew nothing."

He did not admire a well-dressed doctor: "Add to this the indecent finery of usurped garments, of purple mixed with other colors, sparkling rings, gilded spurs, and tell me where is there an eye, healthy as it may be, which can defend itself against such dazzling magnificence?"

The Hippocratic aphorism (Life is short, and the Art long: *vita brevis, longa ars*) which the whole Latin world quoted with approval, received this additional commentary from Petrarch: "Life in itself is short enough, but the physicians with their art, know to their amusement, how to make it still shorter."

The Middle Ages which were successful in quarantining leprosy, failed in their efforts against prostitution. "Theodora, the crowned whore, thought of a way of reforming other prostitutes; she transferred five hundred from the brothels of Constantinople to a peaceful retreat on the Asiatic shore of the Bosphorus; it was a beautiful home, half prison, half convent, entirely safe from male invasion: many of the inmates threw themselves in the sea, and others died from unbearable boredom."

Sexual laxity was the rule, and amiability the fashion. It has been said if Hildebrand had emasculated his clergy instead of merely forbidding them to marry, he would have deprived the middle ages of their choicest scandals.

There were old Parliamentary suggestions to brothel-keepers: "No host shall receive a female from ecclesiastical institutions, nor shall he receive a married woman," and "No host

shall keep a maiden who has the dangerous burning disease."
Iron drawers, known as chastity belts, which could not be removed except with the husband's key, were made for women.
Prudent men, before departing on a journey, guarded the virtue of the wife by thus padlocking the genitalia. These girdles
of chastity were sometimes manufactured from old armor, but
at other times were exquisite samples of the goldsmith's art—
velvet-covered hoops fitting snugly around the waist, from
which projected a sheet of gold anatomically covering the parts
to be protected, with ingenious openings allowing for the performance of the calls of nature, the entire apparatus kept in
place by a lock responding only to a special key.

Mesue, a physician in the ninth century, is noted for his
opposition to the violent purgative medicines which the Greek
and Roman physicians had made common, and he had much
to do with the popularisation, if not with the introduction of,
senna, cassia, tamarinds, sebestens, myrabolans, and jujube. He
modified the effects of certain remedies by judicious combinations, as, for example, by giving violet root and lemon juice
with scammony. He gave pine bark and decoction of hyssop
as emetics, and recommended the pancreas of the hare as a
styptic in diarrhea. He was physician to five successive Caliphs.

The cultivation of medicinal herbs in the monastery gardens during the eighth and tenth centuries laid the foundations
of the science of botany. Their remedies are combinations of
charms, spells, and herb doctoring, such as have always been
prevalent among simple and uneducated peoples. Here is an
example: "For headache take a vessel full of leaves of green
rue, and a spoonful of mustard seed, rub together, add the
white of an egg, a spoonful, that the salve may be thick. Smear
with a feather on the side that is not sore."

During the Middle Ages opium, colocynth, hyoscyamus,
alcohol, turpentine, cold compresses, hellebore and many other
medicaments and procedures were used with commendable discrimination.

THE ROYAL TOUCH

In Great Britain, in 1042, the progress of medicine was clouded by the institution of the "royal touch" under Edward the Confessor, but it was not until the time of Henry VII, in the fifteenth century, that the practice was made into an elaborate church ceremony.

An entry in the diary of Charles II, dated May 29, 1660: "His Majesty began to touch for the Evil according to custom, thus: His Majesty sitting under his state in the banqueting house, the chirurgeons cause the sick to be brought, or led, up to the throne, where they kneel; the King strokes their faces or cheeks with both hands at once, at which instance a chaplain in his formalities says, 'He put his hands upon them, and he healed them'."

What the King was conducting was a tuberculosis clinic; the King's evil was scrofula, tuberculosis of the lymph glands, particularly those of the neck. The disease was once very prevalent, and the people affected were badly deformed by the scars from the chronically discharging abscesses.

Charles II was the busiest of all the royal touchers. One day in 1684 the crowd applying for treatment was so great that six or seven of the sick were trampled to death. It is noteworthy that more people are said to have died of scrofula in the time of Charles II than at any other period of English history.

William of Orange, who came to the throne in 1688, refused to continue the practice of the Royal Touch, and in consequence the people accused him of cruelty. Only on one single occasion was William importuned into laying his hands on a patient. "God give you better health," he said, "and more sense."

Queen Anne, however, who followed him to the throne, was a superstitious woman, and she at once revived the practice, the last of the English royalty to do so. The famous lexicographer, Dr. Samuel Johnson, was one of the last persons touched for scrofula by Queen Anne. On at least one occasion Queen Anne had to issue a royal proclamation postponing the ceremony, for, as a chronicler of the time says: "Her Majesty did not touch, yesterday, for the Evil, as designed, having gout in her hands."

"Even to the last, however, the Royal Touch was an impressive ceremony. On that day in 1775, Louis rode to the Abbey Park, mounted on a beautiful white charger, surrounded by magnificently dressed princes and courtiers, and preceded by a detachment of musketeers and guards. The sick were assembled in a row. The King dismounted and went through the ceremony by touching them."

In 1684, Thomas Rosewell was tried for high treason for speaking disparagingly of the Touch.

In the tenth century the following was used for sea-sickness: "To prevent sea-sickness the traveller had to smear himself with a mixture of pennyroyal and wormwood in oil and vinegar. Peony laid over a lunatic would soon cause him to upheave himself whole; and vervain or verbena if carried on the person would ensure a man from being barked at by dogs."

During this period the following were treatments for harelip, broken leg and anuria:

"For hare-lip, pound mastic very small, add the white of an egg, and mingle as thou dost vermillion, cut with a knife the false edges of the lip, sew fast with silk, then smear without and within with the salve, ere the silk rot. If it draw together arrange it with the hand; anoint again soon."

For the treatment of a broken leg, minute directions are given for the preparation of a salve of bone-wart and egg-white, and it is also mildly suggested that a splint should be applied.

Through all the many leechdoms runs the primitive idea that eating some part of an animal corresponding to that part of the patient which is affected will ward off evil and cure disease. For example:

"In case that a man may not retain his urine . . . burn to ashes the bladder of an unprolific, that is a gelt swine, put it into wine, administer it to drink. For the same, fry a goat's bladder, give it to the man to eat. . . ."

Again:

"If a man cannot mie (pass urine) . . . let him eat a ram's bladder sodden. . . ."

Philon, a physician of Tarsus, invented *Philonium,* a celebrated preparation which was used for centuries. It was composed of opium, saffron, pyrethrum, euphorbium, pepper, henbane, spikenard, honey, and other ingredients. One of its ingredients was "the red hair of a lad whose blood had been shed on the fields of Mercury," and the names of other ingredients are also disguised in mystic language. It was directed to be made into a conserve with the "product of the daughters of the bull of Athens," which meant Attic honey. This theriac of Philon's was originally intended as a remedy for a peculiar form of colic which was epidemic in Rome at that time.

Up to the eleventh century England was under the barbaric domination of the Saxons. The practice of medicine during these times was confined almost exclusively to the use of herbs, incantations, magic and necromancy. After the Norman conquest was in full force however, the English authorities began to recognize the demands of rational medicine by sending their physicians abroad to be educated in the clerical schools that were active during the scholastic period.

THERIAC

Notable among the remedies of the Middle Ages in Europe was Theriac, a name which had been originated by Nicander of Colophon, a compound with a fantastically chequered history. The name is derived from the Greek *theriakos,* pertaining to reptiles, because it contained viper flesh.

According to Pliny, and corroborated by Galen, the formula for the theriac of Nicander was inscribed in verse on stone in the temple of Aesculapius on the island of Cos, the birthplace of Hippocrates.

Among the papers of the vanquished King, Mithridates Eupator, Pompey discovered the formula for the famous confection or electuary which at that time was called *Confectio Mithridates,* and was later improved by Damocrates, physician to Nero, after whom it was subsequently called *Confectio Damocratis.* It is said that the formula, as discovered in the fallen monarch's effects, called only for "twenty leaves of rue, a pinch of salt, two nuts, and two dried figs." This was too ridiculously simple to inspire any confidence in its effect, so a more complicated formula was given out by Damocrates.

The theriac of Venice acquired a supremacy over the other theriacs as made by the rival cities of Genoa, Florence, Bologna, Constantinople or Cairo. It contained 61 ingredients and its manufacture was the occasion of much pomp and ceremony.

In Queen Elizabeth's reign the English apothecaries seem to have been making theriac of their own, which they claimed was superior to the imported product. A controversy had evidently occurred, for Hugh Morgan, Apothecary to the Queen, issued a pamphlet in 1585 in which he emphatically states that his product had been compared with other "theriacle" brought from Constantinople and from Venice, and had received commendation. He goes on to say: "It is very lamentable to consider that strangers do dayly send into England a false and naughty kind of mithridatum and threacle in great barrelles more than a thousand weight in a year and utter the same at a low price for 3 pence and 4 pence a pound to the great hurt of her Majesties' subjects and no small gain to the strangers' purses."

Cairo also had a reputation for very fine theriac. Prosper Alpinus, a physician of Padua, who resided three years in Cairo, gives a graphic account of the ceremony of its preparation in that city. It occurred annually in May in the Mosque of Moreston, under the supervision of the city's chief pharmacist in the presence of all the physicians. At that time purchasers from many European countries visited Cairo for their supplies of theriac.

A celebrated theriac of the seventeenth century was that invented by Sir Walter Raleigh while undergoing imprisonment in the Tower during the reign of James I. It consisted of 40 seeds, herbs, barks, and woods macerated in alcohol, distilled, and the distillate subsequently combined with a great variety of mineral and animal ingredients. This preparation was adopted in the London Pharmacopoeia under the name of *Confectio Raleighana.*

Alfred the Great of England inquired of Helias, Patriarch of Jerusalem, about his Theriaca containing scammony, ammoniac, tragacanth, aloe, galbanum, balsam, petroleum, alabaster, and theriac. Helias sent him the following directions for its use:

"Theriaca is a good drink for all inward tenderness, and the man who so behaves himself as is here said, he may much keep himself. On the day on which he shall drink Triacle he shall fast until midday and not let wind blow on him that day; then let him go to the bath, let him sit there until he sweat; then let him take a cup, put a little warm water in it, then let him take a little bit of the Triacle and mingle it with the water, and drain through some thin raiment, then drink it, and let him go to his bed and wrap himself up warm, and so lie until he sweat well; then let him arise and sit up and clothe himself, and then take his meat at noon, and protect himself against the wind that day; then I believe to God it will help the man much."

Most of the old masters in pharmacy fancied they could suggest some improvement, and the original formula was modified in scores of ways and became to consist of as many as 61 ingredients. It was the addition of vipers to the confection of Mithridates that constituted the principal improvement effected by Andromachus.

The enumeration of the medicinal properties of the antidote left very little room for any other remedy. First it would counteract all poisons and bites of venomous animals. Besides, it would relieve all pains, weaknesses of the stomach, asthma, difficulty of breathing, phthisis, colic, jaundice, dropsy, weakness of sight, inflammation of the bladder and of the kidneys, and plague. Down to the seventeenth century these virtues were almost universally accepted, and many were the learned treatises written to explain its action; how one drug toned down the effect of others, and how the whole formed a sort of harmony in medicine.

Medical men who have studied the formulas of all of the theriacs recorded report that the best that can be said of them is that the balsamic constituents might have a slight antiseptic effect upon the alimentary tract, but that the preparations could have no real remedial value in any but imaginary affections, and certainly no antidotal value in case of poisoning, nor any bactericidal property. It is quite probable that the real popularity of the theriacs, and possibly some of the reputed therapeutic value, was due to the fact that they were usually taken with wine.

Eventually theriac became known as treacle, and when theriac was discarded as a remedy the term treacle was applied to molasses. The sulphur and treacle administered to all young people a generation or two ago as a spring tonic was derived from the old belief in theriac. Charles Dickens referred to the frequent use of treacle in the boys' schools of England.

DANCING MANIA

The dancing mania began and was propagated by the sight of the sufferers from the great Plague, Black Death. It was not a new affliction. There had been isolated outbreaks of this mob excitement previously, but never before had so many people been drawn into the mania. In 1374 a group of men and women who had come out of Germany wandered into the streets of Aix-la-Chapelle. The members of the band formed a circle and then began to dance. In 1418 this mental turmoil reached its highest point in the city of Strassburg.

Saint Vitus became the patron of these sufferers, who in their calmer moments appealed for his aid to keep them from the paroxysms of their mania. This term has survived from the days of the dancing mania. Although we no longer have the mania, the term is applied to a certain nervous disease in which there is twitching of the face and arms; otherwise it has no relation to the mental malady described.

CRUSADES

When Peter the Hermit and Walter the Penniless organized the first crusade, toward the end of the eleventh century, they started a movement that developed into the Renaissance nearly four centuries thereafter. It is said that the emotional appeals of Peter caused multitudes of peasants to follow the hoof-prints of his mule.

What the Crusaders learned from the Saracens supplemented the knowledge gained from the flow of translations, which transmitted all the accepted ideas of many centuries before from East to West.

The crusades were conducted with almost unbelievable cruelty. They represented all types of people and as they advanced by slow marches, begging food and clothing as they went, they spread disease in every community they came in contact with, and prepared the way for countless epidemics.

If a crusader was a man of influence, his bones were boiled and transported home for burial. In 1300 Pope Boniface stopped it with the following: "Persons cutting up the bodies of the dead, barbarously boiling them, in order that the bones, being separated from the flesh, may be carried for burial into their own countries, are by the very act excommunicated."

Indirectly medicine ultimately profited greatly by the commerce which these wars opened up between the East and the West, and the diseases which were spread as the consequence of the intimate association of the unwholesome hordes from all the nations concerned, resulted in the establishment of thousands of hospitals all over Europe.

Constantine Africanus, a professor in the medical school of Salerno, as if with a magic key, opened the world of the East to the West.

THE MEDICAL SCHOOL OF SALERNO

In the science of medicine the Arabians have been deservedly applauded. The School of Salerno, their legitimate offspring, revived in Italy and Europe the precepts of the healing art. An Arab physician had persuaded some Benedictine monks to establish a hospital and medical school near Salerno, Italy. The only institutions of that character were in Spain, Morocco, and Algeria. In Christendom, they had been suppressed for nearly 1,500 years. The monks heeded the Arab's request, because they knew the need of a hospital and medical attention.

The School of Salerno was the principal link between the later Greek physicians and the teaching institutions which remain with us to this day. The origin of the School of Salerno is unknown, but it was certainly in existence in the ninth century.

It was the first institution in Europe to bear any resemblance to a university. Their works were many and various, and among them was the REGIMEN SANITATIS SALERNI. This was one of the most popular medical works ever written. The author was supposed to be one John of Milan, head of the faculty of the School of Salerno at the time it was written.

As indicated in the Regimen, even though it was written after the Salerno school had lapsed from its high estate, pathology was that of the four humors: blood, phlegm, yellow bile, and black bile. Bleeding was done cautiously and fairly rationally.

The school was organized in the ninth century, often spoken of as the darkest of the centuries, reached its highest point of influence at the end of the twelfth century, and was finally abolished by Napoleon on November 29, 1811, after having been in existence for nearly a thousand years.

The decline of the school was as rapid as her career had been brilliant and glorious. Perhaps the most serious blow at her supremacy was the foundation, by Frederick II in 1224, of the University of Naples, an institution upon which that prince bestowed unusual privileges, and in aid of which he and his successors authorized much special legislation, and gave numerous monetary gifts.

There is no doubt that at Salerno, where the influence of the Benedictines was very strong and where the influence of the Popes and the ecclesiastical authorities was always dominant, full liberty of studying and teaching was from the earliest days allowed to the Jews.

Probably the most important representative of the medical school at Salerno, certainly the most significant member of its faculty, if we consider the wide influence for centuries after his time that his writings had, was Constantine Africanus.

Constantine's significance lies in this role of intermediary. Medical literature had become arid. The monastic medical writers had been chewing the same texts for half a millennium. Medicine was in the act of breaking away from the Church.

A friend of Frugardi, one Guido Aretino, published in A. D. 1170 the Practica Chirurgiae, which represented the teaching of Roger as noted down by Guido, partly from lectures and partly from private conversation. Roger was one of the founders of modern surgery.

Roger Frugardi of Palermo was a surgeon of Salerno, and Trotula, a woman physician, was a teacher at Salerno.

The School of Salerno was located at Salerno, a flourishing seaport lying not far to the south of Naples. Norman Duke Robert took Salerno in 1076 and for a time its university was the leading educational center of Christendom. In 1095 the First Crusade began and Salerno acquired additional importance because it was the location of the base hospital for the militant Christians.

The preaching of Peter the Hermit, which marks the close of the eleventh century, was followed by an outburst of crusading enthusiasm that speedily converted Europe into one vast camp. The situation of Salerno on the route of the Western Crusade assisted greatly in extending the reputation of its school of medicine, and the ordinary results of the movement of large bodies of men, together with the casualties of a fierce and bloody contest, enlarged the field of experience of its physicians.

OTHER MEDICAL SCHOOLS

In the twelfth century the medical school of Montpellier began to come to the fore, and the universities of Oxford, Cambridge, and Bologna were founded. During the thirteenth century came the establishment of the universities of Paris and Naples, that of Messina, and above all that of Padua. The foundation of the universities of Prague, Vienna, Heidelberg, Cologne, and Erfurt occurred in the fourteenth century.

Not until 1140 was issued the first European law of medical licensure. It seems rather strange that the above act preceded the establishment of the first medical school by a century—sort of putting the cart before the horse. This law was issued by Grandfather Roger: "Whoever will henceforth practise medicine, let him present himself to our officials and judges to be examined by them; but if he presume of his own temerity, let him be imprisoned and all his goods sold by auction. The object of this is to prevent the subjects of our kingdom incurring peril through the ignorance of physicians."

However, it was not until 1515 that any ordinances were passed for the regulation of the guilds of barbers, bathers and surgeons.

Medical titles change as well as the remedies used and the method of treatment. The title of the medical practitioner is not the same in all countries, and the popular meaning of the words and titles has so changed that the original signification is, in some instances, almost lost. Thus, in English history we have record of the following appellations having been used: Physician, leech, mire or myre, barbers, barber-surgeon, chirurgon, surgeon, doctor. Neither surgeons nor physicians of the present day in Great Britain are called doctors, but are spoken of as surgeon or Mr. In the United States, however, they are almost invariably denominated doctor.

PETRUS HISPANUS

An insight into the practice of medicine in the thirteenth century can be obtained by examining the methods of Petrus Hispanus, a Portuguese physician who was described as "in all things, a scholar; and in medicine a specialist." He practiced both medicine and theology and was so successful that in the same year (1276) he was physician to Pope Gregory X and cardinal-bishop of Frascati. He used the following prescription for hysterical women: "I can say from experience that if a large cupping glass (a common jar will do) be applied to the lower part of the patient's abdomen, with free use of the red-hot iron, it will most thoroughly cure this disease. In hysterical fainting blow pepper and salt up the patient's nose. She will soon come round."

He knew that scabies could be cured in a day by sulphur, and many of his speculations are brilliant. However, we must not praise him too soon, for like the rest of his contemporaries, he believed in witchcraft and demons, advised epileptics to carry a parchment bearing the names of the three wise men of the East, and declared that "wearing the heart of a vulture makes one popular with all men and very wealthy, and that by vivisecting the bird hoopoe and eating its palpitating heart one may learn the future and all secrets concealed in man's minds."

Even in an age when remedies were valued according to their nastiness, Peter managed to distinguish himself as the champion of the therapeutics of dung.

GILBERTUS ANGLICUS

Gilbertus Anglicus' COMPENDIUM MEDICINE is the first complete treatise on general medicine by an Englishman. Valuable passages are clouded by others that are disgraceful. His method of treating sexual impotence follows: "Let a man, twenty years of age or more, before the third hour of the vigil of St. John the Baptist, pull up by the roots a specimen of comfrey (*consolida major*) and another of heal all (*consolida minor*), repeating thrice the Lord's prayer. Let him speak to none while going or returning, not even one word, but in deep silence let him extract the juice from the herbs, and with it write on parchment this charm: The Lord said increase x Utiboth x and multiply x thabechay x and replenish the earth x amath x. If a man wears around his neck a card inscribed with these identical words written in this juice, he will beget a male; conversely, if a woman, she will conceive a female."

Gilbertus has such faith in the potency of this charm that he informs the wearer what to do if it produces satyriasis. In other fields he is not more sensible: he mentions asses' hoofs attached to the patient's leg as treatment for gout, the water in which a murderer has rinsed his hands as an aid in childbirth, and a grunting sow tied to the bed as the cure for lethargy.

Gilbertus indicates that he himself is not favorably disposed toward some of the remedies he describes, but he hesitates to omit what others have included; in places he intimates he would willingly discard the popular complicated formulae of his time for the simple expectant treatment of Hippocrates, but he does not wish his contemporaries to regard him as peculiar.

MOSES MAIMONIDES

A distinguished Jewish physician who lived in the twelfth and thirteenth centuries was Moses Maimonides, "Eagle of the Doctors," a pupil of Averroes.   He was born at Cordova, Spain, on the 30th day of March, 1135 or 1139, the year is in doubt, and died in 1204.   His family was expelled from Cordova in 1148, and his life was one of many vicissitudes.   He achieved such renown in Egypt that his contemporaries said: "From Moses unto Moses there arose not one like Moses."

Correspondence in the Middle Ages was far more important than it has since become, and a letter from Maimonides was an epoch-making event to a Jewish community.   He was the official head of his people in Cairo, but the Jews of the world consulted him on all possible subjects, and his response was practically law.

He published much medical literature, including works in 1168, 1180 and 1190.   His rules of life and health have become part of our popular medical tradition.

He wrote treatises on asthma, hygiene, coitus, hemorrhoids, and on poisons and antidotes.   Maimonides was willing to be guided by Galen until Galen came in conflict with Moses, then he threw Galen overboard.   He was the physician of the emperor Saladin, defender of Acre against the Crusaders.

In addition to the name of Gilbertus Anglicus, already noted, two others of this period, who lived in the fourteenth century, should be mentioned, Bernard de Gordon and John of

Gaddesden. This special mention is made not because of any outstanding accomplishments by any one of these three individuals, but rather for the reason that in noting them, we receive our first formal introduction to English medicine.

BERNARD GORDON

Bernard Gordon, who taught at Montpellier, was probably a Frenchman of Scotch descent and never practiced in England. He entitled his work the Lilly of Medicine. It is a sidelight on the times that physicians, in entitling their books, competed with ballad-mongers; works dealing largely with the therapeutics of excrements bore the poetic names of Flowers of Medicine or Laurels of Practice.

Gordon names the eight diseases which at that time (1305) were considered contagious: acute fever, phthisis, scabies, epilepsy, erysipelas, anthrax, conjunctivitis and leprosy.

Gordon's book contains the first reference in medical literature to eye-glasses, which were first made from the stone beryllus, but he spoils it by adding that whoever uses his eye-salve—the best that God has revealed—will find spectacles unnecessary.

JOHN OF GADDESDEN (1280-1361)

John of Gaddesden was also one of the three Englishmen, all bearing the name of John, who, at varying periods in the fourteenth century made their individual contributions to surgery. The first of them, John of Gaddesden, was more of a physician than a surgeon. John of Arderne was more of a surgeon than a physician. John of Mirfield was neither physician nor surgeon, but rather a priestly bibliophile.

John of Gaddesden, who lived almost a century later than Gilbert Anglicus, was court physician and a fellow and professor at Merton College, Oxford. His main work, compiled in 1314 under the title of ROSA ANGLICA is a hodgepodge of mysticism, superstition, and revolting therapeutics, such as hog's dung for hemorrhage.

In treating smallpox he followed the therapy of Gilbertus Anglicus in the use of red colors: "When the son of the illustrious king of England had the smallpox, I took care that everything about his couch should be red, and his cure was perfectly effected, for he was restored to health without a trace of the disease."

John of Gaddesden is supposed to have been the original of Chaucer's DOCTOUR OF PHISIKE, published in the latter half of the fourteenth century:

"Well could he fortune the ascendant
Of his images for his patient
He knew the cause of every malady
Were it of cold, or hot, or moist, or dry,
And where engendered and of what humour.
He was a very perfect practisour."

JOHN OF ARDERNE

John of Arderne, the second one of the Three Johns, was the first English surgeon worthy to be classed with the men who were recreating surgery in Europe. He was born in A. D. 1307. He was trained in the wars, was a bold surgeon and a shrewd diagnostician. He referred to himself as a surgeon among physicians, and looked down upon barbers who practiced surgery. He was a little in advance of his English contemporaries in that he had more or less abandoned, for example, astrological methods, but he was skilled in leechcraft and still placed some reliance upon charms and spells. The books he wrote, or rather the rolls of vellum that he illuminated, included works on the care of the eyes, on bleeding, on sinuses and fistulae of the anus, on plants and their uses, and on clysters or enemata.

John of Arderne's most important contribution to surgery was the operation he devised for the cure of anal fistula, a condition that most of his predecessors regarded as incurable. His operation was practically identical with the one performed today. He was probably correct in claiming to be the only man of his time, in England or beyond the Sea, who could terminate this tragedy.

He advised his fellows to cultivate modesty, charity, and a studious and chaste mode of life, just as his predecessors had done, but he gave much more detailed instructions to this effect than did the earlier writers. Charity was to be displayed by visiting "poure men," the benefit to the leech being "that thai by their prayers may gete him grace of the holy goste." In visiting the "poure men," however, the leech was not to let his high-mindedness obscure the realities, if we may judge from a general medical treatise of John's. In this he recommended for the treatment of constipation a brew which was really the equivalent of beef-tea, "if he be rich." Then he goes on and adds, "but if he is a pauper he may just drink his own urine." Chastity was enjoined most sternly. The leech was advised to abstain from all harlotry, and he was to be particularly careful in his conduct towards the wives, daughters, and other women in the household of his patients. He gave other advice to physicians which is used elsewhere in connection with similar matter.

JOHN OF MIRFIELD

John of Mirfield, the third member of this fourteenth-century trio of Englishmen known as the Three Johns, was a priestly scholastic keenly interested in medicine and to a less extent in surgery. The date of his birth is not known, nor is it certain whether he ever received any regular medical education. He composed the BREVIARIUM BARTHOLOMEI, a medical work, probably between 1380 and 1395. He tried to present what he had thought good and worthy of quotation from the works of many well-known medical and surgical authorities. His Breviarium is probably a faithful picture of general medical and surgical treatment of that period, a picture which men like John of Arderne were beginning to re-touch.

In the Breviarium are some clinical tests of prognostic significance: "If the right eye of a sick man sheds tears, he will die; in the case of a woman, this applies to the left eye. The sole of a patient's right foot should be anointed with lard, which lard is then thrown to any given dog; if the dog eats it without vomiting, the patient will live, but if the dog returns it or makes no attempt to eat it, the patient will die." Mixed up with these mystic and messy investigations is much sound medicine, and even more common sense. For example, if there is any doubt as to whether a person is or is not dead: "apply lightly roasted onion to his nostrels. If he is alive, he will immediately scratch his nose."

John of Mirfield takes the opportunity of expressing some criticisms, which seems to show that all was no more well with medicine and surgery then than it is today. He indicts first the quacks, and also "what is worse, and is considered by me more horrible—worthless and presumptuous women, usurp this profession to themselves and abuse it." Writing on the attitude to be adopted towards the women of a patient's household, John of Mirfield, the cleric, is not unnaturally less blunt than John of Arderne, the surgeon. He simply suggests that it is not consistent with professional dignity to "speak shamefully to them, or turn bold glances upon them."

According to John of Mirfield "modern physicians" possess three special qualifications, and these are: "to be able to lie in a subtle manner, to show an outward honesty, and to kill with audacity." Perhaps even more crushing is: "the physician if he should happen to be a Good Christian, which rarely chances."

John of Mirfield expressed the following in rhyme:

"When Physick's dearly bought, it doth much healing
bring,
But when 'tis freely given, 'tis ne'er a useful thing."

MUNDINUS

Mundinus, in 1316, wrote a practical handbook of anatomy, which for the next two hundred years was the favorite of all the medical schools. This compendium therefore reveals to us the anatomical knowledge of the fourteenth and fifteenth centuries. He is a landmark in anatomy, and its acknowledged restorer. He taught on the cadaver, and was thus the first inheritor of the Alexandrians, and the forerunner of the anatomists who were to dissect and to see what they dissected.

HOSPITALS IN THE MIDDLE AGES

The first important hospital of western Europe was founded at Fabiola about the year 400. Its purpose, in the words of St. Jerome, was "to gather in the sick from the streets and to nurse the wretched sufferers wasted with poverty and disease." This hospital and the many that came after it extended hospitality to the sick.

The name "hospital" comes from the same Latin source as "hospitality." The word was carried into the English language and either in that form or more commonly as "spittle house" was applied to all institutions of refuge; those that cared for the sick and also those that housed the paupers and insane. It is only in recent times that "hospital" has come to signify a place where the sick receive temporary aid and shelter.

The hospitals of medieval Europe were dark, crowded, and insanitary buildings into which all classes of the destitute were received without discrimination. The inmates were given food, shelter, and religious admonition, but no medical treatment.

Max Nordau has said of the hospitals of Europe in this period: "In one bed of moderate width lay four, five, or six sick persons beside each other, the feet of one to the head of another; children beside gray-haired old men; indeed, incredible but true, men and women intermingled together. In the same bed lay individuals affected with infectious diseases beside others only slightly unwell; on the same couch, body against body, a woman groaned in the pangs of labor, a nursing infant writhed in convulsions, a typhus patient burned in the delirium of fever, a consumptive coughed his hollow cough, and a victim of some disease of the skin tore with furious nails his infernally itching integument. The patients often lacked the greatest necessities. The most miserable food was doled out to them in insufficient quantities and at irregular intervals. The nuns were in the habit of feeding with confectionery those patients who seemed to them pious enough, or at least those who reeled off their rosaries with sufficient zeal, but the body exhausted by disease required not sweets, but cried for meat and wine. Such food, however, the sick never received in profusion, save when it was brought to them by the wealthy citizens from the city. For this purpose the doors of the hospital stood open day and night. Anyone could enter; anyone bring whatever he wished; and while the sick on one day might be starved, on another day they might very likely get immoderately drunk and kill themselves by overloading their stomachs The whole building fairly swarmed with the most horrible vermin, and the air of a morning was so vile in the sick wards that the attendants did not venture to enter them without a sponge saturated with vinegar held before their faces. The bodies of the dead ordinarily lay twenty-four hours, and often longer, upon the deathbed before they were removed, and the sick during this time were compelled to share the bed with the rigid corpse, which in this infernal atmosphere soon began to stink, and over which the green carrion-flies swarmed."

CHAPTER SEVEN

Medicine in Europe in the Fifteenth Century
(THE RENAISSANCE)

W HEN WRITTEN records were begun in England about A. D. 1500, the Massengill family emerged from antiquity in the person of William Mersyngale, rector of the Church of Welbury in the Diocese of York, England, whose will was made September 15, 1472, and probated October 17, 1472. As he was probably an old man when he made his will so shortly before his death, it is likely that he was born about A. D. 1400.

We have now reached the end of what is known as the Medieval Period and emerge upon the period called the Renaissance. However, it must not be imagined that the coming of the Renaissance in the fifteenth century at once meant a brighter and better world. The generation which lived with one foot in the Middle Ages and the other in the Renaissance, did not realize it was straddling two epochs. The children of the Middle Ages who became the fathers of the Renaissance were not conscious of any abrupt break with the past. Agreement is general that the sixteenth century marks the beginning of modern medicine.

At the beginning of the Renaissance medicine was still on a very low plane in England and it was a long climb to modern medicine. Herb-doctoring, quackery, superstition, were parts

of the physician's stock in trade, and through soothsaying and
the intricate pseudoscience of amulets they intrigued the un-
suspecting populace. Uroscopy was a popular art, and consisted in diagnosticating disease by gross visual inspection of the
urinary output of the patient. Gracious lords and masters engaged special physicians-in-ordinary, to make matutinal inspec-
tions of this urine, for prophylactic purposes. Likewise
venesection and purgation were practiced only after the physician had resorted to astrology and determined whether the
conjunction of the stars and planets were favorable. The poor
people were not yet schooled to consult the few properly
qualified physicians, but relied chiefly on vagabonds, quacks
and charlatans. Even in the best walks of society, childbirth
was presided over by ignorant midwives.

The physicians in London were incorporated into a society
in 1518, and in 1540 the barber-surgeons were similarly incorporated.

In the fifteenth century, as before and afterward, purgation
was the strong fort of therapy. According to an old saying:

"Know in beginning of all sharpe diseases,
'Tis counted best to make evacuation."

Evidence of the importance which physicians have always
attached to purgation is the fact that the first medical book
ever printed was a LAXIERKALENDAR in 1457. There was a
great deal of nonsense connected with the giving of purges,
which continued well into the seventeenth century. Reliance
was still placed on the horoscope, and medical practice had not
entirely got away from the purgation calendars of the Middle
Ages, which indicated under each sign of the zodiac the proper
time to administer the cathartic and often forecast awful happenings that were to befall humanity under the various plane-
tary conjunctions.

VENEREAL DISEASES

Jacques de Bethencourt thought a disease should be named according to its cause, hence Venereal disease (*morbus venereus*). Unfortunately for the patients for several centuries syphilis and gonorrhea were usually considered the same disease, or at least that there was a close connection.

In the mid-sixteenth century Brasavolus wrote a book, which was one of those books which should have been left unwritten. For Brasavolus dealt with gonorrhea, not as a distinct disease, but as a complication of syphilis. Others took up the error and the misconception spread everywhere. This erroneous idea of the identity of gonorrhea and syphilis was overthrown by Philippe Ricord in 1838. Ricord was born in Baltimore, Maryland, but studied and practiced in Paris. As a result of his professional experiences he was pessimistic in regard to the morality of the human race and he was outspoken in his pessimism. Oliver Wendell Holmes said he was the "Voltaire of pelvic literature—a skeptic as to the morality of the race in general, who would have submitted Diana to a treatment with his mineral specifics and ordered a course of blue pills (mercury) for the vestal virgins."

Girolamo Fracastoro published in 1530 a medical poem— "Syphilis or on the Gallic Disease." In this poem, Syphilus, the shepherd of King Alcithous of Hayti, enraged at a prolonged drought which causes his flocks to perish, denounces the sun-god and worships his master Alcithous instead, claiming, "At least he will guard our flocks, will lead them to cool shelter and green shades." It was natural enough for a herdsman to speak in this fashion, but Apollo never overlooked an insult to his godhead: "At once upon this criminal earth there arises an unknown plague. Syphilus is the first attacked by it, for he was the first to profane the sacred altars."

Fracastoro, no doubt, derived the name Syphilus from Ovid's Sipylus—Sipylus being one of Niobe's children destroyed by the angry Apollo.   Fracastoro's poem gave syphilis the name by which it has since been known.   He referred to this new disease as the "love-pestilence."

Fracastoro's fame does not rest entirely on his poem, for he recognized the contagiousness of tuberculosis, the specific characters of fevers, the clinical entity of typhus, and has other accomplishments to his credit.

Syphilis, under the name of evil pocks, was first mentioned in print, on August 7, 1495, in the Edict of the Emperor Maximilian, who believed syphilis was sent by God in punishment for blasphemy.   We may never know the date of the disease which has corrupted the blood of the human race—we know only that at the threshold of the Renaissance a new and terrible malady doomed all Europe, impartially attacking cardinals, kings, and peasants.

In the middle of December, 1494, when Charles VIII was invading Naples, syphilis broke out in the French army. Must we agree with Diaz de la Isla, Oviedo, Fallopius and Montanus, that syphilis was imported by the Spaniards from America? Was it possible for the returned crew of Columbus, even if all its members were immoral, to cause an epidemic of such proportions?   Or shall we rather agree with Leoniceno that syphilis is of ancient lineage, and was referred to by Hippocrates himself in the aphorism, "ulcerations of the mouth and mortification of the privy members?"   Upon the other hand, the inquiry has been made, "If syphilis in Europe existed before Columbus, why are we unable to find a single syphilitic bone of pre-Columbian origin?"

John of Vigo mentions the date of the first appearance of the French evil, does not confuse it with gonorrhea, and was among the first to recommend mercury for the treatment of syphilis.   The name of this surgeon survives not in connection with any operation, but in a diachylon plaster and an orange-red powder.

Guy de Chauliac, the dominant surgical figure of the four-teenth century, popularized scorpion oil as a diuretic in venereal disease. Long afterward a medical traveler tells of meeting a convoy of ten mules, all heavily laden with living scorpions—a significant sidelight on the prevalence of gonorrhea.

Casanova, the libertine, was told by a surgeon that he was indebted to him for his present comforts, and when he in-quired why, the surgeon stated: "In this way captain. You had a connection with Don Jerome's housekeeper, and you left her, when you went away, a certain souvenir which she com-municated to a certain friend of hers, who, in perfect good faith, made a present of it to his wife. This lady did not wish, I suppose to be selfish, and she gave the souvenir to a libertine, who in his turn was so generous with it that, in less than a month, I had about fifty clients."

Those who today still look on syphilis and gonorrhea as punishments for sin have not progressed beyond the ideas of medieval Europe. There was an excuse for the Emperor Maxi-milian when he issued his edict in 1495 declaring syphilis to be an affliction from God for the sins of men. The civilization of his time had not progressed beyond such beliefs. Cotton Mather declared syphilis was a punishment "which the Just Judgment of God has reserved for our late Ages . . . ."

BLACK DEATH

From the twelfth to the fifteenth century Europe was vis-ited by frightful plagues that gave the exhausted people scarcely any time for recovery. Black Death and smallpox ravaged them; measles was more destructive than it is today; leprosy spread widely, and those afflicted were torn from their families and banished by Biblical precedent from human so-ciety. The disease of Saint Anthony's fire, now almost for-gotten, was the dread of town and country—a withering, deforming disease that left behind it crippled bodies.

In the years 68 and 79 A. D. outbursts of Black Death, now recognized as bubonic plague, occurred at Rome. The disease raged again in 125 and 164 A. D., and after the later date continued without interruption for sixteen years. This period which Bibbon regarded with envy commenced with a plague which at its height killed ten thousand persons in a single day. Tacitus, the Roman historian, who saw these events, says: "The houses were filled with dead bodies and the streets with funerals." It spread slowly up the Nile; it crept into Asia Minor. It reached Constantinople; there at its height it killed five to ten thousand inhabitants daily. During the fourteenth century it is said to have destroyed in China 13,000,000 of the population, and in the other Eastern countries 24,000,000 more. The loss by death from the plague in Europe only was over 25,000,000.

It continued to recur in Europe, with greater or less severity, for 350 years, or until the end of the seventeenth century. As late as 1630, it killed 500,000 in the Venetian Republic, and during the plague of London, 1665, more than 1,000 died each week. Nearly one-fourth of the population of Europe died of the plague.

In Paris, the learned doctors of the university said that the plague is caused by a "corruption of the atmosphere," caused by malign conjunctions of the planets over the Indian Ocean which have been spread over Europe by "heavy and turbid southerly winds."

SMALLPOX

For many centuries the ghost of smallpox terrorized our forefathers. Plagues came and plagues disappeared, but smallpox was never absent. It was the vastest horror that decimated the human race. No mother counted her children until all had passed through smallpox. In those days the young men sighed, "Oh, for a mistress who is not pock-marked." None were so lowly as to be passed by without notice, none so powerful as to enjoy immunity.   After the Spaniards brought the scourge of smallpox to America, the empire of the monarch of diseases was universal.   No corner of the earth was now safe from the pock-mark.   Falling upon the natives of Mexico, it destroyed six million inhabitants with the same fury that it had decimated China in the pre-Christian era.   The naked savage squatting on the equator, and the fur-clad Eskimo of the arctic circle, were equally apprehensive of its approach.

Today, if a ruler or a prominent statesman were to die of smallpox or even have the disease, it would be a scandalous occurrence.   Yet before Edward Jenner's announcement of the discovery of vaccination in 1798, the presence of smallpox was not a sign of ignorance or neglect.   The disease was inevitable; men were defenseless against it.   Louis XV was one of a long line of kings, queens, and princes who died of the disease.   Perhaps the most pathetic lines written about the disease are in the epigram that Ben Johnson dedicated to it three hundred years ago—a hopeless protest against the inevitable:

"Envious and foul disease, could there not be
One beauty in an age, and free from thee?"

A young apprentice at Sodbury overheard a country-girl say, "I cannot take the smallpox, for I have had the cowpox." Edward Jenner pricked up his ears with interest, for he remembered that the farmers and dairy-girls of his native Gloucestershire had the same notion.   He never forgot the remark. After reflection and experimentation extending over a long period, Jenner was ready for the test.   A dairy-maid named Sarah Nelmes, who had been pricked by a thorn, and became infected with cowpox while milking her master's kine, was his medium. On the fourteenth of May, 1796, Jenner took matter from her hand and inserted it by two superficial incisions into the arm of James Phipps, a healthy boy of eight.   This was the first vaccination.   On the first of the following July, virulent smallpox matter that would have killed any unprotected lad in the world was introduced into his arm, but without the slightest effect, for Phipps had been vaccinated. This was the crucial experiment. The work of twenty-five years was over, and Jenner knew he had closed a gate of death.

Dr. Benjamin Waterhouse of Boston was the first physician to use vaccination in America. In 1802 he vaccinated seven of his children; later he took them to the pesthouse and exposed them to smallpox, but none acquired it.

He even carried the proof of protection further than Jenner. He vaccinated nineteen boys. Twelve of these he afterward inoculated with smallpox matter and at the same time and with the same manner he inoculated two boys who had not been vaccinated. The twelve remained free from the disease; the two unvaccinated boys fell ill with the smallpox.

Thomas Jefferson was our first American President to be vaccinated, and the principle had been discovered then only three years before.

SCURVY

Sir Richard Hawkins stated, in the latter part of the sixteenth century, that he could give an account of ten thousand men who had been destroyed by scurvy in the twenty years that he had been at sea.

The sailor whom Holmes says taught "how to keep off the scurvy" was Captain Cook, the discoverer of the Hawaiian Islands.

ANTIMONY

In the sixteenth century the salt of antimony, tartar emetic, was introduced into medicine as an emetic and purgative and on account of its being a poison was the source of much discussion. A century may inherit a feud in the same manner that a family does. The sixteenth century handed down to the seventeenth century the quarrel about antimony.

Paracelsus had used antimony under the name of stibium, but later the name was changed and the drug popularized by a medical book published in 1604. The origin of the name antimony as given in this book is as follows: The author alleges that he had observed that some pigs which had eaten food containing antimony became very fat. He was led by this observation to try what effect it would have on some monks who had become emaciated as a result of prolonged fasting. He tried the experiment; the monks all died. Hence the name stibium was replaced by antimony, meaning antagonist to monks.

The most interesting of Basil Valentine's books, and the one which has had the most enduring influence, is undoubtedly THE TRIUMPHAL CHARIOT OF ANTIMONY. It has been translated and has had a wide vogue in every language of modern Europe. Its recommendation of antimony had such an effect upon medical practice that it continued to be the most important drug in the pharmacopoeia down almost to the middle of the nineteenth century.

TOBACCO

Tobacco was introduced into pharmacy by Jean Nicot in 1559, and for some years it was advocated as a remedy of almost universal potency. Hariot lauded the healthful qualities of tobacco, "which purgeth superfluous fleame and other grosse humors, openeth all the pores and passages of the body: by which meanes the use thereof, not only preserveth the body from obstructions; but also if any be, so that they have not beene of too long continuance, in short time breaketh them: whereby their bodies are notably preserved in health, and know not many greevous diseases wherewithall wee in England are often-times afflicted." Smokers swore it was an "antidote to all poisons; that it expelled rheums, sour humours, and obstruction of all kinds, and healed wounds better than St. John's wort." Some doctors were of opinion it would heal gout and the ague, neutralize the effects of drunkenness and remove weariness and hunger. It had a very stormy career as a drug, and is now mainly used as an insecticide.

* * *

The physicians of the sixteenth and seventeenth centuries apparently tried to make the deaths of their patients as unpleasant as possible; when Cardinal Richelieu was on his deathbed a female charlatan prescribed for him a mixture of horse dung in white wine, and the cardinal drank it. In the eighteenth century Fauchard, a Frenchman who made notable contributions to dentistry, advised his patients to use their own urine as a mouthwash in case of toothache. Urine was an old remedy, but subject to occasional revival; Madame de Sevigne recommended it highly in the seventeenth century.

SIR JOHN HARINGTON

The forerunner of the modern Chic Sales was Sir John Harington, a godson of Queen Elizabeth, who invented the modern water-closet, which he described under the heading of "A New Discourse of a Stale Subject called the Metamorphosis of Ajax" (London, 1596). A "jakes" was the accepted term for a privy in Elizabethan days. His invention constituted one of the few sanitary innovations that came before the nineteenth century. Its general adoption was slow. A new epoch in the practice of medicine began in 1777, when John Howard published in England his famous books on the sanitation of prisons, hospitals, and quarantine stations.

The medical school at Salerno had produced one of the most popular medical books ever written, REGIMEN SANITATIS SALERNI. Sir John published an English version. The two most quoted couplets in his version of the REGIMEN are probably:

88

"Use three physicians still: first Doctor Quiet,
Next Doctor Merry-man, and Doctor Dyet."

"Joy, Temperance, and Repose,
Slam the door on the doctor's nose."

About the only reference he made to surgery was that it is "that skill which death loves not." The rest is amusing rhyming advice on food and drink and the use of herbs.

Sound common sense and purely Elizabethan ribaldry are mixed throughout the whole of Harington's version:

"Great harmes haue growne, & maladies exceeding,
By keeping in a little blaft of wind:
So Cramps & Dropfies, Collickes haue their breeding,
And Mazed Braines for want of vent behind:
Befides we finde in ftories worth the reading,
A certaine Romane Emperour was fo kind,
Claudius by name, he made a Proclamation,
A Scape to be no loffe of reputation.
Great fuppers do the ftomacke much offend,
Sup light if quiet you to fleepe intend."

The reference to the Emperor Claudius is probably taken from Suetonius, who wrote that the Emperor had in mind at one time the issuing of a proclamation justifying the emission of flatus wherever and whenever the need might exist.

An advertisement of the sixteenth century period: "*Barnaby Factotum*: Draws Teeth, Bleeds and Shaves: Wigs made here; also sausages. Wash Balls, Black Pudding, Scotch Pills, Powders of the Itch, Red Herrings, Breeches Balls and Small Beer by the maker. In *utrumque Paratus*."

CHAPTER EIGHT

Medicine in Europe in the Sixteenth Century

EMERGING from antiquity, when the oldest local records were kept, we find Masongill Hamlet, located in the parish of Thornton in Lonsdale, in the West riding of Yorkshire, England. At present we find Masongill Hall, built early in the twentieth century, and standing nearby, the ruins of the ancient Masongill Hall, whose master is lost in the mists of antiquity. At Whitby, England, we find Gilbert Marsingill, the earliest ancestor with whom the family in the United States has been definitely connected, and whose will was dated August 26, 1592.

In the sixteenth century, which period marked the beginning of modern medicine, the Massengill family in England was still living in the Dogmatic of Empirical age of medicine and awaiting the coming of the Rational age, about the closing of the eighteenth century. It was a century of struggle and conflict, an almost constant battle between the vested doctrines of the past and the aspiring truths of the present.

Great developments in medicine were just ahead. The great Paracelsus became medicine's standard bearer; Vesalius, Eustachio, and Fallopio recast anatomy; Paré restored surgery to a worthy place; ophthalmology was recreated and obstetrics began to be a science and art rather than a murderous occupation. Anatomy, physiology, pathology, medicine, surgery, obstetrics and ophthalmology all underwent transformation. Not only in anatomy and physiology, but in pathology, the Renaissance is the ante-chamber to modernism. The botanists established the study of botany as an independent discipline and thus indirectly rescued pharmacology from the web of alchemy in which it was almost hopelessly entangled.

PARACELSUS (1493-1541)

Paracelsus was born on December 7, 1493, in Einsiedeln, Switzerland, a village near the city of Zurich. He was likely an only child. His father, William Bombast von Hohenheim, an amiable and scholarly burgher, was the physician of the village. He was his son's companion and instructor. The name "Paracelsus" was adopted by the boy himself during his student years as was the custom of the time. Students traveling about to universities tended to take Greek or Latin names, as their own foreign proper names were difficult to pronounce. His family name was Bombast and its connection with Paracelsus did not inspire the modern meaning of the word.

At the age of twenty he began a career of wandering which lasted several years. He served in campaigns as an army surgeon in wars in Denmark, Italy, Belgium, Venice and Constantinople, and visited England, Portugal and France. There is no positive evidence that he ever received the degree of Doctor of Medicine, although it seems unlikely that he could have held his later posts had he not done so.

Paracelsus has been described in appearance as unusually small, delicately built, beardless, powerful nose and a sensitive mouth. If we are to judge by portraits, he became more fleshy and his face puffy and smooth.

Paracelsus was one of the three outstanding physicians of the sixteenth century; the other two were Vesalius, who founded modern anatomy, and Paré, who reformed surgery. Paracelsus was the founder of the Chemical School of Medicine. He enlisted chemistry in the service of therapeutics as never

92

before. He taught the use of sulphur, lead, antimony, mercury, iron, copper, in their various combinations. He condemned the practice of excessive blood-letting as criminal.

He settled down as Professor of Medicine at Freiburg in 1525, for a short time, then was professor at Strassburg and finally became Professor of Medicine at Basel in 1527. His lectures were such as had never been heard before at a university. He began his course by burning the works of Galen and Avicenna in a chafing dish, and denouncing the slavish reliance on authority which at that time characterized medical teaching and practice. He attacked the authority of Galenic and Arabic medicine, pleaded for substituting meditation and thought for dogma, and fairly shouted anathema on outworn texts in such pronouncements as this: "Reading never made a doctor, but practice forms the physician; all reading is merely a footstool to practice, and a mere feather broom."

"The new professor did many astonishing things that day. Instead of using monkish Latin, he lectured in native German, which then seemed 'even to the German emperor, suitable only to address horses.' Paracelsus had with him a pile of books— the works of Galen, Avicenna, Averroes and other medical masters. It was surprising to see the iconoclast in company with the authorities. But Paracelsus did not quote from them. He placed some sulphur in a brazier, set fire to it, cast in the sacred volumes, and burnt up the idols."

"What will you think when I triumph? I am to be the monarch, and the monarchy will belong to me. For I tell you boldly that the hair from the back of my head knows more than all your writers put together; my shoe-buckles have more wisdom in them than either Galen or Avicenna; and my beard more experience than your whole Academy."

Paracelsus left Basel after a residence of less than two years and for the remaining thirteen years of his life he was a wanderer. He was driven from city to city, sometimes by restlessness, more often by bitter persecution. He comments, "I pleased no one but the sick whom I cured."

The complacent cocksureness of Paracelsus was enough to stir the ire of a turtledove: "Tell me, Galenic doctor, he jauntily asks, on which foundation you stand? Have you ever cured podagra, have you ever dared to attack leprosy, or healed dropsy? Truly I think you will be silent and allow that I am your master. If you really wish to learn, listen to what I say, attend to what I write."

He was a giant in the field of therapy. He saw that medical education in his time was defective, and he started a modern revolution which eventually led to a complete upheaval in all departments of medicine. This vigorous, clear-thinking doctor saw that surgeons should practice asepsis. He said to them: "Do not touch wounds, because they cure themselves; it is the external agents which complicate processes of cicatrization." He likewise investigated the therapeutic properties of mercury and mercurial preparations and taught their remedial values and the diagnostic principles suggesting their uses.

Paracelsus believed that there was a specific remedy for each disease if only the remedy could be found. In fact, however, from among all the specifics he advocated only one came very near being a true specific. That one was mercury for the treatment of syphilis. Paracelsus not only supplied a remedy for syphilis, but was the first physician to describe the stages of the disease and its transmission to children.

Paracelsus was several centuries ahead of his time. His contemporaries laughed at him and painted him as an irascible, boasting fool. Today we can fully appreciate his genius and see what an outstanding character he was in the history of medicine. No one man in history exercised such a revolutionary influence on medicine and pharmacy as this erratic genius.

As a physician and a pharmacist Paracelsus deserved some of the very criticisms which he launched at the members of both of these professions, for some of his remedies were repulsive, others were based upon superstition.

During Paracelsus' travels he learned a great deal about medical practice, low company, and mysticism. The mystic views of Paracelsus, or those attributed to him, are curious rather than useful. He seemed to have had as much capacity for belief as he had disbelief in other philosophers' speculations. He believed in gnomes in the interior of the earth, undines in the seas, sylphs in the air, and salamanders in fire.

Paracelsus wrote a poem that his critics called "A study of intellectual egotism." One author said of him: "Paracelsus was an egotist, without doubt. Indeed, egotism seems a ludicrously insignificant term to apply to his gorgeous self-appreciation."

Operinus, who lived with Paracelsus for two years, declared he was almost constantly drunk. He was scarcely sober two hours at a time. He would go to taverns and challenge the peasantry to drink against him. When he had taken a quantity of wine, he would put his finger in his throat and vomit. Then he could start again.

Paracelsus brought the manner of the tavern wine-room into his lecture-room. Within a year after his arrival at Basel he was in conflict with the city authorities and was brought to trial. After abusing the court roundly he fled from the city to avoid the consequences of his impudence. He resumed his wanderings, and in September, 1541, died as the result of an injury received in a drunken brawl at Salzburg.

Perhaps the monument to this great medical revolutionist still stands by the chapel of St. Philip Neri, at Salzburg—a broken pyramid of white marble, with a cavity in which is his portrait, and a Latin inscription which commemorates his cures of diseases.

In making an evaluation of Paracelsus one would have to conclude that he was not an attractive figure. He lacked a balance of mind and a capacity for friendship, and had serious faults of character. But he was possessed of many fine intuitions. He could write these words: "Faith is a luminous star that leads the honest seeker into the mysteries of Nature. You must seek your point of gravity in God, and put your trust in an honest, sincere, divine, pure and strong faith, and cling to it with your whole heart and sense and thought, full of love and confidence."

ANDREAS VESALIUS (1513-1564)

There is not a name of greater renown in the record of professional characters than Andreas Vesalius, who was a native of Brussels, but the precise year of his birth is somewhat indefinite, being stated as April, 1513, and December, 1514.

Vesalius founded modern anatomy. He said in as many words that whatever the older authors had written about the skeletons and internal organs of pigs or monkeys or horses, while true enough so far as horses or monkeys or pigs were concerned, was not necessarily true of the human organism.

When Vesalius was a student, human cadavers were still so scarce that he found it necessary to climb gallows or rob graveyards for material. So difficult was it to obtain a human corpse during the Renaissance that when Rondolet opened his anatomical course at Montpellier, he was forced to dissect the body of one of his own children.

It has been said that the Greek, Hippocrates; the Belgian, Vesalius; the Englishman, Harvey; and the Frenchman, Pasteur, are perhaps the four greatest figures in the history of the medical sciences. The first great contribution to anatomy was made by Andreas Vesalius in 1543. Vesalius actually dissected the human body and made accurate observations unblinded by veneration of Galen.

However, Vesalius was not wholly free from some of the Galenic superstitions of anatomy, for he upheld the idea that the nasal secretion came from the brain. It was two centuries later that its local origin in the mucous membrane of the nose was discovered, and until that time physicians continued to give drugs to increase the flow of mucous, thereby "to purge the brains."

Vesalius was the anatomist who dethroned Galen, though he was not a conscious antagonist of Galen. Before Vesalius finished with the Prince of Physicians, he demonstrated and corrected over two hundred Galenian errors.

In giving birth to modern anatomy in 1543 Vesalius had exhausted himself and in the years following did nothing. He became court-physician of Spain. He took unto himself a wife, made money, and exchanged the intellectual life for the easeful one. He attended the licentious Don Carlos who tripped and broke his head while chasing a girl who ran away.

FALLOPIUS

Fallopius, the great anatomist who named so many anatomial parts, and a pupil of Vesalius, wrote a book. In a leisure moment Vesalius commenced to glance through the volume. A tinge of jealousy crept through his veins. The father of Anatomy read of anatomical discoveries of which he knew nothing. While he had been dawdling away his days in the performance of petty functions, science had been advancing. He determined to quit the court of Spain, and once again devote himself to the pursuit of knowledge.

About this time a nobleman died of an obscure illness and Vesalius performed an autopsy. He and his associates found a beating heart. He was accused of impiety and murder and was sentenced to death. He escaped and went to Palestine. According to a less-known story, Vesalius was thus condemned because while dissecting the mistress of a priest he discovered unmistakable evidence that the bachelor had not kept his vows as to chastity. Still another version is that he took the journey to escape the vigorous tongue of his wife.

Fallopius died young, and the Venetian senate invited Vesalius to again fill the Paduan professorship thus made vacant. Upon his return a storm arose and the anatomist was wrecked. His corpse was found in a hut and it is believed he succumbed to typhus.

AMBROISE PARÉ (1510-1564)

Paré, of France, typified the highest type of medical mind of his time and he was a character of which any generation might be proud. He will be further mentioned in the chapter, Surgeons and Surgery.

MICHAEL SERVETUS (_____-1553)

Michael Servetus, a classmate of Vesalius, a native of Spain, was somewhat of an erratic genius. He began the study of medicine at the University of Paris, under the direction of the celebrated anatomist, Sylvius, where in due time he graduated with honor. Later, he became a pupil of Guinterius, a man who had risen from the depths; he had stood in the streets of Deventer, imploring the passersby for bread. But hunger never prevented Guinterius from studying Greek, and the learned beggar became a professor in the University of Louvain.

Guinterius spoke of Vesalius and Servetus: "Andreas Vesalius, a young man, by Hercules! of singular zeal in the study of anatomy; and Michael Servetus, deeply imbued with learning of every kind, and behind none in his knowledge of the Galenic doctrine. With the aid of these two, I have examined the muscles, veins, arteries and nerves of the whole body, and demonstrated them to all the students."

Servetus published a learned medical work, SYRUPORIUM UNIVERSA RATIO, in which from a therapeutic and physiological standpoint he criticized Galenism and Arabism, and mixed too much theology with his medicine. His book was a distinct advance in the art of prescribing. For the nauseous mixtures —the mere names of which now act as emetics—he introduced more palatable drugs; in these pages we see the first rational attempt to avoid incompatibilities, and we find also the first suggestion of what the pharmacist calls vehicles, that is, pleasant-smelling and sweet-tasting ingredients of no use in themselves, but valuable as carrying other drugs of therapeutic action.

His book aroused bitter antagonism. The Faculty of Paris attempted to impeach him. Dissensions divided the university, riots occurred in the streets, and some of the students were severely injured. Servetus was imprisoned and Calvin labored for a death-sentence.

On October 27, 1553, Calvin's tribunal read the following judgment: "Because in his book he calls the Trinity a devil, and a monster with three heads; because contrary to what Scripture says, he calls Jesus Christ a Son of David; and says that the baptism of little infants is only an invention of witchcraft; and because of many other points and articles and execrable blasphemies with which the said book is all stuffed, hugely scandalous and against the honor and majesty of God, of the Son of God, and of the Holy Spirit . . ."

The following is part of the sentence: "By this our definite sentence which we give here in writing, we condemn thee, M. Servetus, to be bound, and led to the place of Champel, there to be fastened to a stake, and burned alive, with thy book, as well written by thy hand as printed, even till thy body be reduced to ashes, and thus wilt thou finish thy days, to furnish an example to others who might wish to commit the like."

Green wood was used to prolong the agony; to mock him, a crown of straw dipped in sulphur was put upon his head. By his side they tied the book that should have made an epoch.

Thus perished one of the most original thinkers of the sixteenth century; a man who was fully three centuries in advance of the age in which he lived; the discoverer of the pulmonic circulation of the blood; condemned to death for writing the book that contained the most momentous physiological discovery of the time.

LEONARDO DA VINCI

Leonardo da Vinci has been described as the most versatile and intellectually fertile of all the sons of men. It is almost incredible that the same man should have been the greatest artist, the chief engineer and the foremost biologist of his time.

He painted Mona Lisa and the Last Supper.

"He was the illegitimate son, not only of his parents, but of his age. Of unknown antecedents, left-handed, unsexed, he surpassed all men in body and mind. In Leonardo's youth, his physical strength and beauty, his charm of manner, his joyous curiosity in life, his unapproachable skill in music and horsemanship, amazed his contemporaries."

Leonardo da Vinci dissected many bodies for the acquisition of anatomical knowledge, and was the first who drew accurate pictures, including the human skeleton, of these dissections. He was the first of the modern dissectors and the first who drew the human skeleton. He is the real Father of Modern Anatomy. He followed criminals to execution to observe their fear-distorted features, and likewise in the interests of his Art he studied corpses—until the Pope excluded him from the Roman hospital as "a heretic and cynical dissector of cadavers."

Leonardo da Vinci, disinherited by his father, his country and his time, bequeathed to mankind the most precious legacy since the **Greeks.**

VELERIUS CORDUS

Velerius Cordus, a great botanist of this period, died of malaria before he reached his thirtieth year. He examined plants in the forests of Germany and Italy and described 500 species of plants which were unknown to Dioscorides, the father of materia medica. He is of further interest to us from his connection with the discovery of ether, as the author of the first accurate description of nux vomica, and as the compiler of the NUREMBERG DISPENSATORIUM, which is regarded as the first official pharmacopoeia.

100

One of the quatrains of Euricius Cordus, a botanist of the period, has survived among the medical fraternity:

"God and the doctor we alike adore
When on the brink of danger, not before;
The danger past, both are alike requited,
God is forgotten and the doctor slighted."

*   *   *

The earliest botanist of the Renaissance was Niccolo Leoniceno. His countryman Monardes published the first accounts of jalap, sassafras, cebadilla, sarsaparilla, balsam of Tolu and balsam of Peru.

WILLIAM GILBERT

William Gilbert, in a published book, was the first to mention the word electricity. Before Gilbert the twin forces of electricity and magnetism still slumbered in darkness. His studies refuted many of the fables of that time, such as the belief that the lodestone can reconcile quarreling husbands and wives; that there are northern mountains of such magnetic power that they extract nails from the timbers of passing ships; that when a magnet is rubbed with garlic it ceases to attract iron; that if pickled in the salt of a sucking fish it will pull up gold from the deepest wells.

While the scientific advances were being made during the Renaissance much bad doctrine was still being disseminated.

These doctrines remind one very much of Josh Billing's remark that "it is not so much the ignorance of mankind that makes them ridiculous, as the knowing so many things that ain't so."

CORNELIUS AGRIPPA

Cornelius Agrippa sowed the seeds, throughout all Europe, of a doctrine fully as degrading as the demonology of the ancient Egyptians during the mythological age. He believed that everything in nature was the habitation of demons—air, fire, water, land, men, animals, etc. He believed that these demons were the cause of all diseases, and, of course, the treatment prescribed in accordance with that view was necessarily absurd in the same degree. He died at Grenoble, in 1535 A. D.

JEROME CARDAN

Jerome Cardan was another eminent disciple of Cabalistic medicine. He was born at Pavia, in 1501 A. D. He taught that the different parts of the body are under the dominion of different stars. He records the most extravagant stories, visions, dreams, sorceries, etc., and explains them by means of the cabal. He died at Rome in 1576 A. D.

*   *   *

Some of the others who advanced medical science in the sixteenth century are: Pierre Franco, the first to perform suprapubic cystotomy; Francisco Diaz, author of the earliest treatise on urology; Fabricius Hildanus, the first to amputate the thigh; and Tagliacozzi wrote the first monograph on plastic surgery.

We have now come to the end of the sixteenth century, a great period, to many the greatest century of all in the interest of its happenings and the remarkable characters which it produced. The Renaissance was the period of great reformers— Luther in religion, Vesalius in anatomy, Paré in surgery, and Paracelsus in therapy.

CHAPTER NINE

Medicine in Europe in the Seventeenth Century

WHEN THE earliest written records were begun in England in the fifteenth century the Massengill family was there, and they continued to witness the progress of medicine and pharmacy in England and the United States throughout the later centuries.

Daniel Marsingill, great-grandson of Gilbert Marsingill, who was the ancestor of the Massengill family in the United States, "aged neare eighteen being now bound out to sea," made his will January 18, 1645, and in 1653 settled in the colony of Virginia, in that part which later became Charles City County.

Medicine in America in the seventeenth and eighteenth centuries, which was not greatly different from the practice in Europe, will follow in a separate chapter.

In practical medicine the seventeenth century was a period of endless activity. At this period Willis differentiated between diabetes mellitus and diabetes insipidus; Walter Harris wrote about what we now term acidosis; Glisson published an account of rickets; Thuillier showed that ergot was due to corn smut; Bontius described beriberi; Colle and Musitano showed that syphilis could be conveyed by kissing and from drinking-vessels; Guarinoni described gummata of the brain; Ramazzini opened up new medical territory—the immense field of trade-diseases.

The seventeenth century was notable for improved instruments, yet the surgical achievements were not great. The gulf between physician and surgeon was not yet bridged: the physician scorned to think surgically, and the surgeon feared to trespass on medicine.

At this period, although the Grocers were the recognized drug-dealers in England, apothecaries who were associated in their Guild were also recognized. The Act of 1511 incorporating the College of Physicians and giving them the exclusive right to practice physic in London and for seven miles round, was largely used, if not intended, against apothecaries.

The Grocers' Company seceded from the Apothecaries Guild and the feeling between these, and also between the physicians, became very strained. The quarrel ended in the comparative triumph of the apothecaries.

In 1687 the College of Physicians adopted a resolution binding all Fellows, Candidates, and Licentiates of the College to give advice gratis to their neighbouring sick poor when desired within the city of London or seven miles round. But in view of the gross extortions of the apothecaries it was asked, What was the use of the physicians' charity if the cost of compounding the medicines was to be prohibitory? Such was the condition of affairs when in 1696 an influential section of the physicians, fifty-three of them, associated themselves in the establishment of Dispensaries, where medicines should be compounded and supplied to the poor at cost price. Needless to say, the war now waxed fiercer than ever. The physicians were divided among themselves, and the anti-dispensarians refused to meet the dispensarians in consultation.

Witchcraft was the black magic of the Middle Ages. The persecution of witches, which caused the deaths of thousands of innocent children and old women, developed on an enormous scale in Europe in the fifteenth century, and reached its height in Europe and the United States in the seventeenth century. Witchcraft is the exact opposite of faith healing; instead of inspiring health by faith, witchcraft inspires disease.

There were witches in the primitive world, and in the first civilizations; in the early middle ages, Augustine declared that witches indulge in sexual intercourse with the devil, and it is impudence to deny it; the two greatest theologians of the latter middle ages, Albertus Magnus and Thomas Aquinas, were firm believers in witchcraft. Witchcraft was a child of the theologians rather than of the physicians.

In the English colonies, Cotton Mather reasoned as follows: Satan has been in undisturbed possession of America until the Puritan invasion of Massachusetts, hence Satan is seeking his revenge in this vicinity. Cotton Mather, spiritual guide of New England, abetted by his father, Increase Mather, stampeded the courts and was mainly responsible for the witch craze of Salem and the judicial murders.

Men began to appear in court, charged with kissing Satan under the tail, and in giving him four of their hairs in exchange for diabolical knowledge; women were accused of making men impotent with an ointment, and of riding through the air on a broomstick to attend the Witches' Sabbat.

Victims who died under torture were sometimes declared innocent, but the most stubborn resistance was only additional evidence that the devil was hardening them. "Do you believe in witches?" was the inquisitor's first question. To answer Yes meant forbidden knowledge, to answer No meant heresy, and both answers meant death. Women were thrown into the water, with thumbs and toes tied crosswise—if they floated they were guilty, since the water repudiated their baptism. "God reveals the truth through the thumb-screw," was a favorite expression of the witch hunters. The accused were compelled to kneel on spike-covered prayer-stools, and enter cages so constructed as to render existence unbearable; they were chased up and down their cells until exhausted, or whirled around until reason left them; they were fed on salt fish without water, and bathed in quicklime; the jailers flayed the skin and broke body and spirit; every limb was stretched on the rack and every joint dislocated; no sensitive spot escaped a candle-flame or the red-hot iron; pliers extracted the finger-nails with the roots, and bones were crushed until the marrow spurted out. The written records of inquisitors and judges reveal how thoroughly they relished their work in the name of God—the witch hunt enables us to see human nature unmasked.

Not the dark ages, not medieval times, but the enlightened seventeenth century was the Era of the Witch Hunt.

In the seventeenth century the curious theory of telegony —the first male who fecundates a female makes such an indelible impress upon her that subsequent offspring by another man bear the characteristics of the first father—was well known.

The seventeenth century seems to have been the period of the earliest activities of the grave-snatchers or resurrectionists as they were called. The teaching of anatomy demanded a continual supply of bodies, or subjects, for dissection. A few subjects were legally available for dissection, but the legitimate demand was always greater than the legal supply. Edinburgh, which took the lead among the English schools, did not have a skeleton until 1697.

Four gypsies were executed for murder in Edinburgh in 1678 and their bodies were flung into a common grave. Next morning the topmost of the four corpses had disappeared. This is the first record of surgeons having recourse to an unofficial source of supply for anatomical subjects. But however much or however little the supply of anatomical material was increased, the demand outpaced it, and the Edinburgh College of Surgeons in 1711 placed on record the fact that "of late there has been a violation of sepulchres in the Grey Friars Churchyard."

Ten years later, as a sop to growing public indignation, all Edinburgh apprentices had a clause in their indentures to the effect that they were not to violate graves.

The notorious Dick Turpin was hanged at York in 1739. The corpse was allowed to lie in state at the local Blue Boar for twenty-four hours, and was then buried in an unusually deep grave. This did not prevent its being resurrected, but a hue-and-cry was raised and the disinterred Turpin was found in the garden of a surgeon's house. The second interment was successful. The coffin was filled with unslaked lime, buried even more deeply, and relays of watchers guarded the grave. This unsuccessful attempt at resurrection for dissection attracted a great deal of attention, as did more successful sallies, for by this time apprentices and their masters all over the country were going forth in the dead of night to collect the anatomical material that they could obtain in no other way.

In 1751 it was enacted that all murderers executed in London and Middlesex should be either publicly dissected or hung in chains on gibbets. This Act materially increased the supply of subjects for dissection, but still there were not nearly enough. Apprentices went on raiding the graveyards.

There came to light another source of supply. In many districts at that time it was customary to "wake" the dead—that is, the relatives kept vigil over the coffin for the few days that elapsed between death and burial. The rite was losing favor, however, and the bereaved relatives were often very willing to pay the nurse who had attended the dear departed a few pence for continuing to keep an eye on an erstwhile patient. Two women, Helen Torrence and Jean Waldie, made this work their specialty, and as a profitable sideline abstracted from their coffins the bodies they were supposed to watch and sold them to anatomical students.

Later, many murders were committed to obtain the bodies for sale.

In this century John Floyer was the first to count the pulse with the minute watch. William Harvey, the English physiologist, had emphasized the value of the pulse in medical diagnosis, and also suggested the use of the watch in counting the pulse.

Prof. Carl Binz called attention to the fact that more than a century before the birth of either Floyer or Harvey, a distinguished German churchman, who died shortly after the middle of the fifteenth century, had suggested a method of accurate estimation of the pulse that deserves a place in medical history.

There was great faith in deductions from palpation of the radial artery. The pulse lore of the century was tremendous in amount. The fantastic theories of Galen, who wrote sixteen books on the subject and described a pulse for every disease, were still current. According to the hitherto accepted doctrine of the pulse, it was enough to describe the qualities of the beat, which were examined in the utmost detail—often with a good deal of hair-splitting. Descriptions of the pulse were given which were peculiar to different organs affected with different diseases, as the pulse of the heart; the pulse of the liver; the pulse of the kidney; the pulse of the left wrist proper to the heart; the pulse of the joint of the left wrist proper to the liver; the pulse of the right wrist proper to the lungs; the pulse of the joint of the right wrist proper to the stomach; the pulse of the extremity of the right cubitus proper to the kidney, etc.

SANTORIO SANTORIO (1561-1636) said it was much more important to determine the frequency of the pulse, to count the number of beats within a specified time. This is done today with the aid of a watch. But the timepieces that existed at the end of the sixteenth century had no second hand. Santorio, therefore, constructed a special instrument for readings of the pulse, a "pulsilogium."

Santorio was the first man to invent what we now call a "clinical thermometer." This first of clinical thermometers was a primitive instrument. The globular expanded end of a convoluted capillary glass tube (graduated) was placed in the patient's mouth. The other end of the tube dipped into a vessel filled with water. The temperature was estimated from the amount of warmed air that was expired.

It was during the seventeenth century that the microscope was discovered—an instrument which opened new horizons to the antomist's eye. The microscope was perfected through the efforts of the Hollander, Cornelius Drebel (1621) and the brothers Janssen of the Netherlands (1608). Anton van Leeuwenhoek (1632-1723), a great microscopist, was the first one to apply the microscope in the study of medicine, though he himself was not a physician. Enjoying affluence, which his family had acquired in the brewing business, he was able to devote himself enthusiastically to microscopy, accumulating nearly 250 microscopes and over 400 lenses. He was the first to describe the minute structure of the crystalline lens, he furnished a complete description of spermatozoa (discovered by a medical student, Johann Hamm in 1677), made the first adequate morphological study of the red blood corpuscle, noted for the first time the histological details of voluntary muscle, was the first to describe protozoa and bacteria, and demonstrated the capillary network joining the arterial and venous trees.

RICHARD LOWER (1631-1691), an English practitioner, was the first to do a direct blood transfusion from one animal to another (1665). Frederik Ruysch (1638-1731), a Hollander, perfected the method of injecting blood vessels, and a great number of anatomical and histological discoveries were made during this period.

UROSCOPY

From time immemorial the urine has been naturally the subject of medical interest. As practiced in this century it was known as Uroscopy, or "water casting." The urine, usually in a flask, was brought to the physician, who held it to the light with solemn and judicial air, while he read the patient's fate in the uplifted urinal.

"Red Urine signifieth heat of the blood; white, rawness and indigestion in the Stomach; thick, like puddle, excessive labor

109

or sickness; white or red gravel in the bottom threatens the Stone in the Reins; black or green, commonly death."

Molére's Flying Doctor depicts the seventeenth century physician engaged in a urinalysis:

"This urine shows a great deal of heat, a great inflammation of the bowels; it is, however, not so very bad."

"Gorgibus—'Eh, What-Sir, are you swallowing it?' "

"Scanarelle—'Do not be surprised at that, doctors, as a rule, are satisfied with looking at it; but I am a doctor out of the common, I swallow it, for by tasting it I discern much better the cause and the effect of the disease. But, to tell you the truth, there was too little to judge by; let her make water again'!"

Uroscopy, as practiced, continued into the eighteenth century, and love-sickness and female chastity were still diagnosed by a naked-eye examination of a jar of urine held up to the sun. A survey of the medical literature of that time conveys the impression that with the exception of gout, the most prevalent disorder was stone in the bladder. Alkalis were regarded as the remedies, and the leading scientists concerned themselves with the problem.

A great many new remedies came into use in the seventeenth century, some good and some bad, and at the same time, most of the older ones were continued. Clusius, the botanist, gave us the original accounts of Winter's bark, canella bark, vanilla, pimenta, bearberry leaves, gamboge and star-anise. Travelers in all parts of the world sent native drugs to the European botanists: Calumba root, ipecac, copaiba, catechu, cimicifuga, cowhage, pareira brava, Iceland moss, cascarilla and serpentaria.

CINCHONA

Of great importance was a bark that had been brought over from Peru. Cinchona, as this drug was called, had long been used by the Peruvian Indians as a cure for fevers. It was brought into Europe as a secret remedy by the Jesuits in 1632, and later by Juan del Vego, physician to the Count of Chinchon.

A lady's ague was responsible for a medical revolution. Ana, Countess of Chinchon, living in Peru which her husband ruled as viceroy, lay ill with malaria. Other stories varied the details. Thus the fascinating story of quinine being introduced into England with all the necessary elements of adventure, such as Peru, Jesuits, English nobility, a sick countess and the cure of cardinals.

A later discovery throws much doubt upon one of pharmacy's most popular legends. In 1930 the diary of the Count of Chinchon relating to his term of office was discovered. It records the most trivial matters dealing with the daily life of the Count and Countess and yet it makes no mention of the Countess being ill with tertian fever at any time, nor does it describe the discovery of any new drug for the treatment of this disease. On the contrary, it records many attacks of malaria on the part of the Count and states that he was treated by being bled.

It appears that it is not definitely known who introduced cinchona into Europe.

THEODORE TOURQUET, about 1600, a Swiss by birth, who lived in France, wrote a treatise advocating the use of mineral medicines, particularly the antimonials and mercurials. This position, and also the fact that he was a Huguenot, made him unpopular in France. He moved to England, took the name of Mayerne, and was appointed chief adviser to the King and Queen. Mayerne did not, however, confine his medicines to those of chemical origin. He was tinctured with the same credulity which pervaded medicine for hundreds of years, regarding the efficacy of certain animal remedies of disgusting character. The principal ingredient in a remedy for the gout which he frequently prescribed, was the raspings of a human skull of a person who had not been buried. He is also said to have devised an ointment for hypochondria called Balsam of Bats. This contained bats, adders, new-born dogs, earthworms, hogs' grease, stagbone marrow, and the thigh bone of an ox.

About this same time a physician named Besnier was expelled by the Paris Academy of Physicians for having administered antimony to a patient. The Galenists and Paracelsans had another battle in France in 1643 in which the former won another temporary victory in again having the use of metallic salts in medicine prohibited.

In the seventeenth century there was more exact knowledge of poisons than of medicinal drugs. The medical properties of drugs could not be correctly estimated until scientific methods were developed in the eighteenth and nineteenth centuries.

The prescription of medicaments by apothecaries unversed in medicine, and by ignorant old women, was not particularly dangerous to their patients so long as the system of Galen was followed. The vile-tasting mixtures of herbs did not help cure disease, but neither did they do the patient much harm. Physicians used the same drugs. Conditions changed, however, when such poisonous drugs as mercury and antimony were introduced.

Spermaceti was highly regarded as a medicine in this period. Culpepper (1695) says, "Sperma Coeti is well applied outwardly to eating ulcers, and the marks which the small-pox leaves behind; it clears the sight, provokes sweat. Inwardly, it troubles the stomach and belly, helps bruising and stretching the nerves, and therefore is good for women newly delivered."

"The sovereign'st thing on earth was parmceti for an inward bruise." . . . Henry IV. Part I, Act I, Sc. 3.

Usnea was particularly an English drug. It consisted of the moss from the skull of a man who had died a violent death. It was obtainable in England because those were the days when the bodies of criminals who had been executed were suspended in chains at cross roads and in public places as a warning and deterrent to other criminals. This exposure was conducive to the growth of moss on the skull. The skull itself was also used in medicine.

In the seventeenth and eighteenth centuries coral and pearls were considerably used in medicine in the form of magisteries, tinctures, syrups, and arcana. Pearls were used in medicine until the eighteenth century, when it began to be suspected that chalk had the same effect. Emeralds had a great reputation, especially on account of their moral attributes. They were cold in an extra first degree, so cold that they became emblems of chastity, and curious tales of their powers in controlling the passions were told. They declared that the diamond rendered men fearless, that the ruby took away idle and foolish fancies, that the emerald resisted lust, that the amethyst kept men from drunkenness and too much sleep, and so on.

This was the century in which the *pill perpetuoe* was used. This was a pill of metallic antimony which could be used over and over again as a cathartic. One of these would serve a whole family during its lifetime and then could be transmitted as an heirloom to posterity.

THOMAS SYDENHAM (1624-1689), originator of modern internal medication, was born in the year 1624, at Wynford Eagle, in Dorsetshire, where his father, William Sydenham, had a large fortune which became of great advantage to his brilliant son.

Sydenham was one of the great first fruits of the scientific medical schools in England. He studied medicine in Oxford and Cambridge, and then took postgraduate courses at the University of Montpellier, France. He began practicing in London in 1666 and at once demonstrated that in ability, skill, broadness of knowledge and forcefulness, he stood out, not only beyond all other physicians in England, but in Europe. Sydenham was the most distinguished doctor of the seventeenth century. He has been called the English Hippocrates and the Prince of Physicians.

Sydenham was not a distinguished man of science, had not been a professor of a university, nor a voluminous writer. His collected works comprise no more than one volume of moderate size. He was merely an outstanding London practitioner.

Sydenham's reputation and his place in medical history rest solely on his genius as a clinician. When asked once by Sir Richard Blackmore as to the best books for medical reading, he replied, "Read DON QUIXOTE, it's a very good book, I read it myself still."

He grouped symptoms under the three heads of those essentially due to (1) the agent producing the disease, the so-called cardinal symptoms, (2) the accidental symptoms, those resulting from Nature's attempts at cure, and (3) the artificial symptoms, those incident to the application of therapy. On this basis he has furnished capital descriptions of rheumatism, erysipelas, chorea, pleurisy, pneumonia, croup, hysteria and in particular gout, with which he himself suffered for most of his adult life. He popularized the use of cinchona bark, taught the value of diet and exercise and devised the opium mixture that still bears his name.

He taught that morbific or peccant matter was fundamental in the causation of disease. Nature in her struggle to expel such matter produced certain symptoms and signs which were recognized as disease.

Sydenham paid the following tribute to opium. "Without it the healing art would cease to exist, and by its help a skillful physician is enabled to perform cures that seem almost miraculous."

His self treatment for gout and gravel was as follows: "In the morning, when I rise, I drink a dish or two of tea, and then ride in my coach till noon; when I return home, I moderately refresh myself with any sort of meat, of easy digestion, that I like (for moderation is necessary above all things), I drink somewhat more than a quarter of a pint of canary wine, immediately after dinner, every day, to promote digestion of the

114

food in my stomach, and to drive the gout from my bowels. When I have dined, I betake myself to my coach again and when business will permit, I ride into the country two or three miles for good air. A draught of small beer is to me instead of supper, and I take another draught when I am in bed, and about to compose myself to sleep." We have since learned that this is the way not to treat gout.

A medical student, Thomas Dover, residing in Sydenham's house, had the smallpox—and later he told how the master treated him: "First I was bled to the extent of twenty-two ounces; then an emetic. I had no fire allowed in my room, my windows were constantly open, my bed-clothes were ordered to be laid no higher than my waist. He made me take twelve bottles of small beer, acidulated with spirit of vitriol, every twenty-four hours."

The theory of the transference of disease embraced the idea that disease could be transferred from one body to another. Snake bites, for example, were cured by enveloping the punctured site with a freshly bisected fowl. Even the great Sydenham exhibits the tenacious hold of this doctrine. This great clinician fell into the error of subscribing to the *methodus modenai morbos per accubitum junioris*, i e., the method of curing disease in an old person by having him sleep with a vigorous young individual in order to bring about a transference of strength and health. Maybe the many old men who prefer young wives have heard of this doctrine.

After a life thus usefully employed, he died at his house in Pall Mall, on December 29, 1689, and was buried in the aisle, near the south door of the Church of St. James in Westminster. The College of Physicians resolved, in 1809, to erect a mural monument as near as possible to the place of interment, within that church, to the memory of this illustrious man. The title of "English Hippocrates" was of posthumous origin, for Sydenham never heard that pleasing designation. He was not a fellow of the Royal Society or of the College of Physicians, and he was not buried in Westminster Abbey.

THOMAS DOVER of Warwickshire was a student of Sydenham who resided in his house. It has been suggested that after Sydenham treated him for smallpox Dover decided that pirateering was as safe as physic and became the terror of the Spanish main. On an adventurous voyage around the world, he anchored at the island of Juan Fernandez, taking on board its solitary human inhabitant—the immortal Robinson Crusoe; plundered the city of Guayaguil in Peru; combated a plague by making his sailors drink dilute sulphuric acid; sailed past the Cape of Good Hope, and reached home, loaded with wealth, in a Spanish prize. When he grew too old for buccaneering he practiced medicine and wrote THE ANCIENT PHYSICIAN'S LEGACY TO HIS COUNTRY, which contains his diaphoretic prescription of ipecac and opium, still popular as Dover Powder.

WILLIAM HARVEY (1578-1657)

WILLIAM HARVEY, the discoverer of the circulation of the blood, was the most illustrious physician of the seventeenth century.

In the records of Padua there is still extant this entry in Latin: "William Harvey, son of Thomas Harvey, a yeoman of Kent, of the town of Folkestone, educated at the Canterbury Grammar School, aged 16 years, was admitted a lesser pensioner at the table of scholars, on the last day of May, 1593." On April 25, 1602, Harvey obtained from Padua the degree of doctor of physic, and returned to England to receive the doctorate in medicine from Cambridge.

We know little about Harvey himself, of his father we know less, and of his grandfather nothing at all. Harvey married the daughter of the physician Launcelot Browne, but he mentions her only in connection with her pet parrot which he post-mortemed. He had no children. In other words, William Harvey was without ancestry or posterity.

The importance of Harvey's work is all the more appreciated when one realizes that it was done before the microscope was in use. England knew nothing of many of the Italian anatomists, and thought but little of those few it had learned of. There were a few more bodies available for dissection than there had been, but the instruments of investigation were still far from precise. There were no watches with second hands, and time was still quite often reckoned by the interval between the beginning and end of a psalm.

Harvey's discovery of the circulation was the most important event that had occurred in medicine since the earliest rationalizing efforts of the ancient Greeks, and his discovery was the starting point of modern physiology. During the early portion of his career as a lecturer he began to demonstrate his discovery of the circulation of the blood to his classes, but did not publish it to the world until about ten years later.

John Aubrey, the eavesdropper, whom Harvey met after he retired at the age of seventy-three, became his first biographer. Aubrey wrote very frankly of many prominent men of his time. Countless personal traits of the most eminent men of the seventeenth century would be lost, had they not been preserved for us by his prying disposition. He himself knew this and wrote: "How these curiosities would be quite forgott, did not such idle fellowes as I am putt them downe!"

Other quotations from Aubrey are as follows:

"I have heard him say, that after his booke of the Circulation of the Blood came-out, that he fell mightily in his practize, and that 'twas beleeved by the vulgar that he was crackbrained; and all the physitians were against his opinion, and envyed him."

"I remember he kept a pretty young wench to wayte on him, which I guesse he made use of for warmeth-sake as King David did, and tooke care of her in his will, as also of his man servant."

Harvey died of gout, June 3, 1657. His whalebone pointer, tipped with silver, which he used in his lectures, is still preserved by the Royal College of Physicians, and his notes for these lectures are in the British Museum. They are written in a cramped hand, and very hard to read.

THOMAS PARR

Dr. Harvey, at the King's request, performed a post-mortem on the famous case of longevity, Thomas Parr, born in 1483. One hundred and thirty years later, in 1613, he attracted attention because at that age he could thresh grain with a hand flail. His fame, however, did not grow to national proportion until 1635, when he was brought to the attention of Thomas Howard, Earl of Arundel, who took him up to London so that the King might see him. The rich food of the city so disagreed with him that he died of indigestion soon after reaching London in the hundred-fifty-second year of his life.

In his report on the autopsy of Thomas Parr, Dr. Harvey attributed his death to the change from a frugal diet of subrancid cheese, milk in every form, and coarse, hard bread, to the rich feeding he received in London, and to the change from the healthful air of the country to the foggy climate of the metropolis. He also dwelt on the important fact that by his leading such a peasant's life, free from care owing to its simplicity it contributed to his very advanced age; for, as the great Harvey pithily put it, "sorry fare, but free from care."

In a letter from Harvey, himself, to his nephew, published by the Sydenham Society, we find an account of the autopsy: "The body was in such a good condition in a man of 153 that the cartilages of the chest bones were not yet ossified." Harvey put it: "The cartilages were soft and flexible," black hair on the forearms, and the organs apparently healthy. Probably the fact that the testes, as Harvey says, "were sound and large," had something to do with it. He was also an affectionate husband, and to quote Harvey again, "His wife told me that until twelve years ago he never ceased to embrace her frequently;" that is, when he was 140 years old! He had taken on his last wife in his one-hundred-and-twentieth year.

118

Old Parr has been accused of having committed a sexual offense in his 102d year, for which he was found guilty and punished.

Modern historical research has announced that his age is grossly exagerated; that there may have been two Thomas Parrs, father and son, or uncle and nephew, whose overlapping lives have become confused. However, it does not seem reasonable that a mistake would have gone uncorrected at that time, in view of the court record when he was 102 years old, the King's interest, Dr. Harvey's interest, and his burial in Westminster Abbey.

WILLIAM MURRAY

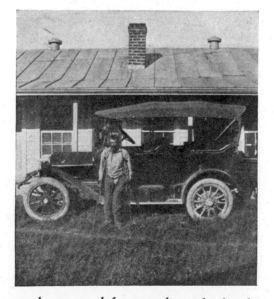

It appears to be natural for people to doubt the age of those who become extremely old, the following being a case of longevity in point:

William Murray (colored), the author being one of "his children", lived to be over 112 years of age, the accompanying picture, including the author's first automobile—an Overland, taken when he was 110. He was born a slave in Eastern Virginia and remained one till his master voluntarily freed him and his other slaves. When a slave he had been a houseboy and carriage driver. Later, he would seldom go to the fields to work and when he did he was of no account, though industrious around the house and stables. As was usual with this class of slaves, he never had any respect for "damn niggers" that worked in the field.

He came to Tennessee in the 1840's in the employ of a stage company as a blacksmith's helper and an extra stage driver, and was a man of middle age at that time. His approximate age was confirmed by substantial people who had known him in Virginia. When he was 80 or 90 years old nobody doubted it, but when he became 100 years old few would believe it.

He was the hostler in our family for many years. When he was 80 he fell through the hay-loft and broke several ribs. Mother took food to his cabin, and on returning announced amid much sorrow that this would be the last of poor old "Uncle Bill." He died March 18, 1917, having lived thirty-two years thereafter to make the world brighter.

"Uncle Bill" could not attribute his longevity to his good habits, for he smoked, chewed, ate vile messes, got on periodical drunks, and consistently violated every rule of correct living, except he did not over-eat. He called taking a drink of liquor "kissing my sister," did so till the end, and accompanied the act with a grimace that left no doubt of his enjoyment.

* * *

MARCELLO MALPIGHI (1628-1694), the father of histology, was an Italian by birth, was a professor at Bologna, Pisa and Messina, physician to Pope Innocent XII, and the greatest microscopist of his time.

Harvey's theory of the circulation of the blood was marred by a notable hiatus. He failed to discover how the blood made its way from the arteries to the veins. This discovery had been rendered possible by Malpighi by the discovery of the microscope. He was the first to discover the capillaries and thus supplied the missing link in Harvey's chain. Malpighi made many important histological discoveries.

ROBERT HOOKE, who published his MICROGRAPHIA in 1665, was the greatest of the English microscopists. He was a mechanical genius and invented many instruments and machines. It has been said of him: "His character was as unprepossessing as his body: he was too miserly to be immoral, but he was crabbed, sour, jealous, vain, and morbid. All this must be admitted, but behind those unfriendly eyes and disheveled locks burnt the fire of genius."

Hooke was not satisfied to make only half the discoveries of his age—he claimed also the other half. That is why a contemporary wrote of him, "Hooke, the most ill-natured conceited man in the world, hated and despised by most of the Royal Society, pretending to have all other inventions, when once discovered by their authors to the world."

JAN BAPTISTE VAN HELMONT (1577-1664) was a man of good family. Born in Brussels, he studied at the University of Louvain. Restlessly, discontentedly, he passed from one faculty to another. Botany led him to materia medica. Then he worked as assistant to a physician. "Soon, however, I became extremely rueful because in the curative art I found nothing to expect but dissatisfaction, uncertainty, and surmise. I could dispute concerning the medical art in connection with every disease, and yet I had no fundamental knowledge how to cure a toothache or the itch."

Medical science, however, was a disillusionment. Abandoning the profession for a time, he traveled to Switzerland, Italy, France, and England. On his journeys, he met alchemists, for in those days there were many of them, bold adventurers, continually on the road. They taught him the secrets of the use of fire. He decided to become a student of natural science.

121

Chemistry would provide true and effective remedies; but, more than this, it would provide a key to the understanding of nature.

The domain of chemistry was very variously enriched by van Helmont's studies. He investigated the various substances having the physical qualities of air, and coined for them a new general denomination, gas. He disclosed their difference from (visible) steam; and he discovered carbonic acid, thus becoming the founder of pneumatic chemistry. Previous to his discovery chemists had no clear perception of a distinction between the various gases; they reckoned them all as air.

The closing years of van Helmont's life were harrassed. A small work of his in manuscript, directed against a Jesuit and discussing the magnetic treatment of wounds, fell into the hands of a stranger, was printed against his wishes, and attracted the unfavourable attention of the Inquisition. A charge was brought against him, and for a time he was imprisoned. An interminable trial dragged on. Van Helmont recanted, but this was of no avail during his lifetime, and he was not acquitted until two years after his death, the ground for the acquittal being that he had always led so pious a life.

FRANZ DE LE BOE (Sylvius) (1614-1672), sprang from a French Huguenot family which had originally been known by the name of Dubois, and had migrated into the Low Countries. War had driven his parents thence into Germany, so that Sylvius was born at Hanau. He studied in German and Dutch universities, and took his degree in medicine at Basle in the year 1637. Later he went to Paris to improve his medical education, removing thence to Holland, where he gave botanical and anatomical lectures in Leyden, attracting many students. It was especially as an anatomist that he excelled. He wrote an anatomical work, and a fissure in the brain bears his name.

Sylvius had no regular post at Leyden. He merely gave lectures there as any doctor might. When his friends urged him to start a practice in Amsterdam, he followed the call, and soon became one of the most highly esteemed physicians in that city.

His contemporaries describe him as an extraordinarily handsome, imposing, witty man, who could laugh merrily on occasion, thus fulfilling his favorite motto of *"bene agere ac laeteri."* All the same, he was a man of exquisite manners. His jokes were never offensive; and, one of his biographers tells us, he was never seen intoxicated—which was not to be said of many men in seventeenth-century Holland. Nor was he a stickler for fees, being ready to do his best gratuitously on behalf of the poor who were members of the Protestant Walloon Church.

Sylvius carried on a successful practice in Amsterdam for seventeen years. Then, in 1658, when the chair of medicine fell vacant in Leyden, he was unanimously appointed professor.

His inclination was to attach especial importance to anatomy and physiology; but with the anatomy and physiology of that time the phenomena of health and disease could not be adequately explained, and therefore his speculations ran also into other fields, such as that of chemistry, for which he showed a predilection.

Fermentation was the process by which one substance changed into another. By such a process, by fermentation, through the influence exerted by the glandular secretions, what was ingested as nutriment was converted into blood. The ultimate products of these changes were acids and alkalis. If the balance between the acids and the alkalis was rightly maintained, the individual was healthy. On the other hand, a disturbance in body-chemistry led to the formation of "acrimoniae," which might be either acid or alkaline, which made their way into the blood, and there gave rise to illness. The aim of treatment must be, "to maintain the energies of the organism, to drive away the illness, to remove the causes, to mitigate the symptoms." Acids were counteracted by alkalis, and alkalis by acids. The bodily juices—bile, mucus, etc.,—were evacuated by emetics and purgatives both of vegetable and of mineral origin.

Van Helmont and Sylvius both thought in chemical terms, and both turned chemistry to account for the purposes of medicine. Yet how different were the two men. Van Helmont was a Catholic and a mystic; Sylvius was a Huguenot and a rationalist. Van Helmont lived a lonely life, was misunderstood, and ultimately persecuted. Sylvius was a cheerful fellow, surrounded by thankful patients and admiring students, and secured immediate success. Still, van Helmont's work has been more enduring; the problems he mooted are those which still exercise our minds today. Sylvius' mission has become no more than a memory of a distant past.

"Short-lived is the work of the happy man. He only who has eaten his bread with tears, knows the heavenly powers."

If we stop here to take stock, we shall see that three fundamentally important advances were made by scientific medicine during the early seventeenth century. The circulation became a proved fact, the phenomenon of generation was unravelled in large part, and the microscope was discovered. Two other important advances must also be noted as beginning during this century—the development of chemistry, and the birth of histology.

CHAPTER TEN

Medicine in Europe in the Eighteenth Century

WITH THE coming of Daniel Massingill to the colony of Virginia in 1653 the main interest in the Massengill family is transferred from the Old World to the New.

The division of medical history into centuries is a purely arbitrary and artificial classification that lends itself better than any other to the purposes of a general résumé. The Rational age in medicine begins where dogmatism leaves off; viz., about the close of the eighteenth century and the beginning of the nineteenth.

The field of medicine was wide and ill defined, cluttered, particularly in the eighteenth century, with an enormous variety of theories. Facts discovered in the seventeenth century frequently produced theories in the eighteenth. The eighteenth century is still spoken of as the "Period of Theories and Systems." There were so many theories, physicians did not know what to do. This confusion is apparent in MELCHIOR ADAM WEIKARD's PHILOSOPHICAL PHYSICIAN which resulted in his ostracism. Weikard later admitted it was not tactful of him to have written the book, and he likened himself to the young girl who said, when she became pregnant, "But what doesn't one do when one is discontented."

On the threshold of the eighteenth century there was a remarkable change in the outlook of medical men. Everywhere there was great activity in study and experimenting. In the eighteenth century the minds of men were free to think as liberally as they wished on any subject as a result of the Reformation, and now modern medicine was beginning to take shape under the revival of the scientific spirit. Except in respect to smallpox, medicine had really made little practical progress in the treatment or prevention of diseases up to the beginning of the nineteenth century. Anatomy continued to advance and physiology, pathology and histology were developed intensively for the first time in medical history.

Some of the substances introduced into the practice of medicine during this period were glycerin, citric, gallic, melic, tartaric and hydrocyanic acids.

In the eighteenth century when a girl was married, she received as a portion of her dowery a big medicine-spoon, and it was taken for granted that it would be filled frequently.

William Withering in 1785 gave the first accurate knowledge of Fox-glove. He began to collect plants for a young woman patient, and by the time he married her, he was a leading botanist; he confesses he received his hint about digitalis from an old woman's recipe, and the result was his pharmacological classic on the most valuable drug since the discovery of Peruvian bark. Digitalis, "the opium of the heart," was named by Fuchs, and was the most important addition to materia medica in the eighteenth century.

In the eighteenth century the fact that small doses of ergot caused the uterus to contract forcibly without poisoning the women to whom it was administered became known to some of the physicians of Europe.

Phlebotomy was a therapeutic sheet anchor which enjoyed wide popularity during this century. It was a very ancient method and its efficacy was as yet unquestioned by most physicians. There was hardly a disease for which it was not used. John Coakley Lettsom, a young Quaker physician, is remembered by Lord Erskine's neat rhyme, prompted by the way in which he signed himself "I. Lettsom":

"Whenever patients come to I,
　　I physcis, bleeds, and sweats 'em.
If, after that, they choose to die,
　　What's that to me? I. Lettsom."

JOHANN GOTTLIEB WOLSTEIN, a director of the
Vienna Veterinary Institute, may be considered the founder of
veterinary science in German-speaking countries. He published books in 1787 and 1791 and pointed out that fever by
itself is not a disease, but nature's best weapon for the combat
of disease. "Blood," he said, "is no water—it is the juice of
life; a juice which after each venesection nature replaces rapidly, but in a raw, unprepared, watery, spiritless state." The
bloodletters of the day did not listen to Wolstein, but kept on
bleeding their patients white.

JOSEPH-JACQUES DE GARDANE in 1774 was critical
of the profession's treatment of diseases, especially venereal
diseases: "There is nothing more surprising than the methods
hitherto followed. In all the seasons of the year, all subjects
presenting themselves, without regard to their sex or their age,
and without any other preparation than that given to every-
body, go through the same trials: all are bled, purged, bathed
and rubbed. In such a case the application of the grand remedy becomes a business affair, a money matter. He who treats
makes a bargain, pledging himself to cure the patient in the
space of a short and often limited time, with the result that,
when the time of treatment has expired, the patient is pronounced cured. It is in vain that the sequelae of the disease
give evidence against the supposed success; one tries to persuade
the patient that he is well, and reassuring him with further
promises, discharges him: in such a manner the majority of
those much vaunted cures are brought about.

"It is true that such conditions are demanded by the patient
himself who negotiates for his health within a fixed time, but
they are never fulfilled by those who do not blush to receive
his money in advance. Hence arises that quackery so char-

acteristic of those who treat venereal diseases. In the end, one always resorts to trickery, because one has promised more than one can do. But enough of those who in fear of losing their prey, snatch a fee from the hand of a patient in pain. A physician should promise nothing to his patient."

The eighteenth century is the period when Moliere, the French author, so caustically holds up to ridicule the pedantry and ineptitude of the French physician. The army surgeons in Prussia during this same century were ranked slightly above the drummers and beneath the chaplains, and were required to shave the officers upon request.

QUACKS AND NOSTRUMS

"From powerful causes spring the empiric's gains,
Man's love of life, his weakness, and his pains;
These first induce him the vile trash to try,
Then lend his name that other men may buy."
Crabbe:—The Borough.

A story is told of a famous quack of the eighteenth century. His name was Rock, and he sold a cure-all remedy from an open-air booth near Saint Paul's Cathedral, London. He succeeded famously. One day an old friend of his chanced to pass, and after mutual greetings the two went to a nearby inn to pledge their friendship. The visitor made a statement of his surprise at the quack's success in these words: "Thee knowest thee never had no more brains than a pumpkin." Instead of becoming indignant, the quack took him to the window and bade him count the passers-by. When twenty had passed, he asked his visitor, "How many wise men do you suppose were among that twenty?" "Mayhaps one," was the reply. "Well," returned the quack, "all the rest will come to me."

There have always been quacks and always will be, but the eighteenth century was the "Golden Age" of picturesque and successful quacks, with high infantile and adult mortality, devastating epidemic diseases, the worst hospital management on record, brutal mishandling of the insane, the deaf, the dumb, the blind and the poor.

Medical ethics were less rigid in those days, and every one quacked it a little. There must have been some physicians among them who became discouraged and turned to quacks, who based their diagnosis on showy guesses or made none at all and gave treatment, useless treatment, with all the confidence of ignorance.

Rhazes, in the Middle Ages, had knowledge of the quacks: "The heart of the public is further turned from the capable physician and towards fools because the ignorant sometimes succeed in curing complaints where this has not been done by the most famous physicians. The causes are manifold, luck, opportunity, etc. Sometimes the qualified physician effects an improvement which is not, however, yet visible; the patient is then placed under another doctor who rapidly brings about a cure and obtains the entire credit.

"Many a quack is experienced in the treatment of a single complaint, or two, according to his practice, or because he has seen the treatment of an intelligent physician. Ignorant people, therefore, think that he has equal dexterity in everything and entrust themselves to him. It is a great mistake to think that, because he has a genuine remedy for one complaint, he has one for all. I have myself learnt remedies from women and herbalists who had no knowledge of medicine."

"There are so many little arts used by mountebanks and pretenders to physic, that an entire treatise, had I a mind to write one, would not contain them; but their impudence and daring boldness is equal to the guilt and inward conviction they have of tormenting and putting persons to pain in their last hours, for no reason at all."

The culmination of quackery in the eighteenth century was due largely to the poor examples of royalty, male and female, who sat on the throne and patronized charlatans. Queen Anne, suffering from weak eyes, insulted the medical profession by transforming a mountebank into Sir William Read, principal oculist to her majesty. As an advertiser, Read was more aggressive than his predecessor John Case, who inscribed under the Sign of the Golden Ball:

> Within this place
> Lives Doctor Case.

The TATLER maintained that Case made more money by this couplet than Dryden by all his poetical works put together; Addison wrote also a note about Read:

"There was an epigram current, that Sir William could hardly read, but he seldom suffered any periodical to make its appearance in public without some testimony under his own hand that he could hardly write. It appears he was a very comely person and a man of fashion, rich and ostentatious. . . . He kept an excellent table and was noted for his special brew of punch, which he served out to his guests in golden goblets."

It is probable that cosmetics were used then much more extensively among all classes than they are today. Even in bygone days there were ardent reformers in the field, for a bill introduced into the English Parliament in 1770 contains the following provisions: "All women of whatever age, rank, profession, or degree, whether virgins, maids, or widows, that shall, from and after such Art, impose upon, seduce, and betray into matrimony, any of His Majesty's subjects, by scents, paints, cosmetic washes, artificial teeth, fake hair, Spanish wool, iron stays, hoops, high heeled shoes, bolstered hips, shall incur the penalty of the law in force against witchcraft and like misdemeanors and that marriage, upon conviction, shall stand null and void."

Joshua Ward, known as "Spot" because of a birthmark on his face, took up medicine when he failed in business as a drysalter. He invented a "Pill" containing antimony, and by administering this remedy and at the same time practicing faith healing with the "laying on of hands," he developed a great reputation and became popular in the courts of King George II.

Franz Anton Mesmer, of Suabia, came to Vienna to study medicine. Numerous discoveries in electricity had been made and charlatans have a flair for exploiting scientific progress. Mesmer promulgated the theory that the sun and moon act upon living beings by means of the subtle fluids known as animal magnetism, analogous in its effect to the properties of the lodestone. He claimed that he could magnetize trees, so every leaf contributed healing to all who approached. Vienna knew him and did not believe him, and he went to Paris. He erected a temple to the god of health, and here thronged the afflicted.

"The patients sat around a magnetic baquet, and waited; the majority were women, and for them a special set of handsome young men had been provided. Each selected a woman and stared her in the eye; no word was spoken, but from somewhere softly sailed the music of an accordion, and the voice of a hidden opera-singer sweetened the incense-laden air. The young Apollos embraced the knees of the women, rubbed various spots, and gently massaged their breasts. The women closed their eyes, and felt the magnetism surge through them. At the critical moment, the master magnetizer, Mesmer himself, appeared on the scene. Clad in a lilac gown, with lofty mien and majestic tread, he advanced among his patients, making "passes" and accomplishing miracles. If a lady had a "crisis," Mesmer lifted her up and carried her to his private crisis-chamber. Nor were male visitors lacking at these seances, though as a rule they came not for Mesmer's medicine, but to observe the fainting girls who often fell into convulsions. It must have been a pleasant form of hypnosis, for as soon as a patient recovered from one crisis, she begged for another."

Mesmerism became a sensation. It seemed as if all the world wished to be magnetized. The French government offered Mesmer a pension and the Cross of the Order of St. Michael for his secret; he refused, because he was already making a fortune.

Mesmer's disciple, Charles D'Eslon, a leading member of the Faculty and physician to Comte d'Artois, received a visit from a man in uniform: "In my capacity as lieutenant-general of police, I wish to know whether, when a woman is magnetized and passing through the crisis, it would not be easy to outrage her." D'Eslon answered in the affirmative, but explained that only the colleagues of Mesmer, physicians of probity, were entitled and privileged to produce a crisis.

Finally a commission was appointed to investigate the phenomenon; among the commissioners were some of the most illustrious scientists of the eighteenth century: the first name signed to the report is Benjamin Franklin, who was then located in Paris. They reached the verdict that magnetism is due to the imagination. They prepared also a secret report, "not adapted for general publication," which is more curious than the official version.

Benjamin Franklin, America's intellectual giant of the eighteenth century was one of the authors of the following extracts:

"It has been observed that women are like musical strings stretched in perfect unison; when one is moved, all the others are instantly affected. Thus the commissioners have repeatedly observed that when the crisis occurs in one woman, it occurs almost at once in others also. . . .

"Women are always magnetized by men; the established relations are doubtless those of a patient to the physician, but this physician is a man, and whatever the illness may be, it does not deprive us of our sex, it does not entirely withdraw us from the power of the other sex; illness may weaken impressions without destroying them. Moreover, most of the women who present themselves to be magnetized are not really ill; many come out of idleness, or for amusement; others, if not perfectly well, retain their freshness and their force, their senses are unimpaired and they have all the sensitiveness of youth; their charms are such as to affect the physician, and their health is such as to make them liable to be affected by him, so that the danger is reciprocal. . . .

"The magnetizer generally keeps the patient's knees enclosed within his own, and consequently the knees and all the lower parts of the body are in close contact. The hand is applied to the hypochondriac region, and sometimes to that of the ovarium, so that the touch is exerted at once on many parts, and these the most sensitive parts of the body.

"The experimenter, after applying his left hand in this manner, passes his right hand behind the woman's body, and they incline towards each other so as to favor this twofold contact. This causes the closest proximity; the two faces almost touch, the breath is intermingled, all physical impressions are felt in common, and the reciprocal attraction of the sexes must consequently be excited in all its force. It is not surprising that the senses are inflamed. The action of the imagination at the same time produces a certain disorder throughout the machine; it obscures the judgment, distracts the attention; the women in question are unable to take account of their sensations, and are not aware of their condition....

"The commissioners' experiments, showing that all these results are due to contact, to imagination and imitation."

Well-meaning but misguided legislative bodies have purchased remedies quite as illogical as the one bought by the State of New York:

Pursuant to the directions of an act, entitled, "An act for granting a compensation to John M. Crous, for discovering and publishing a cure for the canine madness, passed the second day of February, 1806."

For his remedy, Mr. Crous was rewarded by the State of New York with $1,000, a considerable sum in 1806. And what was the valuable remedy of Mr. Crous? I fear the laudable desire of the New York Legislature to spare the citizens from a frightful disease was stronger than the medical discretion of that body; the prescription calls for a mixture made from the pulverized jawbone of a dog, the ground-up false tongue of a newly foaled colt, and the green rust scraped off the surface of an English penny of the reign of George I.

The Englishman, in the seventeenth century, who variously called himself Robert Tabor, Talbor and Talbot was shrewd enough to see the merits of Peruvian bark, advertised he possessed a secret remedy that triumphed over disease and kept death at bay. His successful treatment of Lady Mordaunt's daughter brought him to the chamber of Charles II, who "for good and acceptable services performed" appointed him royal physician, although he was not any sort of physician. Charles warned the College of Physicians not to interfere with Talbor's medical practice, and His Majesty further showed his gratitude by conferring knighthood upon him.

Sir Robert Talbor, under the name of Talbot, next appeared in France. "Nothing is talked of here but the Englishman and his cures . . . when his remedy is published, all physicians will be superfluous." Talbot's great opportunity came when the Dauphin was sick: "The English physician has promised the King, at the price of his head, to cure the Dauphin in four days. If he should fail, I really believe they will throw him out of the window, but if he succeeds I say a temple should be erected to him as to a second Aesculapius.

"D'Aquin, Louis XIV's chief physician, who is driven to his wit's end, at not being possessed of this panacea; and the rest of the tribe, who are overwhelmed with despair at the experience, the success, and the almost divine prognostications of this little foreigner. The King will have him make up his medicines in his presence, and trusts the management of the Prince wholly to him. The Dauphiness is already much better; and yesterday the Count de Grammont saluted D'Aquin with the following:

> "D'Aquin can no longer withstand
>   Talbot, victorious over death;
> The princess owns his healing hand,
>   Let each one sing with joyful breath, etc."

D'Aquin insisted the Dauphin had been bilious and never in serious danger; his words were drowned in the flood of praise that greeted "the Englishman's cure." Louis XIV deigned to request him to remain on French soil, as an ornament to the nation. As Talbor declined, the King purchased his formula with the understanding that it would not be divulged during the inventor's lifetime. Aside from an annual pension, Talbor received two thousand guineas, and the title of Chevalier. The world had not long to wait for the "Wonderful Secret for Cureing of Agues and Feavers," for upon the heels of his royal triumphs, Talbor died at the age of forty (1681). Talbor's method was immediately translated into English "for Publick Good." The formula consisted of rose leaves soaked in water with lemon juice, to which was added a strong dose of Peruvian bark (a synonym for Cinchona bark).

Talbor advertised that his secret remedy did not contain Cinchona, and he even went so far as to point out the dangers of using Cinchona bark in the treatment of malaria.

Here is the story of a widow who fooled a nation. She claimed to have a cure for stone in the bladder and became a celebrity. The following announcement appeared in the GENTLEMEN's MAGAZINE, in 1738: "Mrs. Stephens has proposed to make her medicine publick on consideration of £5,000 to be raised by contribution." The church and peerage of England responded generously, yet the £5,000 could not be raised.

Joanna Stephens determined to keep her secret, but such was the public clamor that an Act of Parliament appointed a commission of investigation, which included the three leading surgeons of the metropolis: William Cheselden, of Chelsea Hospital, who could incise the bladder and remove the stone in fifty-four seconds; Sir Caesar Hawkins, of St. George's Hospital, inventor of the cutting gorget; and Samuel Sharp, of Guy's Hospital, whose treatise on surgical operations passed through ten editions and a French translation in his own lifetime. Their unanimous decision was as follows: "We have examined the said medicines and her method of preparing the same, and are convinced by experiment, of the utility, efficacy, and dissolving power thereof." Whereupon the British Government gave Mrs. Stephens the £5,000 and in return Mrs. Stephens published (June 19, 1738) a "full discovery" in the London Gazette. Her prescriptions were a decoction, containing boiled herbs and soap, with swine's-cresses burnt to blackness, "but this was only with a view to disguise it;" pills, consisting of wild carrot and burdock seeds, hips and hawes, reduced to ashes with alicant soap and honey; powder, composed of roasted egg-shells crushed with garden-snails in the month of May.

The "Act for providing a Reward to Joanna Stephens," bore not only the names of the surgeons, but the greater name of Stephen Hales, England's chief physiologist since Harvey. The prime minister, Sir Robert Walpole, swallowed the saponified snails by the pound. After his death, Sir Caesar Hawkins performed the autopsy, and discovered several stones in his bladder. It is calculated that in the last few years of his life an otherwise intelligent Prime Minister had consumed 180 lbs. of soap and not less than 1,200 gallons of lime-water.

Aetius was a Greek of the fifth century, who was an authority on plasters, and who was said to have first made use of the magnet in medicine. He was the first physician-pharmacist to embrace Christianity. In the works of Aetius, reference is made to several celebrated nostrums, one of which, a collyrium, sold for the equivalent of $500, and was scarce at that price; another was modestly named "isotheos" (equal to God).

During Sir Walter Raleigh's twelve years' imprisonment in the Tower in the earlier part of the reign of James I, he was allowed a room in which he fitted up a laboratory, and divided his time between chemical experiments and literary labors. It was believed that Raleigh had brought with him from Guiana some wonderful curative balsam, and this opinion, combined with the knowledge that he dabbled largely with retorts and alembics in the Tower, ensured a lively public interest in his "Great Cordial" when it was available.

The composition of the "Great Cordial" was given September 20, 1662:

"The cordial then consisted of forty roots, seeds, herbs, etc., macerated in spirit of wine, and distilled. With the distillate were combined bezoar stones, pearls, coral, deer's horn, amber, musk, antimony, various earths, sugar, and much besides. Vipers' flesh, with the heart and liver, and 'mineral unicorn' were added later on the suggestion of Sir Kenelm Digby."

Quacks abounded in London at this time. The three greatest, and perhaps the last of the great quacks, were a German, an Italian Jew, and a Scot—Myersbach, Count Alessandro Di Cagliostro (the Quack of Quacks), and James Graham.

Myersbach was an M. D. of Erfurth in Germany. The degree was not hard to get at that time. A young man traveling in Germany had no difficulty in obtaining it for one Anglicus Ponto. After paying the necessary fees and receiving the degree, he revealed the fact that Ponto was his favorite mastiff.

Myersbach's specialty was urinoscopy or water-casting. In the Middle Ages the urinal was the emblem of medical practice, and was even used as a convenient sign-board device. Ancient water-casters claimed no difficulty in forecasting the sex of an unborn child from the prospective mother's urine.

Myersbach reached London about 1774, and proceeded to accumulate a fortune. After two years of immunity from all criticism, he was attacked by John Coakley Lettsom, one of the founders of the Medical Society of London. Lettsom and his friends got a great deal of amusement out of Myersbach. They submitted a flask of port wine to him, and were assured that the case from which it came was one of serious disease of the womb. From the urine of a gelding the omniscient doctor deduced that the patient was a lady, and that she had a disorder of the womb, two children, and a bad temper. A cow's urine distressed him greatly. He explained that it obviously came from a young man who had been much too free with the ladies of the town.

137

Dr. Lettsom made the following public statement in regard to Myersbach:

"Dr. Myersbach knew less of urine than a chambermaid and as little of medicine as most of his patients." Myersbach discreetly packed up his bags and retired to the Continent for some twelve months. Then he returned and had as great a success as ever.

Cagliostro, the Quack of Quacks, started life as Joseph Balsamo and graduated early as a sneak-thief and forger. He came to London in 1771 with his wife Lorenzo because there was more scope for his natural genius in capital cities, and also because he was wanted by the authorities, for forgery and kindred activities in many other places. Soon the London police were seeking him as earnestly as their colleagues in Italy, Spain, and Portugal, but by that time Joseph was in Paris, as the Marquis de Balsamo, rejuvenating the aged, healing the sick, softening marble, making gold, transforming cotton into silk, and generally benefiting mankind at large.

He traveled extensively, modestly confining his activities to making beautiful the very ugly, and causing diamonds and pearls to grow to twice their original size. He returned to London, but this time as Captain, later Colonel, and soon afterward Count, Cagliostro. Unfortunately he was found out while indulging in his favorite relaxation of swindling the very wealthy, and languished for a while in an English prison. On being released he must have resolved to turn over a new leaf. He was soon established in popularity as a nobleman, an illustrious scientist, and a great philanthropist.

He started traveling again in a magnificent private carriage, surrounded by couriers, lackeys, and valets. His claims were as modest as ever. He could, for a considerable consideration, raise the dead, restore lost youth, foretell the future, and perform miracles. In Russia, Poland, and Germany he was received with acclamation and showered with presents. He would never take fees for healing the sick—and never refuse presents. Wherever he went the troops had to be called out to control the crowds. He was an honored guest of every other princely family in Europe.

He returned to Paris in 1785, to be promoted immediately to the pedestal from which Mesmer had just toppled. Cagliostro and his wife were mixed up—for perhaps the first time in their career innocently—in the affair of Marie Antoinette's diamond necklace. They were sent to the Bastille, but acquitted after trial. Their release provoked great popular demonstrations in their favor, but the King ordered them both to leave Paris within a week. The one crime of which he was not guilty ruined Cagliostro. London would have none of him. Switzerland drove him from its frontiers, and he returned at last to Rome. There was no market even there for his love-philtres and elixirs. He took up again Freemasonry, in which he had long dabbled, and this soon brought him into the hands of the Inquisition. Five years later he died in prison.

James Graham, born in 1745, the third of this trio, was the son of an Edinburgh saddler. He studied medicine there for a short time, but it is doubtful if he ever took a degree or obtained a qualification of any kind. After practicing for a short time at Pontefract, he went to America as a sort of itinerant specialist in diseases of the eye and ear. There he became acquainted with Benjamin Franklin's discoveries and quickly saw the possibilities of using electricity for the exploitation of the public. He returned to England, and after practicing for a while in the neighborhood of Bath and Bristol he established what might be termed an electro-therapeutic practice in London. This first venture was not very successful, and so he returned to Bath, and soon had great numbers of patients waiting to spend a few minutes sitting on his "magnetic throne" or lying in an "electrical bath."

Graham knew how to keep his followers interested, whether lecturing on the "Preservation and Exaltation of Loveliness," or publishing a pamphlet on sex, "as delivered by Hebe Vestina at the Temple of Hymen." He vended a remedy, so rare and valuable, that he demanded for this Elixir of Life the payment of £1,000 in advance; whoever took it would reach 150 years at the minimum, and in fact would live as long as the medicine was renewed, a process which could go on indefinitely.

Graham later went to Paris and treated many aristocratic patients. He built a Temple, the door of which was always open, so that the poor might enter as freely as the rich. All that was demanded of the poor was a fee of £6, which was paid to one of two regally dressed porters. Once this trifling formality was over, rich and poor males were alike conducted to the Great Apollo Apartment. Soft music always preceded his discourse, and at appropriate moments his audience received mild electrical shocks from the carefully wired chairs in which they were seated. As a grand finale an enormous spectre came up through the floor and handed to Graham bottles of his famous "aetherial balsam," which was guaranteed to promote fertility.

The Goddess of Health who officiated at the ceremonies was the bewitching shawl-dancer, Emma Lyon, who was familiar with many beds, later famous as Lady Hamilton and as the enchantress of Lord Nelson.

If, despite the guarantee, the aetherial balsam did not promote a successful conception and lead to the production of the loveliest possible children, Graham placed at the disposal of his clients his wonder of wonders, the innermost mystery of the Temple of Health. This was his Celestial Bed, which assured conception to the occupants.

To quote from an article written at the time and reprinted in the British Medical Journal for 1911: "A sumptuous bed in brocaded damask supported by four crystal pillars of spiral shape festooned with garlands of flowers in gilded metal is its essential feature; and for a fee of fifty guineas Dr. Graham offers couples, old and young, the means of getting offspring. On whatever side one gets into this bed, which is called 'Celestial,' one hears an organ played in unison with three others, which make agreeable music consisting of varied airs which carry the happy couple into the arms of Morpheus. For nearly

140

an hour that the concert lasts one sees in the bed streams of light which play especially over the pillows. When the time for getting up has come, the magician comes to feel the pulse of the faithful, gives them breakfast, and sends them away full of hope, not forgetting to recommend them to send him other clients."

Other claims made for the Celestial Bed: If the young lay in this bed, they would retain their good looks; if the old experienced its effects, they would be rejuvenated; if married or unmarried slept in it, their progeny would be healthy, beautiful, and virtuous. The price for a night in this bed was from £50 to £100.

This vogue lasted for three most profitable years, at the end of which time Graham returned to his native Edinburgh, there to preach the virtues of the mud bath and a fasting cure. In his declining years he became first religious and later maniacal. He died suddenly in 1794. Graham's cure was to assure life for a century, but he died before he was fifty.

In 1796 Dr. Perkins patented his "tractors", consisting of two short metallic rods which were used for the treatment of disease by being drawn over the skin. They created much interest and were largely sold. A Perkins Institute was established in London. It was demonstrated that patients recovered just as well when two pieces of wood were used, provided they were told that it was the Perkins tractors that were being used.

Usnea was an official drug in the pharmacoea until the nineteenth century and there were many testimonials to the relief it had brought to patients with nervous or wasting diseases. It was a moss scraped from the skull of a criminal who had been hung in chains.

The counterpart of Usnea for external application was a piece of the rope with which a man had been hanged. The rope was the property of the hangman; he cut it into as many pieces as possible and auctioned them off to the highest bidders.

HERMANN BOERHAAVE (1668-1738)

Hermann Boerhaave was one of the most celebrated physicians of the eighteenth century. He was born in the village of Voorhout, near Leyden, on December 31, 1668. His father was a clergyman, well skilled in the Hebrew, Greek, and Latin languages, who destined his only son, Hermann, to succeed him in the church. Soon, however, he found that mathematics, chemistry, botany, and medicine were far more to his taste, and in the end he made up his mind to transfer to the medical faculty. In 1693, he took the degree of Doctor of Medicine. He occupied most of the chairs in the University of Leyden and was known as the Batavian Hippocrates. His practice was a form of eclecticism, claiming to accept what was good in all the theories of the time.

Boerhaave made no discoveries; he did not contribute any new ideas of moment to medicine. Nor did he belong to any school. Yet that was what gave him his strength. He adopted what seemed to him good, no matter the source. The secret of his successes is to be found, not so much in his scientific writings, as in his personality, in his alluring personality as physician and clinical teacher. He was generous and devoid of professional envy.

Boerhaave's practice increased from year to year. Haller writes: "From ten till twelve his consulting-room was thronged by those who sought his advice, for pressure of work now made it impossible for him to visit patients in their homes. Often enough the morning consultations outlasted the fixed hours, so that lecture time had come before he had had a moment in which to eat his dinner. At three in the afternoon additional patients began to arrive. What remained of his day was spent in an extensive correspondence and in his long-continued labours upon the writings of the Greek physicians."

He became so famous that a letter mailed in China by a mandarin addressed "Boerhaave in Europe," was placed on his desk; one night he kept Peter the Great waiting because he recognized no distinctions among patients; his practice was so extensive that he left millions of guilders to his daughter.

In spite of his mildness and kindness, Boerhaave could assert himself. Knowing the history of medicine, he felt impelled to say, "Galen has done more harm than good." In a similar strain, Boerhaave declared: "If we compare the good which a half dozen true sons of Aesculapius have accomplished since the origin of medical art upon the earth, with the evil which the immense mass of doctors of this profession among the human race have done, there can be no doubt that it would have been far better if there had never been any physicians in the world."

This reflection did not cost Boerhaave his general popularity, since all physicians believed they were among the six exempted Asclepiads.

In 1725 he suffered from severe inflammation of the joints, which deprived him completely of sleep. These attacks of gout became so violent and so frequent that Boerhaave had to cut down his work, and in 1729 he resigned the professorships of chemistry and botany. He continued, however, to give clinical instruction until in 1738, in the seventieth year of his life, when he was finally relieved of his sufferings.

ALBRECHT VON HALLER (1708-1777), a scion of an old Swiss family at Berne, was Boerhaave's greatest pupil. He was an infant prodigy, explaining the Bible at four, outlining a Chaldee grammar, compiling two thousand biographical sketches, preparing a Greek and Hebrew vocabulary, and writing a Latin satire on his tutor, before his tenth birthday. His contemporaries regarded him as a man of universal learning, as one who was interested in every domain of human knowledge.

He wrote poems and novels that were read at the time. He had nothing in common with the vigorous young associates of his own age, till he became a student at Tubingen. The merry life of the students, the influence of frivolous comrades, and association with the pretty ladies of Tubingen "who were by no means coy," continued to break down the barriers between young Haller and the life of the everyday world.

Tubingen, however, was not a place for serious studies, so in the spring of 1725 Haller removed to Leyden. There he found all that his heart could desire: a dissecting-room in which there were human bodies; a botanical garden; a clinic. Above all in Albinus and Boerhaave he found teachers who were to exert a decisive influence upon his career. It was in Leyden that he received the impetus which made him a man of science. Devoting himself to his medical training with the utmost zeal, he was able as early as 1727 to take his degree as doctor of medicine with a dissertation upon an anatomical topic.

After an additional term as Basle, spent mainly in anatomical studies, in the spring of 1729 Haller returned to Berne and settled down there as a doctor. It is easy to understand that in the narrow surroundings of the Swiss capital he felt extremely unhappy. Then, when he was beginning to lose heart, in the spring of 1736 he received a call to the recently founded University of Gottingen as professor of anatomy, surgery, and botany.

Haller's versatile genius revealed itself best in physiology. Before his time there had never existed a complete treatise on physiology. From 1759 to 1766 he published a great work ELEMENTA PHYSIOLOGIAE CORPORIS HUMANI, in eight quarto volumes, thus establishing modern physiology and earning for himself the lasting title of father of physiology.

Rumor has it that one day an English ship was seized by pirates who found on board their prize a box of books directed to Haller. Noticing the inscription, the pirate captain hastened to the next port and left the box to be forwarded, feeling that it would be insufferable to rob so famous a man of learning as Herr von Haller.

In 1759, a student of twenty-six, a Berlin tailor's son working for his doctorate, attacked the preformation doctrine in his thesis, THEORIA GENERATIONIS, which he dedicated to Haller,

144

whom he called "glorious man." Haller was polite, but remained convinced. Between Haller, potentate of physiology, and this unknown Caspar Wolff, there could be no argument. Haller simply laughed, and no one read the young doctor's thesis. Caspar Wolff is now "justly reckoned the founder of modern embryology."

FRANCOIS XAVIER BICHAT (1771-1802). As one contemplates the wonders of eighteenth century medicine, he barely emerges from the captivating influence of Haller, before encountering the striking genius of Bichat, also the founder of a new branch of medical science—Francois Xavier Bichat, a Frenchman, the son of a French physician. Bichat is regarded as the founder of modern histology.

Bass called Bichat the Napoleon of medicine, because like the great general, he "placed facts in the first rank and banished ideas and ideologists." We are reminded of Paracelsus when Bichat writes, "If I have gone forward so rapidly, the result is that I have read little; books are merely the memoranda of facts. But are such memoranda necessary in a science whose material is ever near us, where we have so to speak, living books, in the sick and the dead?"

GERHARD VAN SWIETEN (1700-1772) was one of Boerhaave's pupils, and perhaps the favorite of them all. Van Swieten certainly had merits as a medical man: when he was called over from Holland, the Austrian throne had no heir; van Swieten drew the husband aside, and gave him some private instruction, with the result that Maria Theresa became pregnant sixteen times. He was now forty-five years of age. Had it not been for Maria Theresa's summons he would probably have remained for the rest of his life a general practitioner in a small Dutch town. History would have taken little notice of him, regarding him as no more than one among the very large number of Boerhaave's pupils.

For years Boerhaave and van Swieten had lived and worked side by side in the friendliest way, closely linked though there was so much difference between their ages. Van Swieten practiced in Leyden, and was a very successful lecturer at the university.

But he was a Roman Catholic, and as such he could not occupy a professional chair in Leyden. There was no possibility of his becoming Boerhaave's successor. When the latter died, van Swieten had to quit the university. The students rose in rebellion, but without avail. Van Swieten himself had to pacify them, explaining that there was no choice but to obey the law.

We have a contemporary description of van Swieten's daily work: "He rose at five and went to court at half-past six. Returning home at eight or nine, he shut himself up in his study and worked there until two o'clock in the afternoon. Then he had his dinner, which occupied an hour. After that he devoted an hour to giving free medical advice to the poor and then went on working in his study until seven in the evening. At this hour he paid a second visit to the court. At nine he ate a frugal supper and went to bed at half-past ten."

ANTON DE HAEN (1704-1776) was the successor of van Swieten at the Old Vienna School. He was a clinician of ability who left eighteen volumes behind him, and in these treatises we find his defense of witchcraft. This incongruity later struck Virchow, who in his survey of a century of pathology, exclaimed: "With the fanaticism of a monk, de Haen defends magic and miracles, and attacks the philosophers as atheists. He prepared the soil in which soon were to sprout animal magnetism and somnambulism. What contrasts in one man! The same physician who introduced the thermometer into the observation of the sick, and dissection into clinical investigation, believes in witchcraft and persecutes witches."

It was only to be expected that two such strong personalities as van Swieten and de Haen should found a school. Van Swieten died in 1772; de Haen in 1776; and Haller in 1777. Thus the great generation of the disciples of Boerhaave came to

146

an end, but their work lived after them. An admirable new university had come into being at Gottingen.

GIOVANNI BATTISTA MORGAGNI (1682-1771) established pathological anatomy in the eighteenth century. The founder of histology, Bichat, was a Frenchman, whose work was ended by death in his thirty-second year; the founder of pathology, Morgagni, was an Italian who compiled his great work when he was within hailing distance of eighty. He was in his ninetieth year when he died.

LAZZARO SPALLANZANI was the indolent kinsman of Laura Bassi, professor of experimental physics at the University of Bologna. He was fifteen before he finished his grammar school course. Spallanzani is one of the great names in physiology. His early idleness was replaced by an incessant and effective activity. In his experiments on digestion, he swallowed linen bags containing food, perforated wooden tubes, and was enough of a scientific martyr to obtain gastric juice by making himself vomit on an empty stomach. He supplemented his self-experimentation by experiments on a surprising variety of animals.

Spallanzani found the fertilizing power of the spermatic fluid is lost when it is filtered, though he left the correct interpretation for later workers; by putting male frogs into trousers during cohabitation, he noted the ova remained unfertilized; he found that fertilization does not occur unless there is contact between sperm and egg. He was the first who artificially fecundated the eggs of frog and toad, and the first who empregnated a bitch by injecting warm semen into the vagina.

THOMAS FULLER, a country practitioner of Sevenoaks in Kent, gave a clear conception of specificness in infection and immunity of eruptive fevers in anticipation of the modern doctrine: "Many varieties are to be met with in books, of other diseases mixed in with the smallpox, but nobody ever yet saw a miliary fever, or measles, or any of its sub-species beget a true smallpox, or any of its sorts; nor on the contrary; and nobody was ever defended from the infection of any one sort by having had another sort. To every seed its own body; and therefore the pestilence can never breed the smallpox, nor the smallpox the measles, nor they the crystals of chicken pox, any more than a hen can a duck, a wolf a sheep, or a thistle figs; and consequently one sort cannot be a preservative against any other sort."

STEPHEN HALES was a physician and a parson. In 1733 he wrote a book on the force of blood in animals. A century after Harvey's demonstration of the circulation, Hales discovered how to investigate its dynamics. When Hales fastened glass-tubes into the arteries and veins of horses, he devised a crude pressure-gauge which in his hands gave remarkable results. Thus to the old story of the pulse, Stephen Hales added the new chapter of blood-pressure. This busy clergyman stands among the pioneers of experimental physiology, and as the Father of Blood Pressure he initiated a method which is now of primary importance in the diagnosis and treatment of disease.

JAMES CURRIE, a Scotsman, spent several years in America, where he had been informed it was easy to acquire a fortune. Ill-luck in business and the Declaration of Independence drove him home, where he graduated in medicine, and in his spare time introduced cold douche-baths of sea-water in typhoid, including verification and tabulation of results with the clinical thermometer.

Valvular disease of the heart ended a career of constant misfortune and glory; and he sleeps beneath the appropriate epitaph:

"Art taught by thee shall o'er the burning frame
The healing freshness pour and bless thy name."

THOMAS ROBERT MALTHUS, a clergyman, argued that "the realization of a happy society will always be hindered by the miseries consequent on the tendency of population to increase faster than the means of subsistence," and thus became the father of the birth-control movement and began a controversy which is still mooted.

Praise and obloquy were showered upon the author in profusion. Unswayed by the adulation, and untouched by the abuse, he quietly kept on revising successive editions of his epoch-making book. According to Malthus, only when time had cooled the passions and partial impotence supervened, should man and woman repair to the altar. He looked upon the lusty bridegroom and the blushing young bride as a menace to society—his ideal was the decorous middle-aged couple content with Platonic relations.

WILLIAM CULLEN, an Edinburgh professor, made many comments upon the use of drugs which are worth reading even today, for the spirit of criticism is modern. He suggested that the use of certain drugs be restricted and the use of others abandoned. Cullen's century witnessed the origin of American medicine, and before this country wrote its own manuals of materia medica, his works were gospel.

JOHN BROWN (1735-1788), a Scot, founded the "Brunonian system." Brown was a very remarkable man, at once a genius and a rogue. He entered the medical profession after having been a minister of religion and then a schoolmaster. A heavy drinker, he became deeply burdened with debt, and thereby found his way into prison. Nevertheless his ELEMENTA MEDICINAE, published in 1780, created much interest. He set out from the doctrines of Cullen, in whose house he had lived for a short time as private tutor. He differed in various respects from his patron. According to Brown's teaching, the decisive factor in bringing about disease was not excess or defect of nervous energy, but the stimulus, the exciting factor, which set nervous energy in motion.

WILLIAM HEBERDEN of London first described angina pectoris, and the fingers in arthritis deformans still known as Heberden's nodules.

England in particular was the country where clinical medicine seemed to thrive most actively during this period. The two Hunter Brothers, William (1718-1783) and John (1728-1793), have become fixtures in medical history.

WILLIAM HUNTER, the elder of the brothers, settled in London in 1740. He had studied medicine in Glasgow, was a successful surgeon, was devoted to anatomy, and was the pride of the family.

JOHN HUNTER was born at Long-Calderwood, in the county of Lanark, on February 14, 1728. In childhood he was the despair of the elders of his household, and no one ever anticipated for him a great career. At school he was an unsatisfactory pupil, so that his schooldays were short. Capricious and ill-tempered, when he could not get his own way he would howl for hours in succession. The only things he really liked doing were playing practical jokes or wandering in the woods in search of birds' eggs.

What was to become of him? Perhaps William would help him, could find a use for him. John wrote to London, and William agreed to give his young brother a trial. Wonder of wonders, the ne'er-do-well proved his mettle as William's assistant! He worked all day and far on into the night, kept the dissecting-room in good order, and showed himself an adept at securing the requisite bodies. Soon, moreover, he became a skilled dissector.

On William's recommendation, John Hunter entered as surgeon-apprentice at Chelsea Hospital, and after a few years he had mastered the craft. William wanted John to make up for the defects of his general education, so he sent the young man to Oxford, but John stayed only a few months, saying when he returned: "They wanted to make an old woman of me, or that I should stuff Latin at the University; but these schemes I cracked like so many vermin as they came before me."

For a time he became an army surgeon, and then a naval surgeon. England was at war with France and Spain. Hunter

was present at several engagements, and acquired a great deal
of experience. When the army was disbanded Hunter returned to London and settled down as a surgeon.

Hunter was perpetually on the look-out for rare beasts.
If a gypsy passed by with a dancing bear, Hunter would make
a bargain with the man to bring the creature for dissection
when it died. The Irish giant cost him much labor and a great
deal of money. He was absolutely determined to have
O'Bryan's skeleton for his collection. When the giant fell
sick, Hunter had him kept under observation. But the Irish-
man scented danger, and, regarding with horror the thought
that his body would be cut up, he made his friends promise that
when he died they would never lose sight of his corpse until it
had been sealed up in a leaden coffin and sunk in the sea. We
are told that bribery and corruption to the tune of £500 were
needed before Hunter could get his way. The upshot was that
the skeleton is in the Royal College of Surgeons' museum, and
that O'Bryan's name has become immortal.

In Hunter's time, physicians were still discussing whether
syphilis and gonorrhea were two manifestations of the same
disease, or different diseases. To settle the problem, John
Hunter, on a Friday in May, 1767, inoculated himself on the
prepuce and glans with gonorrheal pus; unknown to him, the
subject from whom he took the poison had also a hidden
chancre within his urethra, and Hunter contracted not only
gonorrhea but syphilis. He was now convinced that "matter
from a gonorrhea will produce chancres," and there is but a
single venereal virus. It is one of the tragedies of science—the
master of the experimental method being led hopelessly astray
by an heroic experiment.

John Hunter was the first investigator since the days of
antiquity to advance the theory of inflammation a stage. "Inflammation in itself is not to be considered as a disease, but as
a salutary operation, consequent either to some violence or some
disease. Inflammation is not only occasionally the cause of
diseases, but it is often a mode of cure, since it frequently pro-

duces a resolution of indurated parts, by changing the diseased action into a salutary one, if capable of resolution."

In the eighteenth century, medicine and surgery were two distinct provinces. John Hunter was one of the most successful surgeons of his time. Along this path he was a pioneer hastening greatly in advance of his time, and he constructed the first bridge between surgery and medicine.

CARL VON LINNÉ, whose name is better known in the Latinized form of Linnaeus, was a Swedish botanist and was probably the greatest one who ever lived. He served as a link between European and American medicine.

Linnaeus, who completed his medical studies in order to wed the daughter of a practitioner who would accept only a physician as a son-in-law, wrote a work on materia medica.

CHAPTER ELEVEN

Medicine in America in the Seventeenth and Eighteenth Centuries

IN AMERICA, by the middle of the eighteenth century, the Massengill family pioneered from Virginia into North Carolina and later farther westward. Henry Massengill in 1769 was the second permanent white settler in what is now Tennessee. Later, in the wilderness west of the Alleghany mountains, he and his neighbors formed the Watauga Association, which adopted the first written constitution for the government of American-born freemen.

Medicine in America during the seventeenth and eighteenth centuries is not greatly different from medicine in Europe at the same period. Clinical medicine was evolved in the eighteenth century, after attention had been given to the importance of pathology and post-mortem examinations of diseases, and this work led to better diagnostic practices.

Physicians in the new world, as a rule, either compounded their own prescriptions or else employed apothecaries as assistants. They imported such European drugs and preparations as they needed and used the indigenous drugs whose properties they learned from the Indians.

The medical schools of the United States came into existence in the following order: Philadelphia, 1765; Columbia, 1767; Harvard, 1782; Queen's, 1792; Dartmouth, 1798; Transyl-

vania, 1799; College of P. & S., 1807; Maryland, 1807; Middle-
bury, 1810; Brown, 1811, 1828; Yale, 1813; Castleton, 1818-
1861; Bowdoin, 1820; Univ. of Vt., 1822; Berkshire, at
Pittsfield, Mass., 1823-1867; Colby, at Waterville, Maine, 1830;
after this time the private and sectarian medical schools sprang
up over night.

The financial support of these early medical schools came
in the main from the students and therefore there was more or
less necessity to attract as many students as possible by means
of popular teachers and practitioners, and these men were
obliged to carry on their private practice both to earn an income and to have illustrative cases for their lectures. Their
fees were generally inclusive of medicines made from plants
which they or their pupils raised or collected in the fields. For
bleeding the charge was six pence, a dozen cathartic pills cost
a shilling, and often bills were paid in vegetables or meat, two
quarts of corn, for example, being equal in value to "one portion of Pink Root, two portions of Physic, and calling to visit
your child, June 16, 1799."

Dr. Ramsay was brought to Dartmouth from Edinburg
at a salary of $500 a year and Dr. Nathan Smith had half that
sum.

MEDICINE IN VIRGINIA

The first doctors to practice in Virginia were picked and
sent over by the London Company. They were English physicians transferred to Virginia soil. Their medical education
was obtained like that of other English physicians of that day.
To understand properly the seventeenth century practice of
medicine in Virginia one must visualize the doctor and chirurgeon practicing side by side, often confused with one another,
with no clearly defined differentiation unless it were one of
education. There were no obstetricians, only mid-wives; no
dentists, except perhaps an occasional traveling one, the emergency dentistry being in the hands of the physicians.

154

Henry Kenton was the first English physician to land upon the American continent (1603) and the first to lose his life in line of duty.

When the colonists in 1607 landed at Jamestown among their number were two "chirurgeons." At that time there was no very sharp distinction between surgery and barbering. One of the chirurgeons was Will Wilkinson. He was classed with "Will Garret the Bricklayer" and "Tho: Cowper the Barber" and was manifestly not a "gentleman." The inclusion of a barber in the personnel of the adventures at a time when there was no very sharp distinction between surgery and barbering leads us to believe that the early Virginia chirurgeons were relieved of this distasteful sideline of their profession. The term "barber-surgeon" does not appear in the Virginia records, and it is to be inferred that the cleft between the two professions, which had occurred in England, was real and permanent in the colony. The gentleman chirurgeon was Thomas Wotton.

The following year, 1608, 120 additional settlers reached the colony and with this supply came Dr. Walter Russell, physician, Post Ginnat, chirurgeon, and two apothecaries, Thomas Field and John Harford. Walter Russell was the first physician, as distinguished from the chirurgeon, to come to this country.

When Lord Delaware came to Virginia in 1610, he brought with him a physician, Lawrence Bohun, "Doctor in phisick." He is the second physician mentioned in the colonial records as coming to Virginia, and is said to have been "a long time brought up amongst the most learned surgeons and physicians in the Netherlands." Sickness and a dwindling medical supply stimulated "Mr. Dr. Bone (Bohun)" to investigate the medical properties of native plants. He experimented with sassafras, galbanum, mechoacon, or rubarbum album, "in cold and moist bodies, for the purginge of Fleame and superfluous matter."

In 1621 Dr. Bohun was succeeded by Dr. Pottes, a Master of Arts and as he affirmed "well practiced in Chirurgerie and Phisique, and expert also in distilling of waters."

In August the Council in England wrote Governor Yeardly in Virginia that "they had sent . . . Dr. John Potts for the phisition's place with two chirurgions and a chest of Physicke and Chirurgery."

During Dr. Pott's first year, news reached England that the colonists, after making a treaty of peace with the Indians, had poisoned a great many of them, and that Dr. Potts was said to be "the chief actor in it." He was much blamed in England and lost the position he had held in the Council. The Earl of Warwick objected to his appointment, because he was "the poysoner of the salvages thear."

A glimpse of the convivial disposition into which Pott appears to have retreated on occasion is given in a letter from George Sandys at Jamestown to a friend in London: "I have given from time to time the best councell I am able, at the first, he (Dr. Pott) kept companie too much with inferiours, who hung upon him while his good liquor lasted. After, he consorted with Captaine Whitacres, a man of no good example."

In 1625 a petty quarrel brought the Doctor into court. "At a Court, May 9, 1625: Mrs. Elizabeth Hamer sworne and examined sayeth, yt (that) Mrs. Blany did miscary with a Childe, ut sayeth she doth not know whether Mrs. Blaynie did request a peece of hog flesh of Mr. Doctor Pott or nott, or that the wante of the peece of flesh was the occasione of her miscaryinge with Childe, but sayeth yt Mrs. Blany did tell this Emamt (Examinent) yt she sent to Doctor Pott for A peece, and was denied."

Pott came to the colony with excellent professional recommendations. His greatest enemy, Governor Harvey, wrote that he was "skilled in the epidemical diseases" of the planters. The court records contain frequent references to his fees for medical attendance. In 1625 John Jefferson is ordered to pay

Dr. Pott "for Curynge of henry booth's Eye." The next year
we find Stephen Tailor "being sicke an brought home to Dr.
Pott's his house." The hospitalization of patients in the homes
of physicians runs through the whole century.

Dr. Pott was the first to locate land at the present site of
Williamsburg. His place there was called Harrop after the
family estate in Cheshire, England.

Edward Gibson was apparently a physician, for in 1622,
just before the massacre, he made a professional trip to Falling
Creek: "Capt. Nicholas Martin sworne and examined saith
that Ed: Gibson camm upp to the fallinge Creeke, administered Phisick to ev'y of the p'sons specified, then went & did
that Cure upon Fossett who was farre spent with the droppsie
and not one of these his patients misc(arried)."

"SEASONING"

The immigrant who survived his passage from England had
to face what was known in Virginia as the "seasoning." This
usually came in the summer and was attributed to many causes.
According to DeVries, during "June, July and August people
that have lately arrived from England die like cats and dogs,
whence they call is the sickly season." Immigrants soon
learned that to avoid the "summer sickness," as the seasoning
was sometimes called, it was best to reach Virginia in the fall
and winter.

Beverly explains the "fluxes, fevers and the bellyache" that
greeted newcomers by the fact that they "greedily surfeit with
their delicious fruits, and are guilty of great intemperance
therein, through the exceeding plenty thereof, and liberty
given by the inhabitants; by which means they fall sick, and
then unjustly complain of the unhealthiness of the country."

The diseases that afflicted the colonists were beriberi (the
early settlers were warned to avoid localities in which the
natives showed large bellies and strange swellings), scurvy,
malaria, influenza, pneumonia, pleurisy, smallpox, measles,

fluxes, fevers, calenture (yellow fever), and, no doubt, many others.

On account of the number of immigrants who suffered from scurvy at sea, Dr. John Woodall, the medical adviser to Sir Thomas Smith, gave it his special attention. He was a "Master in Chirurgerie," and in 1636 published THE SURGEON'S MATE, the earliest book in which lemon juice was prescribed for scurvy.

April, 1688: "A fast for ye great mortality (the first time the Winter distemper was soe very fatal . . . the people dyed, 1688, as in a plague—bleeding the remedy, Ld. Howard had 80 ounces taken from him)."

Smallpox, unknown to America until after the advent of the Spaniards, was first recorded in the West Indies in 1507. The first recorded epidemic of smallpox in the colony occurred in 1667. In that year a sailor with smallpox landed at Accomack. He was isolated by the chirurgeons but escaped to a nearby Indian town and infected two tribes. The disease spread all over the Eastern Shore with fearful mortality.

Lord Delaware, who was himself a catalogue of seventeenth century diseases, complained that among other ailments "the Flux surprised me, and kept me many daies; then the cramp assaulted my weak body, with strong paines . . . & afterwards the Gout . . . afflicted me . . . "

Percy, speaking of the diseases of 1607 and 1608, mentions "Flixes" among the serious disorders of the first years. In 1618 the Neptune and the Treasurer were said to have "brought a most pestilent disease (called the bloody flux) which infected almost the whole colony. That disease, notwithstanding all our former afflictions, was never known before amongst us."

Most of the Virginians referred to in the colonial records as "doctor" probably had no academic right to such a title. Yet a few undoubtedly did hold degrees in medicine.

Many physicians were at one time indentured servants. Patrick Napier and Francis Haddon are known to have come to Virginia under terms of indenture, paying their passage money by a period of servitude. John Williams was a Dutchman and a chirurgeon who was punished in 1640 for an attempted runaway while serving an indenture. John Inman is another example.

The more common type of indenture was the apprentice-ship of a young man to an established physician to learn his profession. As there were no medical schools in America until 1776, this was the usual method of becoming a doctor.

An interesting contract between Charles Clay and Stephen Tickner, chirurgeon, appears in the Surry County Records: "This Indenture made the ffourth day of . . . in the yeare of or Lord God 1657: Between Charles Clay of the one ptie: & Stephen Tickner Chyrurgion of the other ptie: Witnesseth That the sd Charles Clay doth hereby Covenant, grant & prom-ise to & wth the sd Stephen Tickner, to serve him or assigns in Such Imploymts as the sd Tickner shall Employ him about in the way of Chyrurgerye, or Phissicke, ffor & duringe the terme & time of seaven yeares & the sd Tickner is to use his best skill & Judgmt to (teach) him his Art, & what Cloathes the sd Charles doth bringe, the sd Tickner is to returne to him at the Expiration of the time afforesd. Signed: Charles Clay."

In the eighteenth century we find William Byrd II writing to Sir Hans Sloane: "Here be some men indeed that are call'd Doctors: but they are generally discarded Surgeons of Ships, that know nothing above very common Remedys. They are not acquainted enough with Plants, or other parts of Natural History, to do any Service to the World, which makes me wish that we had some missionary Philosopher, that might instruct us in the many useful things which we now possess to no pur-pose."

The following are some of the remedies used in Virginia in the seventeenth and eighteenth centuries: "Rock alum, plain alum, a kind of clay called wapeib which the inhabitants used "for the cure of sores and woundes," sassafras, which he considers better than guaiacum, and sweet gums and tobacco."

In June 1613 Sir Samuel Argoll writes of his voyage to Virginia: "In this Journie I likewise found . . . a strange kind of Earth, the vertue whereof I know not; but the Indians eate it for Physicke, alleaging that it cureth the sicknesse and paine of the belly. I likewise found a kind of water issuing out of the Earth, which hath a tart taste much like unto Allum-water, it is good and wholesome: for my men did drinke much of it, and never found it otherwise. I also found an earth like a Gumme, white and cleere; another sort of red like Terra sigillata; another very white, and of so light a substance, that being cast into the water, it swimmeth.

"We conceive it to be Terra Lemnia and it is exceeding good for the flux, youe shall therefore do well to bring it into use in the Colony: we desire youe Captain Newce therefore to send us over three or foure Tunne of the said white earth. . . . "

Terra Alba Virginensis was said to possess absorbent and alexipharmic (poison expelling) properties. It was described as "both aromatical and cordiall, and diapharetick" and was recommended in pestilent and malignant fevers. Argoll found that the gum of white poplar and of another tree very much like it was clear and odoriferous and not unlike turpentine. He at once perceived that it would make a good balsam and so applied it. The result was thoroughly satisfactory, and it was said to "heale any green wound." Another interesting tree on Jamestown Island was "small of leaves, armes, and fruict, like the mirtle tree." The fruit tasted like the myrtle, but was found to be much more "bynding." "These trees growe in greate plentie, round about a standing pond of fresh water in the middle of the island, the pill or rind whereof is of a great force against inveterate dissentericall fluxes."

A different type of apprenticeship was that entered into by young men already educated in medicine, who came to this country as indentured servants, completed their period of servitude and were later admitted to the ranks of practising physicians.

That it was possible to acquire a good reputation as a physician without even the benefits of an apprenticeship seems to be indicated by the obituary of Dr. Jordan Anderson. Upon his death at his country seat in Chesterfield County on October 20th, 1805, in his eighty-fourth year, it was said of him: "Although he was not regularly bred to the Faculty, yet by his long studies and practice, he had acquired a good share of knowledge both in physick and surgery."

"The French relations of their Voyages to Canada, tell us that the Indians and themselves falling into a contagious disease, of which Phisitians could give no Reason or Remedy, they were all in a short space restored to their health meerly by drinking water, in which Saxifrage was infused and boyled." Sassafras was said to be useful in skin diseases, gout, rheumatism and syphilis. At one time it was commonly sold at daybreak in London under the name of Saloop, and until fairly recently saloop venders were found there.

Snake root (serpentaria) was said to have a tonic, diuretic, diaphoretic and stimulant effect and was popular in typhoid and digestive disorders. Blacksnake root (radex serpentaria nigra) was a remedy for gout, rheumatism and amenorrhea. Mr. Thomas Glover, who is described as "an ingenious chirurgeon that hath lived some years in that country," sent an account of Virginia to the Royal Society in 1676. He notes that "here groweth the Radex Serpentaria Nigra, which was so much used in the last great pestilence, that the price of it advanced from ten shillings to three pounds sterling a pound. Beverly years later wrote, "There is the snake root so much admired in England as a cordial and being a great antidote in all pestilent disorders," and "There's the rattlesnake root, to which no remedy was ever yet found comparable; for it effectually cures the bite of a rattlesnake which sometimes has been mortal in two minutes. If this medicine be early applied, it presently removes the infection, and in two or three hours restores the patient to as perfect health as if he had never been hurt."

Thomas Glover describes four other popular simples—dittany, turbith, mechoacon, and the fever and ague root.

"The Jamestown weed, called *datura stramonium,* is at first sedative and antispasmotic, in larger doses a narcotic and poisonous."

Beverly extolled the wild cherry bark as a substitute for cortex peruviana and the powdered bark of the prickly ash as a specific in "old wounds and long running sores."

Ipecac, a medicine much prized by Colonel Byrd in the next century, was a secret remedy for dysentery until 1688, when the French Government paid 20,000 francs for it.

In an appeal to the colonists in 1621 to send home specimens of the native simples the Company furnished "a valuation of the Commodities growing and to be had in Virginia." Mastic was said to bring three shillings a pound, wild sarsaparilla five shillings a hundred, domestic sarsaparilla ten shillings a hundred, while "red earth allenagra" brought three shillings a hundred. Red alum, called "carthagena allum," and "roach" alum, called "Romish allum," brought ten shillings the hundred.

"Out of this search for health-giving and health-restoring plants and minerals very little of permanent value resulted, though the virtues of snake-root, dittany, turbith and mechoacon, fever and ague root, senna, lemnian earth, alum, sweet gums and tobacco continued to be extolled and enthusiastically advocated."

In December, 1620, Captain George Thorpe wrote to England that he was "persuaded that more do die here of the disease of their minds than of their body . . . and by not knowing they shall (have to) drink water here."

Every age has its fashions. In medicine that of the seventeenth century was the clyster. The clyster, an enema for opening the bowels, was administered not by the gravity method but by a large and formidable syringe. The new fashion was widely advocated and obtained an extraordinary vogue.

The ibis is said by Pliny to have demonstrated its use to the Egyptians: "By means of its hooked beak it laves the body through that part."

In colonial Virginia, clysters, or "glysters," probably enjoyed the same popularity. There are many references to them in the itemized accounts of doctors, preserved in the county court records. The clyster was apparently administered by the physician, and the fee was thirty pounds of tobacco.

Phlebotomy was very popular at this period. There was always, however, some stigma connected with it. In the Middle Ages medicine was largely in the hands of the clergy, who regarded blood-letting, surgery and dissection as phases of medicine to be farmed out to the more menial barbers and barber-surgeons. Blood-letting was, therefore, more particularly the function of the chirurgeon or barber. It will be recalled that Washington in his last illness had himself bled by his overseer before sending for a physician, indicating the menial character of the procedure.

It was an old saying:

> "By bleeding, to the marrow commeth heat,
> It maketh cleane your braine, relieves your eye,
> It mends your appetite, restoreth sleepe,
> Correcting humours that do waking keepe:
> All inward parts and senses also clearing,
> It mends the voyce, touch, smell & tast, & hearing."

> "To bleed doth cheer the pensive, and remove
> The raging fires bred by burning love."

Cupping, also, a form of bloodletting, which is as old as the animal horn with which it was executed by primitive peoples,

163

was commonly resorted to. Among other popular therapeutic procedures were vomiting, sweating and blistering.

In seventeenth century Virginia roads were little better than bridle paths, in spite of county surveyors, laws, orders and indictments. "Until after the middle of the eighteenth century there were but few roads save bridle paths, and such as there were became impassable in rainy weather. It was often necessary for the traveler to swim across a stream."

Throughout most of the counties a bridle path led to the doors of most of Virginia's citizens. Over such highways the colonial doctor made his way on horseback. With him he carried a full equipment in instruments and drugs in his saddle bags, which distinguished the physician of pioneer America.

The colonial physician of the seventeenth century has been described as follows:

"It does not require great imagination to see our seventeenth century doctor dressed in knee breeches and jerkin, perhaps adorned with periwig and cap; not given to church-going, but fond of ale, horse-racing and cuss words; husband of a multiparous wife; owner of a log cabin home or at best a frame cottage which he guarded with gun, pistol and scimitar; his road a bridle path and his means of conveyance a horse or boat. We find him caring for his patients in his own house; tutoring apprentices; reading old Latin text books by candle light, without spectacles; writing with a goose quill pen; sitting on a rough stool or bench; eating at a crude table from pewter dishes, without fork or table knife; having no knowledge of bath tubs; keeping his clothes in trunk or chest; sleeping, night-capped, on a flock bed in a bedroom shared by others; dividing his time, which he measured with hour-glass and sundial, among medicine, politics and farming; often in court, often a justice, member of Council or Assembly, and subject, like his neighbors, to military service."

164

MEDICAL FEES

Lanfranchi said, "Do all you can for the poor, but get all you can from the rich."

It was in Babylon itself, not quite 2250 years before Christ, that the great law-giver Hammurabi drew up his Code. In it he regulated, among innumerable other things, the exact fees that a surgeon was to receive for certain operations. Hammurabi wrote:

If a physician operate on a man for a severe wound (or make a severe wound upon a man) with a bronze lancet and save the man's life; or if he open an abscess (in the eye) of a man with a bronze lancet and save that man's eye, he shall receive ten shekels of silver (as his fee).

If he be a free man, he shall receive five shekels.

If it be a man's slave, the owner of the slave shall give two shekels of silver to the physician.

If a physician set a broken bone for a man or cure his diseased bowels, the patient shall give five shekels of silver to the physician.

If he be a free man, he shall give three shekels of silver.

If it be a man's slave, the owner of the slave shall give two shekels of silver to the physician.

It is clear that where the Code speaks of a "man" a gentleman or a nobleman is meant. The variation in fees according to the social status of the patient has persisted to this day. Certain penal clauses calculated to discourage the rash surgeon have not survived. They laid it down that if, as a result of an operation, "a man" lost his life, or his eye, the surgeon should have his hands cut off by way of retaliation.

In rural regions the physician's fee was often paid, if paid at all, in farm produce, and his remuneration was so uncertain that he was frequently obliged to combine farming with his professional vocation. This was also true of the clerical profession at that period, as farm or glebe lands were attached to nearly all the colonial churches.

Through all times Socrates will be recalled as the man who, even at the end, remembered his doctor's bill. He had been accused of corrupting the ethics of young men, found guilty and condemned to drink the poisonous hemlock. He drank the potion and soon fell into a stupor, but near the end he roused long enough to say: "We owe a cock to AEsculapius."

The first fee bill passed by any of the colonies was enacted by the Virginia Burgesses in September, 1736. It sought to remedy the abuses of excessive fees and "unreasonable prices" for medicines. It clearly recognized the difference between surgeons and apothecaries who had only been through apprenticeships and "those persons who have studied physic in any university and taken a degree therein."

Virginia had practically no specie in the seventeenth century, and a primitive system of barter prevailed. Debts were paid with anything that had value, even with hens and beaver skins. There are many instances of corn being used. In 1636 Dr. John Holloway was awarded a barrel of corn in a law suit, and in 1642 Dr. Stringer paid a debt in corn. The real medium of exchange was tobacco.

From the number of times the physicians appear in court to demand their fees one would infer that collections were not always good. There was a wise thirteenth century observation to young physicians: "It is always surer, however, to receive payment while the ailing person is not as yet entirely well, otherwise there is always some risk of not being paid."

Under the London Company the Physician-General was paid by the Company. Dr. Bohun was allotted "500 acres of land and 20 tenants to be placed thereon, at the Company's charge," and Dr. Pott came over under the same arrangement. Earlier physicians, Wotton and Russell, undoubtedly received their pay through the company, for during the first years everything was in common, and medical attention was furnished free. Yet even before 1624 doctors had probably begun to render personal bills for their services.

Bargaining between doctor and patient was common. The patient wanted assurance of a cure. The expenditure of a doctor's time and skill was considered worth something, but the cure was worth more, and it was often so stipulated. In 1683 Dr. William Poole, of Middlesex County, was promised 2,000 pounds of tobacco for curing a case of blindness. If he failed he was to have only "reasonable satisfaction for his trouble."

Dr. Peter Plovier made a bargain with Thomas Kirby and family, of "Warrwicke County." He promised to adminster "such Phisick, Medicines and Chirurgery as hee or any of his family shall have occasion to make use of" during their natural lives, in exchange for 100 acres of land.

His bill to John Gosling, March 22, 1658:

"For 2 glisters	040
" a glister	030
" a potion Cord.	036
For an astringent potion	035
For my visitts paines & attendance	------
For a glistere	030
For an astringent potion	035
For a cord. Astringent bole	036
For a bole as before	036
For a purging potion	050
For a cordyall Iuleb	120
For a portion as before	036

	1284	(pounds of
Allowed	1084	tobacco)

(Signed) John Cluloe"

William Fleming's account book for 1768 illustrates the more usual surgery of the day:

167

Drawing tooth for Negro Wench	0—2—6
Opening a Tumor & Dressing	3—0—0
Opening his breast & Extracting pin	2—8—2
Amputating leg & dressing	8—0—0

The following items are of a bill rendered by Dr. Haddon, of York County Virginia, about 1660, for performing an amputation:

"They included one highly flavoured and two ordinary cordials, three ointments for the wound, an ointment precipitate, the operation of letting blood, a purge per diem, two purges electuaries, external applications, a cordial and two astringent powders, phlebotomy, a defensive and a large cloth."

"On another occasion the same doctor prescribed 'a purging glister, a caphalick and a cordial electuary, oil of spirits and sweet almonds, a purging and a cordial bolus, purging pills, ursecatory, and oxymell. His charge for six visits after dark was a hogshead of tobacco weighing 400 pounds.'"

It took men of strong constitutions to withstand the hardships and heroic treatments of the times:

"...The old Gentleman who departed in his eighty eight year, has had a rupture about forty years, a secret, till his last Illness, to every Body save one Acquaintance, for that Mortifying he was forced to confess it: And such was his strength of Constitution, he struggled with the Conquerour for tenn days, after the Doctors had declared he could not live tenn Hours..."

After death came the next step was to arrange for the funeral, which was usually a gala occasion. A specimen of a funeral bill:

	lbs. tobacco
Funeral sermon	200
For a briefe	400
For 2 turkeys	80
For coffin	150

2 geese	80
1 hog	100
2 bushels of flour	90
Dunghill fowle	100
20 lbs. butter	100
Sugar and spice	50
Dressing the dinner	100
6 gallon sider	60
6 gallon rum	240

Some of the colonists did not approve of the usual excesses at the wakes and funerals:

Ralph Langley, "being very weak & Crazie," concludes his will in 1683 with a mild protest against such excesses: "I beseech yr honor that there be noe more charge at my funerall than what the plantation will aford onlly 6 gallons of strong Drink."

Another protest is voiced in the will of Captain George Jordan, a leading planter of Surry County, in 1677; he requests that he be buried in "Major Browne his Orchard, & that at my buriall there may be no Drunckeness nor Gunns, but a good and decent funerall to Entertaine my ffriends & Neighbors ... "

PARISH MEDICINE IN VIRGINIA

The colony of Virginia was divided into parishes to which were delegated social and political responsibilities and the care of the poor of each parish often devolved upon the vestry, who employed paid physicians to board and treat the sick and often to bury the dead.

The following are examples of this type of practice:

In 1708 this vestry ordered that John Gibbs "be Allowed Ye next levy Seven hundred pounds of Tobaccoes provided he make a perfect Cure of Christopher Kelshaw's Legg. If no Cure to be Allowed nothing." In 1717 the same Gibbs re-

169

ceived "for keeping Cha; MckCarty 6 months... 1200" (pounds tobacco), and Dr. Baker was paid "for a visit to Fran: Horne... 00-200" (pounds tobacco).

The entries in the vestry book of St. Peter's, New Kent County, are equally interesting. In 1711 the vestry "Ordered that the Church wardens Agree with some Doctor to Cure Mary Wild of her Ailement, & if she think herself able to undergo a Course of phisic, the Church wardens are to agree with ye Doctor for ye same." In 1744 they paid "To George Taylor for keeping Catherine Taylor in Child bed... 400" (pounds tobacco), and "To Sarah Broker as part of her fee for bringing Cath. Taylor to bed... 30"; in 1745 "To Sarah Broker for curing Jo'n Moone's Leg & Washing the surplice... 459;" "To Hannah Pearson for curing Amey Binns... 300;" "To Hannah Pearson for curing Andrew Farney's Leg... 300;" "To 5 lb. to Capt. Doran for Salivating Eliz'th Taylor a 14 P ... 715."

The Cumberland Parish vestry book (Lunenburg County) records that at a meeting of the vestry on November 7, 1754, Benjamin Clements was paid pounds 5-10s. "for doctoring J and Mary Brown" and pounds 4 "for doctoring M. Young." On December 5, 1757 Dr. Crawford was paid pounds 1-12s. "for Medisons given Nancy Keney." There are three references to Dr. Joseph Dodson. On November 29, 1758 he was paid pounds 5 "for his Accot for curing Elizabeth Taylor," on November 12, 1759 pounds 6-10s., and on November 3, 1760 pounds 3 "for curing Agatha Dodd." Dr. Clack Courtney's account of pounds 6-10s. was paid on November 12, 1759. On November 15, 1775 Dr. Walter Bennett was paid for "attending Geo. Simmons" pounds 20, and on February 26, 1776 pounds 2-10s. One woman was paid for medical services. At a meeting held November 28, 1769 the vestry "Allowed Mrs. Mourning Hix for cureing Joel Gunter... 4-00-0."

In 1799 Dr. Foushee, who lived in Richmond, advised "those who apply to him in the way of his profession (Physick) that his charges are as formerly, i.e. a visit in town in the day five shillings; an emetic, two shillings, sixpence; either in commodities that he needs or in tobacco at 20 shillings per hundred weight or money." In 1822 he became the second president of the Medical Society of Virginia.

On August 19, 1787 Francis Taylor wrote: "Send some of my urine to C. Taylor to carry with him to the Dutch Doctor in Shenandoah." A week later, "C. Taylor got home last night from Dr. Neaves and brought some directions for my disorder, which the Doctor says is the gravel in the Kidneys, his charge was 2/6."

LAY MEDICINE IN VIRGINIA

Plantation and parish medicine was largely practiced in Virginia. The Virginian was fond of exchanging his medical knowledge with his neighbor, and the plantation with its large population of dependent blacks gave him ample opportunity to put his learning to practical purpose. Agrarian Virginia with its scattered estates and expensive medical service was a field in which medical folk-lore flourished. Newspapers and almanacs constituted a sort of experience meeting where home-concocted preparations, nostrums and unscientific therapy were passed from one individual to another, and the receipts were carefully copied into diaries and letter-books for preservation.

Lord Bacon observed that "in all times in the opinion of the multitude, witches, old women and impostors have had a competition with physicians." This type of credulity has not been confined to the multitude. We expect better things of the educated and enlightened but, as Sir William Osler pointed out, "in all things related to disease credulity remains a permanent fact uninfluenced by civilization or education."

In the ante bellum south slave practice formed a large part of the doctor's daily work. For many reasons the best physicians were glad to engage in it. Wealthy masters demanded the best medical attention for their slaves and were willing to pay well for it.

But there were other ways of meeting sickness on the plantation. The practice of prescribing for one's self and family, at least in minor ailments, was common in colonial Virginia, and the physician often was not summoned until the complaint had become serious.

When all is said, however, the health of the slaves rested largely in the hands of the overseers. Most plantation owners gave explicit directions governing the management of sickness among their negroes.

Colonel Corbin in his instructions to the manager of his plantations in 1759 directed "the children to be well looked after and to give them every Spring & Fall the Jerusalem Oak seed for a week together, & that none of them suffer in time of sickness for want of proper care. Jerusalem oak seed was a plantation remedy for worms.

Perhaps the most fantastic remedy was one said to be "infallible against the Cramp." It required the patient to enclose between two rags a good quantity of powder of brimstone, which must then be fastened at bed-time to the instep by means of a tape or ribbon. The cramp would certainly disappear by morning.

Francis Taylor's invaluable diary also gives evidences of the home treatment of slaves. Hearing that a snake had bitten his negro, Frank, he promptly applied "salt & dough & weed," remarking, "I staid till evening when he was easier & could walk though still swelled." When Molly scalded her hand, he "sent for linseed oil." Two days later he noted, "Frank is sick. Gave him dose of saltz." On March 14, 1788, the diary records Taylor's treatment of Moses, who was thought to have pleurisy: "I gave him 25 grains of ipecac, but understand it operated downwards. Also gave Milly the same quantity for vomit, I gave her last Monday a dose of salts. She complains of pain in the head for about a week." A few days later, "I gave a vomit to Davey this morning—he has complained of a lax for several days." By way of commentary on his treatment of Moses' pleurisy the week before, he wrote on August 21, "set Moses to getting rales for yard." We soon find him prescribing for Frank again: "Gave Frank jalap." Some time afterward: "Davey complained of Pain in his side and breast—I gave him 24 grains of jalap & 8 of ipecac." Again, "Moses was taken very unwell. Gave him purge of jalap." Later, "gave Sarey a dose of castor oil." A few days later, "Sarey complained of being worse. I sent for C. Taylor." Still later, "Sarey says she is worse. Gave her two doses of Bark & Rhubarb. 20 Bark, 5 Rhubarb."

"Brother Tom," a negro coachman owned by Robert Carter of Nomini Hall, had considerable fame as a doctor and was borrowed by neighboring planters to treat their slaves. A letter from William Dawson, asking that Tom be sent to see a sick child, explained, "The black people at this place hath more faith in him as a doctor than any white doctor; and as I wrote you in a former letter I cannot expect you to lose your man's time, etc., for nothing, but am quite willing to pay for same."

The famous Capt. John Smith, Virginia colonist, practiced medicine when the occasion demanded. Once an Indian prisoner at Jamestown was almost smothered to death in his dungeon and so "pittiously" burnt that little hope was held out for his recovery. Smith promised the man's brother to "make him alive again." This he did by filling the sufferer full of aqua-vitae and vinegar and putting him before a fire to sleep. The treatment worked wonders. In the morning the wounds were dressed, and the prisoner and his brother "went away so well contented, that this was spread among all the Salvages for a miracle, that Captaine Smith could make a man alive that is dead."

P. C. Weston in 1856 ordered: "All sick persons are to stay in the hospital night and day. The nurses are never to be allowed to give any medicine without the orders of the Overseer or Doctor. In all cases at all serious the Doctor is to be sent for. The Overseer is particularly warned not to give strong medicine, such as calomel, or tartar emetic; simple remedies such as flaxseed tea, mint-water, No. 6, magnesia, etc., are sufficient for most cases, and do less harm. Strong medicines should be left to the Doctor; and since the Proprietor never grudges a Doctor's bill, however large, he has a right to expect the Overseer shall always send for the Doctor when a serious case occurs."

The contacts of female slaves with the sick were varied and much more important than those of the male. There was an occasional negro "doctoress" who flourished under a good reputation for cures. Usually these women combined the duties of midwife with skill in preparing and administering medicinal herbs. "Elsey is the Doctoress of the Plantation. In case of extraordinary illness, when she thinks she can do no more for the sick, you will employ a Physician."

Thomas Jefferson was greatly interested in botany and was probably better versed in medicine than the average doctor of his day. In his library were many books bearing on medicine, and he read them intelligently. Jefferson undoubtedly practiced on himself and his "family" of negroes. We find an instance in a letter to Madison. "I am sorry to hear of the situation of your family," he wrote, "and the more so as that species of fever is dangerous in the hands of our medical boys. I am not a physician & still less a quack but I may relate a fact. While I was at Paris, both my daughters were taken with what we formerly called a nervous fever, now a typhus, distinguished very certainly by a threadlike pulse, low, quick and every now and then fluttering. Dr. Gem, an English physician, attended them."

He once treated himself for a "stricture of the ilium" and expressed the opinion that he would soon have been well "but that a dose of calomel and jalap, in which were eight or nine grains of the former, brought on a salivation."

An interesting case of lay medicine in Europe, in the nineteenth century, is that of Vincenz Priessnitz, a Silesian peasant boy, who sprained his wrist and crushed his thumb, which injuries he healed by pumping cold water over them and applying wet compresses; later, a cart passed over his body, breaking his ribs, and when he overheard gloomy prognostications from his medical attendants, he tore their bandages from his body, applied wet ones in their place, and pressing his abdomen against the window-sill, he breathed deeply.

Gifted with natural clinical insight, and a first-class organizing ability, Priessnitz established an hydropathic institute at Graefenberg, which was soon crowded with health-seekers from all parts of the world. In time many well-known physicians of standing sojourned at Graefenberg to learn from the untutored Priessnitz such practical thermotherapeutic procedures as the douche, the plunge, the dripping sheet, the dry blanket pack, the wet sheet pack, the foot bath, the sitz bath, and the warm bath.

CLERGYMEN

In New England drugs were carried by itinerant preachers, who sold their wares to grateful parishioners for whom frontier isolation made purchasing difficult. There is no record of such a method of distribution in Virginia, though there is nothing to indicate that it did not occur.

The clergymen and the parish authorities in colonial Virginia entered into the practice of medicine.

The Reverend John Clayton, minister at Jamestown, 1684-86, shows great alarm in a letter, probably written to Dr. Boyle, over "the Distemper of the Colick that is predominant and has miserable sad effects it begins with violent gripes wch declining takes away the use of limbs. Their fingers stand stiffly bent, the hands of some hang as if they were loose at the wrists from the arms, they are sceletons so meagre & leane that a consumption might seeme a fatning to them, cruelly are they distracted with a flatus, & at length those that seemeingly recover are oft troubled wth a sort of gout."

The Rev. Clayton has left an illuminating account of the elaborate methods of treatment he himself used, particularly in the matter of dogbites. For hydrophobia he prescribed the volatile salts of amber, ten grains in treacle water every half hour. To this was added "posset drink" (sour milk) with sage and rue. Clayton said that a doctress of his acquaintance treated snake bite with "Oriental Bezoar shaved and a decoction of dittany." He recommends chalybeates, decoctions, carminative seeds and aromatic spirits. "But," he says, "their (Virginia) Doctors are so learned, that I never met with any of them that understood what Armoniack Spirits were: Two or three of them one time ran me clear down by Consent, that they were Vomitive, and that they never used any thing for that Purpose but Crocus Metallorum, which indeed every House keeps; and if their Finger, as the Saying is, ake but, they immediately give three or four Spoonfuls thereof; if this fail, they give him a second Dose, then perhaps Purge them with fifteen or twenty Grains of the Rosin of Jalap, afterwards Sweat them with Venice treacle, Powder of Snakeroot, or Gascoin's Powder; and when these fail conclamatum est."

Joseph Doddridge was born in Pennsylvania in 1768 and died in Virginia in November 1826. He first came to Virginia in 1787 as a Wesleyan Methodist missionary, but later went back to Philadelphia where he was ordained an Episcopal minister in 1792 and also studied medicine under Benjamin Rush. In a chapter on medicine he states that the children of the frontier suffered chiefly from croup and worms. Croup (diphtheria) was extremely fatal. The juice of roasted onions was a supposed cure. For the worms large doses of common salt, scrapings of pewter spoons or sulphate of iron were given.

176

The itch, a common frontier disease, was usually cured by lard and brimstone. Rheumatism was prevalent and a natural sequel to a life of exposure. The oil of geese, wolves, bears and pole cats was a favorite remedy. Malaria occurred and was treated chiefly by sweating. Pleurisy was the only disease which demanded bleeding. Accidents were frequent. For burns, poultices of slippery elm and Indian meal were used. For snake bite, besides cupping and sucking the wound, deep incisions were made and a number of native plants employed for poultices. To gunshot wounds poultices of slippery elm bark and flaxseed were applied.

QUACKS IN VIRGINIA

The historian, William Smith, of New York, declared in 1757 that "quacks abound like locusts in Egypt. We have no laws to protect the king's subjects from the malpractice of pretenders. Any man at his pleasure sets up for physician, apothecary and chirurgeon. No candidates are either examined, licensed or sworn to fair practice."

The same conditions obtained in Virginia. In 1761 the Virginia students studying medicine in Edinburgh, "beholding with inexpressible concern the unguarded state of physic in our native country which lies open to the intrusion of every pretender to the medical art," memorialized the House of Burgesses. They demanded laws to remedy the public evil and asked that no one in the future be allowed to practice medicine without being "properly licensed and honored with a doctor's degree." Arthur Lee wrote from Edinburgh to his brother in Virginia, suggesting the registration of diplomas in the county courts as the surest method of preventing irregular practice.

The practitioners of medicine in eighteenth century Virginia fell naturally into three classes: those who had a university education and a medical degree, those who had served apprenticeships, and those who were quacks. The proportion

177

of doctors with degrees to those without them was about one to nine. At the end of the century there were probably five hundred physicians in the State of Virginia. About fifty-five of them held degrees.

In Rind's Virginia Gazette for November 1, 1770, the sheriff of Loudon County advertised for the capture of William George, "by profession a doctor, and practiced as such for more than two years in these parts," who had "run away from his bail" the previous July. The sheriff judged, from notes in George's prayer book, that he was born July 20, 1746, and came from Gloucester, England. He "carried with his some instruments belonging to surgery, which I believe he understands. As he has several fine ruffled shirts no doubt he will endeavour to pass for a Gentleman, being a pretty good scholar."

"This is to give notice that Mr. Richard Bryan, living in King George County, is most excellent at curing the Iliack Passion, or the Dry-Gripes, the cure of which he is dextrous into Admiration; for he has often performed the Cure with one Dose, after the Patient had been given out as incurable, by some very eminent Physicians, and never has yet failed of any he took in Hand."

"Dr. Rowan, from London, now at Mr. Robinson's in York, cures the Scurvy, leprosy, ulcers, cancers, blotches, evil, old sores, green wounds, piles, fistulas, inside or out, without cutting, also deafness, and all inflammations of the head or eyes; he discharges all rheumatick and gouty pains of the body and nerves, cures fevers, agues, yellow jaundice, scald heads, straightens crooked limbs, cures the headache in a few minutes, cures the venereal with or without physick, discharges worms out of men, women and children, and many other disorders too tedious to be inserted, though incurable to others. No cure no money."

The comment on Georgia physicians made by Dr. Archibald D. Alexander, a Virginia doctor who traveled in Georgia

178

in 1802, describes a condition which must have prevailed in
Virginia earlier in the eighteenth century, though medical
standards here had improved at the time he wrote: "It is a
charming country for Physicians, there are but few qualified
for the practice, but a numerous train of empirics who well
deserve this devise, a coat ornamented with three Ducks heads,
and the motto Quack, Quack, Quack—I have been solicited
by a number of the first Characters in a variety of places to
settle in this Country, there are a great many situations where
a person might accumulate a large fortune in a short space of
time at the practice of Medicine."

Colonel Byrd, stopping at Tuckahoe on one of his excur-
sions up the James, used the flux as a topic of conversation to
"bring (Mrs. Randolph) to the Use of her Tongue." "I discover'd she was a notable Quack," he explains, "and therefore
paid that regard to her knowledge, as to put some questions to
her about the bad distemper that raged then in the Country.
I mean the Bloody Flux, that was brought us in the Negro-ship
consigned to Colo. Braxton. She told me she made use of very
simple remedies in that case, with very good success. She did
the Business either with Hartshorn Drink, that had Plantain
Leaves boil'd in it, or else with a Strong decoction of St. Andrew's Cross, in new milk instead of water. I agreed with her
that those remedies might be very good, but would be more
effective after a dose or two of Indian Physick."

In 1711 the first American patent medicine appeared. It
was called "Tuscarora Rice," and was sold by a Mrs. Masters
as a consumption cure. This was the period of traveling Indian medicine men and peripatetic quacks. The New Jersey
State Medical Society in 1772 had a law passed prohibiting both
the practice of the healing art and the sale of medicines by
"mountebank doctors."

A little less offensive are the repeated advertisements in
eighteenth century newspapers by really reputable physicians.
The medical profession of that day availed itself of the public

press to announce a new partnership, a change of residence, a particular method of therapy, or a new line of drugs, just received from England; and when they could get a hearing physicians took the advocacy or defense of their medical theories before the bar of public opinion.

During the seventeenth century, the young crown colonies enjoyed only the most primitive medical facilities and put forth no academic efforts. This state of affairs changed to some extent during the eighteenth century, especially during the latter part of the century.

Many Virginia youths during the eighteenth century took advantage of opportunities for study abroad and as a result acquired a preeminence in their profession upon their return to practice in America.

Although the eighteenth century Virginia doctor was better educated than his predecessor of the seventeenth century, although he had a more intelligent clientele, more books and better means of communication, he was seriously handicapped by his devotion to theory, and it is doubtful if his notions of medical practice or his therapy were greatly in advance of those of the preceding century. In fact he had nothing upon which to base any improvement. His method of examination of patients and his conception of the cause and mechanism of disease were fully as faulty as they had been a hundred years before. The Virginia doctor continued to sweat, blister, purge, vomit and bleed his patients with the same traditional faith and the same inevitable results.

Medicine was not taught systematically in this country until the latter part of the eighteenth century. In 1765 William Shippen and John Morgan founded the medical department of the College of Philadelphia, which soon became the University of Pennsylvania.

A medical department existed at William and Mary for a short time during this century. With the reorganization of the college in 1779 and the appointment of James McClurg as professor of anatomy and medicine, opportunities were offered to Virginians similar to those in other colonies. The school, however, functioned only three years.

Virginia doctors of the eighteenth century were interested in agriculture, and many of them made contributions to agricultural literature. From medicine to farming was not a far cry. The training in botany given physicians of this period not only increased their interest in the cultivation of the soil but made them really capable of intelligent approach to the problems involved.

Before 1800 there were but four medical periodicals published in England and only one in America, the MEDICAL REPOSITORY, established in New York in 1797. The first issue of this American journal contained two items from Virginia. In one "A correspondent of the NORFOLK CHRONICLE recommends as a means to restore infectious air to purity, to wet a cloth of any kind in water mixed with quick-lime, and to hang the cloth so steeped in a room till it becomes dry; after which to renew the operation as long as appears needful."

The mainstays of treatment in the eighteenth century continued to be calomel, opium, ipecac and the famous rattlesnake root. Each had its indications and was given by plantation owner and doctor alike with confidence. "Copious bleeding and the use of mercury" were described by a Virginia doctor as late as 1805 as having cured a case of hydrophobia. When erysipelas was believed to be "fixed on the stomach," it was brought to the surface by tartar emetic plasters.

A letter from Thomas Jones written during an illness in 1725 shows him resigned to the inevitable: "It seems before ye Doctor proceeds any further on his part, he wants ye operation of Nature, who I am afraid will treat me very roughly, and who I suppose is taking her rounds this sickly time. . . . I may suppose I am to wade through Rivers of water gruel, & Chicken Broth strengthened with mollasses with no other support than ye yolks of four poached eggs once a day without bread or salt . . . "

Epidemics did not threaten the lives of Virginians in the eighteenth century as they had in the preceding hundred years. Those that occurred are more easily defined and were limited chiefly to yellow fever, typhoid fever, smallpox, malaria and dysentery. Many of the prevalent diseases were not, strictly speaking, epidemic, though they were called so by contemporary writers. The sicknesses of the colony formed a large part of the table talk and letter writing of its people, and every diary of the period contains endless notations of the prevailing symptoms.

Dysentery was still known in the eighteenth century as "the flux" and was a dreaded distemper. The same George Hume who described his suffering from ague and fever wrote in 1723 to relatives in Scotland: "We had no sooner landed in this country but I was taken immediately w'th all ye most common distampers y't attend it but y't most violent of all was a severe flux of w'ch my uncle died being the governour's factor at a place called Germawna."

A fairly good idea of the medical treatment which Virginians of this century received may be had from an inspection of the list of medicines ordered by George Washington in 1767 from his London factors, and intended for the negro slaves and his family at Mount Vernon:

"2 best Lannets (lancets) in one case.
6 common Do. each in sepe.
25 lb. Antimony.
10 lbs. flour of Sulphur.
2 Oz. Honey Water.
3 Quarts Spirits of Turpentine.
2 lb. best Jesuit's Bark, powdered.
3 Oz. Rhubarb Do. and put into a bottle.
1 pint Spirit of Hartshorn.
6 oz. Do. of Lavendar.

6 Do. Do Nitre.

1 lb. Blistering Plaister.

4 Oz. Tincture of Castor.

8 Do. Balsam Capivi.

¼ lb. Termerick.

GENERAL WASHINGTON'S ILLNESS AND TREATMENT

In 1799 Dr. Dick was summoned to Mount Vernon, to find Washington *in extremis,* attended by his friend, Dr. Craik. Dr. Brown arrived soon after, and the three made frantic efforts to save their illustrious patient.

Drs. Craik and Dick issued the following statement:

"Some time in the night of Friday, the 13th inst., having been exposed to rain on the preceding day, General Washington was attacked with an inflammatory affection of the upper part of the windpipe, called in technical language, cynanche trachealis. The disease commenced with a violent ague, accompanied with some pain in the upper and fore part of the throat, a sense of stricture in the same part, a cough, and a difficult rather than painful deglutition, which were soon succeeded by fever and a quick and laborious respiration. The necessity of blood-letting suggesting itself to the General, he procured a bleeder in the neighborhood, who took from the arm in the night, twelve or fourteen ounces of blood; he would not by any means be prevailed upon by the family to send for the attending physician till the following morning, who arrived at Mount Vernon at eleven o'clock on Saturday morning. Discovering the case to be highly alarming, and foreseeing the fatal tendency of the disease, two consulting physicians were immediately sent for, who arrived, one at half past three and the other at four in the afternoon. In the interim were employed two copious bleedings; a blister was applied to the part affected, two moderate doses of calomel were given, an injection was administered which operated on the lower intestines, but all without any perceptible advantage, the respiration becoming still more difficult and distressing. Upon the arrival of the first of the consulting physicians, it was agreed, as there were yet no signs of accumulation in the bronchial vessels of the lungs, to try the result of another bleeding, when about thirty-two ounces were drawn, without the smallest apparent alleviation of the disease. Vapours of vinegar and water were frequently inhaled, ten grains of calomel were given, succeeded by repeated doses of emetic tartar, amounting in all to five or six grains, with no other effect than a copious discharge from the bowels. The powers of life seemed now manifestly yielding to the force of the disorder. Blisters were applied to the extremities, together with a cataplasm of bran and vinegar to the throat. Speaking, which was painful from the beginning, now became almost impracticable, respiration grew more and more contracted and imperfect, till half after eleven o'clock on Saturday night, when, retaining the full possession of his intellect, he expired without a struggle."

Dr. Brown later wrote to Dr. Craik in regard to Dr. Dick:

"You must remember he was averse to bleeding the General, and I have often thought that if we had acted according to his suggestion when he said, 'he needs all his strength—bleeding will diminish it', and taken no more blood from him, our good friend might have been alive now. But we were governed by the best light we had; we thought we were right, and so we are justified."

Washington's death was followed by a wave of calumny that spent its fury chiefly upon the medical profession. Wells, who has ably weighed all the evidence, has come to the physicians' defense in a thoroughly convincing argument. He discusses the possibilities of acute laryngitis, quinsey, laryngeal diphtheria and inflammatory oedema of the larynx, showing that the latter was unquestionably the cause of Washington's death.

"In their treatment of Washington his doctors followed the accepted rules laid down by the best authorities of that day. As bleeding was then practised, the amount of blood withdrawn was not unusual. From the nature of the illness death was a foregone conclusion. The vigorous therapy resorted to by his physicians may have hastened Washington's death, but it could in no way have caused it."

AMERICAN SURGERY

(See additional data in Surgeons & Surgery Chapter)

In America surgery can hardly be said to have existed until the Revolutionary War. Several factors were responsible for this improvement. There was the example of the superior surgery practiced by the surgeons attached to the foreign armies operating in this country during the Revolutionary War. The war moreover furnished a wealth of surgical material. "No wonder bold surgeons developed out of such training. John Warren of Boston in 1781 amputated the shoulder joint, John Bard of New Jersey in 1759 performed laparotomies for extra-uterine pregnancy, William Baynham of Virginia in 1791 and 1799 performed the same operation, and Wright Post of New York in 1796 operated for femoral aneurism by the Hunterian method."

Among the prominent physicians in the Colonial War were Drs. William Flemming, Thompson Sawyers and Dr. Thomas Walker, who also was a noted explorer. Dr. Walker has been credited by at least one authority with having been one of the earliest to trephine bone for suppurative osteomyelitis. Andrew Robertson, native of Scotland, graduate of the University of Edinburgh, and military surgeon attached to the British army in Flanders, came to America with Braddock in 1755 and took part in the ill-fated expedition against the French and Indians. Shortly afterward he quit the army and settled in Lancaster County, Virginia.

In Virginia the "chirurgeon" finally had disappeared. In his stead we have the surgeon—a much more respectable member of society, but one still not quite able to shake off entirely the unpleasant aura of the barber, bone-setter and stone-cutter from whom he had sprung. In the old world, where proprieties and conventions counted for much, the opprobrium attached to the surgeon continued to linger.

The exigencies of life in the new world did not make for the sharp cleavage and distinction between physicians and surgeons that obtained in Europe. In America it was more convenient as well as more profitable to be a jack of all trades, and more and more doctors began to advertise themselves as physicians and surgeons, some adding a third profession, that of "man mid-wife."

The extent of the lack of supplies during the Revolutionary War may be gathered from a report of Dr. John Morgan, July 17, 1776. Among the fifteen regiments, "All the instruments were reported to be private property, and amounted to six sets of amputating instruments, two of trepanning ditto, fifteen cases of pocket instruments, seventy-five crooked and six straight needles. Amongst the whole fifteen Surgeons, there were only four scalpels, or incision knives, for dilating wounds, or any other purpose; three pair of forceps for extracting bullets; half a paper and seventy pins; and but few bandages, ligatures, or tourniquets, and as little old linen, lint or tow, but what they had procured from the General Hospital; and only two ounces of spunge in all."

The sanitary measures during the Revolutionary War are described as follows:

"The Commander in Chief is inform'd that notwithstanding his Orders, the carcases of dead horses lay in & about Camp. And that the Offil of the Commissarys Stalls, still lay unburned. That much filth, etc., are spread among the Huts, which are or will be soon adjuced to a state of putrification & Occation a sickly Camp. The Commanding Officers will immediately see

there Respective Incampments cleaned, There old vaults filled
& New ones dugg once a Week, all filth and Nastyness buried
& that fresh earth be put into the Vants every day."

HOSPITALS IN AMERICA

"Hospital management was bad in the seventeenth century
the world over. It was worse in the eighteenth. There was
the same overcrowding, several patients occupying one bed or
pallet, the same absence of ventilation, the same presence of
vermin and filth, the same lack of appreciation of the need for
isolation of contagious diseases, the same misdirected effort at
nursing, the same fatal issue following every attempt at major
surgery. The mortality in the general hospitals of the period
could not have been less than twenty per cent."

Dr. Tilton declared that "it would be shocking to humanity
to relate the history of our General Hospital in the years of
1777 and 1778 when it swallowed up at least one-half of our
army owing to a fatal tendency in the system to throw all the
sick of the army into the general hospital, whence crowds infection, and consequent mortality, too affecting to mention.
I have no hesitation in declaring it as my opinion that we lost
not less than from ten to twenty of camp diseases for one by
weapons of the enemy."

The fearful mortality that accompanied hospitalization in
America at this time received further comment from Dr.
Thatcher, who wrote, "it has been estimated that the loss of
lives in the various armies of the United States during the war
is not less than 70,000. The number who died on the horrid
prison ships of the enemy cannot be calculated. It is however
confidently asserted that no less than 11,000 of our brave soldiers died on board the one called Jersey Prison Ship only."

THE FIRST MARINE HOSPITAL IN AMERICA

On April 15, 1708, the Council ordered "that a house be
hyred for the accommodation of the sick men belonging to her

Majesty's Ship the Garland and that the Rent of the said house be paid out of her Majesty's Revenue of two Shils per hogshead and it is recommended to Collo William Wilson to provide a house accordingly." However, it was not until 1780 that steps were taken to establish a permanent marine hospital.

THE HOSPITAL FOR THE INSANE AT WILLIAMSBURG

On November 15, 1769, a committee was instructed to prepare a bill "to make Provision for the Support and Maintenance of Ideots, Lunatics, and other persons of unsound Minds."

The act to care for the insane, as it was finally passed by the Burgesses on June 27, 1770, took cognizance of the fact that "several persons of insane and disordered minds have been frequently found wandering in different parts of this colony."

Within, the building was fitted out as madhouses always had been, with cells and chains. In 1773 the building was completed, and on September 13 the trustees advertised in the Gazette that "the hospital will be ready by the twelfth of next month for the reception of such idiots, lunatics, and persons of unsound minds as may be sent thereto."

During the sixteenth, seventeenth and eighteenth centuries the treatment of the insane was at its worst. No sympathy was extended to them; unspeakable atrocities were committed upon them; they endured incredible suffering. They were chained in dungeons, beaten, tortured, or exhibited as curiosities to the people of a Sunday afternoon.

Virginia enjoys the reputation of having established at Williamsburg in 1773 the first insane asylum in America. In the seventeenth century, however, the barbarous ideas current on the Continent in regard to the management of the insane prevailed here also. The violent were chained or caged, the harmless were allowed at large. These poor creatures were drugged with camphor, opium or belladonna; purged, vomited and bled; kept in prison and in mechanical restraints, until

188

Philippe Pinel introduced the modern humane treatment. It was late in the eighteenth century before the change came.

In spite of all the therapeutic extremes in Virginia during the eighteenth century there were many worth-while physicians:

William Baynham was born December 7, 1749, in Caroline County, Virginia. His father, Dr. John Baynham, had long practiced in that community and served as both magistrate and vestryman. Like many other sons, William followed in his father's footsteps and at an early age was apprenticed to Dr. Thomas Walker, of Castle Hill, Albemarle County, one of the most eminent men of his day.

William Baynham was the finest anatomist of the century in America. He was not attached to one of the five medical schools started in this country before the turn of the century, nor was he a resident of a large northern city. He practiced surgery and medicine in rural Virginia and affords a striking example of pioneer surgery outside of the principal American medical centers. He studied in Europe and in 1785 returned to America, settled in Essex County and set up as a practitioner of surgery and medicine. He was now thirty-six years of age and with sixteen years of experience in London behind him became at once a man to be sought after. He was called here and there, to large cities and to other states. Though he continued to reside in a remote Virginia county until his death December 8, 1814, he enjoyed a reputation that was national in scope.

Jessee Bennett, in 1794, successfully performed on his wife the formidable operation of Caesarean section, at the same time removing both ovaries. This was the first operation of its kind in America, done thirty-three years earlier than that by John Lambert Richmond, who, according to Garrison, performed the first Caesarean section in this country at Newton, Ohio, on April 22, 1827. Bennett did not report the operation, therefore, he has not been given a place of honor in the medical history of America. When asked why he did not report his case

189

in some medical journal, Bennett replied that "no doctor with any feelings of delicacy would report an operation he had done on his own wife," and added that "no strange doctors would believe that operation could be done in the Virginia backwoods and the mother live, and he'd be damned if he would give them a chance to call him a liar."

William Cabell, in 1744, was a justice of Albemarle. Later he became coroner and assistant surveyor. By 1753 he had acquired 26,000 acres of land. He was an interesting frontiersman, described as "ready to turn his hand and mind to whatever turned up, dispensing justice, surveying lands, amputating a limb, curing a wound, physicking his neighbor, bartering or fighting with Indians, or what not." Importing his medicines, he dispensed them in his own apothecary shop, along with medical products concocted from native plants. His materia medica included Turlington's Balsam, Bateman's Drops, Stoughton's Bitters and Anderson's Pills. He frequently prescribed rhubarb but used very little calomel. Near his home he conducted a private hospital where he performed major operations, patients paying for board and necessities but usually not remunerating the doctor unless cured. Charges for cures ranged from five to one hundred pounds. If the patient died, Dr. Cabell's artisans supplied the coffin and buried him. An item in his account book reads: "To coffin, sheet and interment, pounds 2- 11s.-6d." This remarkable man, whose sayings were long quoted in the neighborhood, died April 2, 1774, "after a long and tedious illness" and is buried at the present Liberty Hall estate.

Arthur Lee (1740-1792). He studied in England, having graduated in 1764. After graduation Dr. Lee traveled through Germany and Holland. He returned to America and began the practice of medicine at Williamsburg in 1766, where he gained considerable reputation and practice. Later he suddenly gave up the practice of medicine and studied law.

190

Walter Jones (1745-1815), "The luminary of the Northern Neck," as he was styled by his admirers, was born in Northampton County, Virginia.

From William and Mary College Jones went to the University of Edinburgh to study medicine. There he did exceptionally well, enjoying the friendship and esteem of many of his professors, especially of Dr. Cullen. In fact, he was regarded as "the most shining young gentleman of his profession in Edinburgh and one who would make a great figure wherever he went." His studies over, he returned to Virginia in 1770 and established himself at Hayfield, in Lancaster County. Here he quickly gained a reputation as a physician and a scholar and enjoyed a large practice.

Theodorick Bland (1740-1790), described by a well-known historian of the Revolution as poet, soldier and legislator, went through a long and thorough medical training in the best universities of Europe and for seven years practiced his profession in the colony. In 1765 he returned to Virginia.

At the end of seven years he abandoned the practice of medicine and made the following explanation:

"With a constitution weak and infirm from my cradle, I buffeted the winds and faced the weather in all its extremes from the severest cold to the most intense and scorching heat; I exposed myself to every inclemancy both by night and by day; and have for near seven years undergone all the distresses, cares and anxieties, which are the constant and unremitting attendants of a conscientious practitioner of physic, and all this in direct opposition to my leading and strongest inclinations to a calm, quiet, and philosophical life in a rural situation, and with a loss of every social and domestic enjoyment; for what enjoyment of time can a man have who is subject to perpetual alarms? My resolution to renounce the practice of physic is not the effect of whim or caprice, but of absolute and cogent necessity."

James McClurg, though he could not support his family from his profession, made medicine his mistress and adhered to it with a devotion that won the respect of his contemporaries all over the country.

Arthur Lee, Walter Jones, John Mitchell, Elisha Dick, William Brown, George Gilmer, James Greenway, John M. Galt, William Foushee, Robert Wellford and others, were recognized beyond the confines of the colony for their attainments in medicine, while there were many lesser lights who were highly esteemed by their fellow Virginians.

MEDICINE IN THE NEW ENGLAND SECTION

Samuel Fuller (1580-1633), the doctor of the Mayflower, was born and baptized at Redenhall Parish Church in Norfolk County, England, January 20, 1580. In the negotiations and preparations for fitting out the "Speedwell" and the "Mayflower" (1617-20) Fuller was an active and influential party.

In the list of passengers sailing on the "Mayflower" the occupation of Samuel Fuller is given as physician, "and the vocations were as far as ascertained the callings the individuals who represented them had followed before taking ship." Dr. Thacher in his memoirs says, "The first physician of whom we have any account among the Colonists was Dr. Samuel Fuller. Whether he had enjoyed a collegiate education is uncertain; but he is said to have been well qualified in his profession, he was zealous in the cause of religion, and eminently useful as a physician and surgeon."

It has been said that the "Mayflower" had a surgeon (Giles Heale), but nothing is recorded about him other than his signature to William Mullins' will. Mullins died February, 1621, on the "Mayflower." There is no other mention of this surgeon either as a passenger or sailor on board the "Mayflower."

In June, 1630, Doctor Fuller wrote: "I have been to Matapan (now Dorchester) and let some twenty of these people's blood." Again, in August, 1630, while at Charlestown, he writes: "There is come hither a ship (with cattle and more passengers) on Saturday last which brings this news out of England; that the plague is sore, both in the city and country, also there is like to be a good dearth in the land by reason of the dry season; the sad news here is that many are sick and many are dead; I here but lose time and long to be at home. I can do them no good, for I want drugs and things fitting to work with."

In the epidemic of smallpox which prevailed in 1633 many fell sick and about twenty died, men, women, and children, including many of the old settlers from Holland, among whom was Samuel Fuller (after he had much helped others) and "had been a great help and comforte unto them; as in his faculties, so otherwise, being a deacon in ye church, a man godly, and forward to doe good, being much missed after his death: and he and ye rest of their brethren much lamented by them, and caused much sadness and mourning amongst them." This disease also was very fatal among the Indians from all adjoining places. A curious fact in relation to this epidemic was that it had been prophesied by the Indians in May on account of the great quantities of a sort of fly, about the size of wasps or bumblebees, which came out of holes in the ground, and filled the woods, eating the green things and making a constant yelling noise, deafening to hear. These insects (locusts?) were unknown to the English. The epidemic followed in June, July and August, during the heat of the summer.

Notwithstanding the many trials, hardships, and toils to which a physician is subjected even in these days of conveniences and luxuries, it is both gratifying and significant to find this early physician, Samuel Fuller, acting as the guardian of the future welfare of the community by perpetuating learning among children. In his will, the first one probated in this country, he mentions four youths entrusted to his care who were to be returned to their parents at Charlestown and Dorchester.

In New England drugs were sold by itinerant preachers to their parishoners. It has been said: "New England medicine in the seventeenth century is as dreary as its literature and as repellent as its theology."

The following advertisement appeared in THE BOSTON GAZETTE, June 19, 1744. The advertiser, Mr. Gardiner, was not only the most noted druggist in New England, but also an accomplished physician and surgeon:

"Just imported in the Ship from London, And to be Sold By Mr. Sylvester Gardiner, At the Sign of the Unicorn and Mortar in Marlborough Street.

"All sorts of Drugs and Medicines, both Chymical and Galenical; where all Doctors, Apothecaries or others, may be supply'd with the very best and freshest of Either at the lowest Price; and Captains of Ships with Doctor's Boxes put in the neatest and best Manner; with printed Directions: Likewise all Merchants may be furnished at the same Place with Surgeons Chests put up in the same manner, and at the same Price, as they are for the Royal Navy, at the Apothecary's Hall in London; where only are to be sold by appointment of the Patentees, the true Doctor Bateman's Pectoral."

In "The Boston Gazette, or Weekly Advertiser," December 18, 1753, is a long communication covering two pages of newspaper, setting forth "Examples of Great Medicines Drawn from Unpromising Bodies." It is made up of extracts from a work printed at Oxford, England, in the year 1664. The article is printed with the following subheadings: "Medicines out of Soot;" "The Use of Horse-dung;" "Medical Virtues of Human Urine;" "Medicines out of Humane Blood;" and "The Great Effects of Sow Buggs." Under the second subheading the writer goes on to show that "there are not any Medicines to be taken into the Body more cheap and contemptible than the Excrements of Men and Horses, and than Insects; and yet even these want not considerable Medical Virtues." He furthermore asserts that "the juice of Horse-dung, especially of Stone-horses," . . . i.e. stallions, . . . is good for the stoppage of urine, and certain other complaints."

The following advertisement is taken from the New England Courant of December 17, 1772. The substance of it is much like the quack notices of the period:

"For the good of the publick, a certain person hath a secret medicine which cures the gravil and cholick immediately, and dry belly ach in a little time; and restores the use of the limbs again (tho' of never so long continuance), and is excellent for the gout. Enquire of Mr. Samuel Gerrish, bookseller, near the Brick Meeting House, over against the Town-House in Boston. N. B. The poor who are not able to pay for it, may have it gratis."

For many years before the Puritans came to this country, being subjected to bitter persecution, and foreseeing the possibility of an ejectment, a considerable number of their ministers studied medicine. They saw the probable needs of the future, and fitted themselves as best they could for any emergency that might arise in a new settlement, hence they formed a large proportion of the early physicians of Massachusetts. History repeats itself, and we see today American missionaries who first study medicine as a partial preparation for their new duties.

Among those who came over in Winthrop's fleet was Richard Palgrave, a physician, from Stepney, London.

Another passenger in the same fleet was William Gager, one of the deacons of the Charlestown Church, whom Governor Dudley styles "a right godly man, skillful chyrurgeon," but who unfortunately died soon after his arrival.

John Winthrop, Junior, having prescribed buttered musket balls for a disease, added that they should be taken on the full of the moon, and that if a bit of a lion's mane could be obtained and hung under the left arm, it would also help!

Another among the early settlers of Massachusetts who practiced medicine was Giles Firman, "a godly man, an apothecary of Sudbury, in England," who came to this country in the year 1632.

In the year 1649, a law was passed to regulate, within certain limits, the practice of medicine and surgery, and required the practitioner to act according to the most approved precepts of the art in each domain.

A female physician named Margaret Jones, according to Gov. Winthrop (1648) possessed "such a malignant touch, as many persons were taken with deafness or vomiting, or other violent pains or sickness; her medicines, though harmless in themselves, yet had extraordinarily violent effects; such as refused her medicines she would tell that they would never be healed, and accordingly their diseases and hurts continued with relapses against the ordinary course, and beyond the apprehension of all physicians and surgeons."

She was executed for witchcraft, the first execution in the colony.

Dr. Oliver Wendell Holmes occupied the chair of anatomy at Harvard for thirty-five years. His humor was often carried over to his medical labors. Small, smiling, asthmatic, Holmes was always ready to battle for science.

The following is his opinion of materia medica as used at that time:

"Throw out opium, which the Creator himself seems to prescribe, for we often see the scarlet poppy growing in the cornfields, as if it were foreseen that wherever there is hunger to be fed there must also be pain to be soothed; throw out a few specifics which our art did not discover, and is hardly needed to apply; throw out wine, which is a food, and the vapors which produce the miracle of anesthesia, and I firmly believe that if the whole materia medica, as now used, could be sunk to the bottom of the sea, it would be all the better for mankind—and all the worse for the fishes."

The first coroner's inquest was held in New Hampshire in January, 1655, by a jury of twelve men, under the direction of Dr. Fernold. Following the death of Dr. Fernold this colony was without a physician for many years. During this period the sick were attended by the more capable women of the group. In fact, during the early Colonial days these women attended to nearly all of the obstetrical cases, and they became expert in this line for the time. General neighborhood nursing was the only resource of the sick of this colony for several years.

The second physician to come to New Hampshire was John Fletcher, in 1669. He lived a life of mixed activities and died September 5, 1695. John Fletcher, as was true of many of the physicians of early Colonial days, was a minister as well as a physician. He is given the credit of founding the first church in Portsmouth in 1671.

Next in order came John Buss, who was also a minister. Dr. Buss settled at Dover in that part now known as Durham in 1684. He practiced medicine and preached from that date until 1718.

During those early days the ministers, who were often doctors as well, were very expert in phlebotomy and they always resorted to bleeding, as well as praying, in all severe cases of sickness.

John Clarke appears to have been the first physician to arrive in Boston in 1631, and resided there till 1638. He then removed to Portsmouth, in the northern part of Rhode Island, and the following year to Newport.

Robert Jeffries was authorized "to exercise the function of surgery" by the government of the Island in 1641, and soon after, Dr. John Cranston was also licensed, with the privilege of dealing in drugs and medicines; and after him, in 1687, came Dr. Samuel Ayrault, a Huguenot from New Rochelle, who practiced a few years.

Thomas Rodman arrived in Newport, 1680, and performed professional duty until his death in 1727, being then eighty years old.

Norbent Felicien Vigneron, native of Provence d'Artois, in France, arrived in 1690, and died in 1764, at the age of nearly ninety-five years.

John Brett came from Germany. He was a pupil of Boerhaave.

William Hunter arrived in this country from Edinburgh in 1752, where he had been a pupil of the elder Monro. He practiced in Newport, and was the first male accoucheur in the colony.

There were great numbers of prominent physicians in New Hampshire and Rhode Island during colonial and later days, too numerous to mention here.

In the early days of New England, it was not customary to address or speak of a physician by the title of Doctor. Perhaps one reason for this was that there were so very few persons who had ever taken a medical diploma. The custom of giving the title has literally grown up by degrees.

The earliest date at which we find the title Dr. substituted for surgeon and physician in America is in New England about 1769. Since that period it has become common throughout the United States, and the popular appellation of "doctor" is now almost exclusively given by the people to the medical practitioner when speaking to him, and the term physician used more generally when speaking of him.

Benjamin Rush (1745-1813), the "American Sydenham," as he was termed by Lettsom, was born in Byberry Township, Philadelphia County, on December 24, 1745. Rush is the outstanding figure in early American medicine. His family were English Quakers, but, curiously enough, both his father and grandfather were gunsmiths.

Upon the death of Dr. John Morgan in 1789, Rush succeeded him as professor of the theory and practice of medicine in the College of Philadelphia. When, in 1791, that institution was merged with the University of the state of Pennsylvania, to form the University of Pennsylvania, Dr. Rush was appointed professor of the institutes of medicine and clinical medicine.

When he was a young man he wrote: "Medicine is my wife; science is my mistress; books are my companions; my study is my grave, there I lie buried, the world forgetting, by the world forgot." In the latter part of his life, after having married a wife and begot thirteen children by her, he writes in treating of the causes of insanity, "celibacy is a pleasant breakfast, a tolerable dinner, but a very bad supper. The supper is not only bad, but eaten alone, no wonder it sometimes becomes a predisposing cause to madness."

Some of his admirers called him the "Hippocrates of Pennsylvania."

SEE AMERICAN PHARMACY CHAPTER FOR DR. JOHN MORGAN

SEE AMERICAN PHARMACY CHAPTER FOR DR. HUGH MERCER

William Shippen (1736-1808), was an army surgeon with Washington. He, with Morgan, has the distinction of being the founder of the first medical school in America, that which is now the medical department of the University of Pennsylvania. Shippen, Rush and Morgan, practicing mostly in the eighteenth century, were the three men responsible for the lusty start of medicine in America after the revolution. Besides them there were no outstanding men in American medicine during this period.

We can partially visualize them through their joint accomplishments. There were, for example, before the close of the eighteenth century, five worthy medical schools in America—University of Pennsylvania, Kings College in New York, Harvard University, College of Philadelphia and Dartmouth College.

Dr. John Jones was the first American physician to publish a medical book. In 1775 he issued his PRACTICAL REMARKS

ON THE TREATMENT OF WOUNDS AND FRACTURES in New York City.

James Thacher, the earliest medical biographer, began his first series of biographies in 1827, and, in 1813, Dr. James Tilton published his famous OBSERVATIONS ON MILITARY HOSPITALS.

Herman van de Bogaerdet was the first physician mentioned in connection with the life of New Amsterdam, later New York. These company physicians as a rule were not permanent members of the colonies, but from 1650 onwards medical men became fixtures in the new colonies.

In the New England group John Fisk, Thomas Oliver, Samuel Seabury and many others became prominent in medicine.

MEDICINE IN PHILADELPHIA

Since early colonial times Philadelphia has been a center in the development of the medical arts.

It was after the arrival of William Penn in 1682 that the barber-surgeons were definitely displaced by serious practitioners. The Welsh Quaker medical men were among the latter; in fact, they have, to a great measure, set the standard which Philadelphia was to follow and adhere to in the years to come.

Some of the names of striking figures who have played such an important role in the medical world in general, and, more particularly in the development of Philadelphia as a medical center, follow: Samuel Jackson, clinical medicine; William W. Gerhard, who discovered the difference between typhus and typhoid fevers; Robley Dunglison; Joseph Pancoast, anatomy and surgery; R. M. Huston, materia medica; T. D. Muetter, surgery; J. K. Mitchell, practice of medicine; Charles D. Meigs, obstetrics; Franklin Bache, chemistry;

George McClellan, surgery; S. D. Gross, surgery; S. D. Gross, Jr., genito-urinary diseases; J. K. Mitchell, practice and chemistry; S. W. Mitchell, son of J. K., nervous diseases; Franklin Bache, great-grandson of Benjamin Franklin, chemistry;

G. B. Wood and Joseph Carson, materia medica and therapeutics; Joseph Leidy, anatomy; D. H. Agnew, surgery; William Pepper, Sr. and Jr., clinical medicine; F. G. Smith, physiology; Alfred Stille, practice of medicine; J. M. Da Costa, diagnostitian.

MEDICINE IN NORTH CAROLINA

Medicine in North Carolina during this period was, on account of its proximity, practiced the same as in Virginia.

The following are some of the eighteenth century advertisements:

"Dr. Ward wishes to thank the public for the kind reception given to his purging cake. Ward's Anodyne Pearls 16 in a paper for only 1s and that to be returned to any buyer who shall say they have not answered the character here given. . . . To preclude the attempts of imposture, by any imitation, Doctor Ward will sign his name with red ink, on every paper of printed directions that will be given along with them." (The Cape Fear Mercury, Dec. 29, 1773.)

"To be sold. . . . Stoughton's excellent London Bitters, being a grand Preventative against the Ague and Fever, and giving Strength and Digestion to the Stomach: Also some Cases of genuine Cordials." (North Carolina Gazette, Feb. 24, 1775.)

"For sale, . . . Dr. Stephany's incomparable gold tincture, also his infallible ague pills (sold by no other person in this state)." (The State Gazette of North Carolina, March 2, 1788.)

"Any person that will dispose of their Front Teeth (slaves excepted) may receive Two Guineas for each, by calling on Doctor Laymeur. For further particulars enquire of the Printer." (North Carolina Gazette, Feb. 16, 1786.)

MEDICINE IN SOUTH CAROLINA

Dr. William Bull was the first native South Carolina physician of note, and the first American who received the degree of M. D. This was granted at Leyden in 1734, his thesis being on "Colica pictonum." He died July 4, 1791, aged eighty-two.

Dr. John Moultrie was the next South Carolinian who received the degree of M. D., which was granted in 1749, from Edinburgh. He commenced practice in Charleston as early as 1733, and for forty years was the most celebrated physician and popular obstetrician in the state or in the South. It is probable that his devotion to obstetrics antedates that of any other physician in America.

The following physicians of South Carolina served in a professional capacity in the Continental Army:

Samuel J. Axon, Robert Brownfield, Nathan Brownson, John Carne, Peter Fayssoux, Henry C. Flagg, Oliver Hart, James Houston, Charles Lockman, James Martin, William Neufville, Joseph Prescott, Jesse H. Ramsey, William Read, Sylvester Springer, William S. Stevens, Frederick Gunn, Benjamin Tetard, Thomas T. Tucker, Samuel Vickers, and John Wallace.

MEDICINE IN CALIFORNIA AND THE
SOUTH-WEST

The scalpel marched step by step with the cross and sword in all the explorations of the early Spanish settlers and this close association was kept until the time of the American settlement of California.

Fathers Kino and Salrua-Terra of the Jesuit Order started missions in Lower California in 1697. Coronado and Juan de Onate established missions in New Mexico prior to 1598, and Vizcaino in 1602 visited Alta California, now known as California, to prepare the way for missions.

202

Californian Indian medicine with its most interesting, fantastic, and weird practices yielded slowly to the Old World's white physician's methods of bleeding, blistering, cupping, and physicking. The advent of the white man in California was really when the Spanish padres came up from Baja (Lower) California in 1769 to found missions among the Indians.

Therefore, the white man's history of California goes back to the cradle of the new Spanish province when the sword, cross, and scalpel proceeded hand in hand. Dr. George Lyman wrote, "Had it not been for the presence of Dr. Pedro Pratt, it is probable that the projected province would have miscarried and never withstood the travail of its birth."

The complete list of surgeons-general who resided at Monterey, the medical center, and carried on during the Spanish reign in California were ten.

While myth surrounds the representatives of Indian medicine, real facts come down to us, through written Spanish mission records, concerning these ten doctors who were of such stellar stuff that they were recipients of king's commissions.

Pablo Soler (1791-1800), was the outstanding medical authority during the days of the Spanish rule in the province called California. Of him the written records state, "He made long, arduous horseback rides, visiting the presidios and caring for the sick officers, soldiers, Indians, settlers, and priests." Starvation and sickness were a common lot.

That Spanish doctors were aware of the contagiousness of pulmonary tuberculosis, or phthisis as they called it, is shown by the following: "Morelos caused to be burned the bedding, clothing, and house (after the plaster was removed) of a man who died from this disease."

Benites was a medical writer as well as an observer, for he furnished (1804), at the suggestion of the Mexican Viceroy, an able and exhaustive report of the diseases he encountered and their treatment, to the authorities in the capital of Spain.

Wounds (dueling was frequent), scurvy, fractures, dysentery, sore eyes, dropsy, gonorrhea, syphilis, dementia praecox, varicose veins, fevers, plethora—thus the record runs.

The first doctor on Rich Bar on the Feather River was Fayette Clappe. A few weeks later he had twenty-nine associates and all had plenty to do, for a page from his wife's diary reads: "In one period of twenty-four days we have had several murders, many fearful accidents, bloody deaths, whippings, a hanging, an attempt at suicide, and a fatal duel—these are stirring times!"

SPANISH, MEXICAN AND AMERICAN PRACTITIONERS

The history of medicine and the medical men of this portion of the United States falls naturally into three petty distinct periods, namely, the Spanish, the Mexican, and the American eras. The settlement of Upper California by the Franciscan friars and the Spanish Government in 1769 may be regarded as the beginning of the Spanish medical era.

The Spanish Medical Era was marked more especially by the activities of the Franciscan friars. Father Junipero Serra, the president and leader of the Franciscan missionaries and the founder of the Missions, a native of Spain, was an early and earnest student of the medical value of the flora of this region. Largely through his influence, the padres became more or less adept in the use of the indigenous drugs in the treatment of human ills. Father Serra's work in the control of scurvy by the use of the juice of the citrus fruits was a service well worthy of commendation.

The Mexican Medical Era (1822-1846) was distinguished by the arrival of three pioneer physicians—Dr. John Marsh, who came to Los Angeles in January, 1836; Dr. Richard S. Den, who arrived in California in 1843; and Dr. John S. Griffin, assistant surgeon, U. S. A., who arrived in 1846.

The American Medical Era began with our war with Mexico, in 1846. During this period, the growth of the medical profession kept pace with the rapid increase of population and advance of civilization in this region.

Tularemia has the distinction of being the first truly American disease. It was discovered by the United States Public Health Service and nearly all of the knowledge concerning it has been elucidated by the physicians of that organization. They also named it.

The name goes back to the time when California was a Spanish possession. In certain marshy places there grew a variety of bullrush called by the Spaniards and Mexicans *tule*. The areas where these reeds grew abundantly were named *tulares*. The story of the disease tularemia commences shortly after the San Francisco fire of 1906.

AMERICAN INDIANS

One may measure the state of civilization by the quality and character of medical practice. One of the best examples of the stoicism of the savage is his ability to take terrific doses of obnoxious medicines. The American Indians furnished an example of the medicine of primitive persons, and we have considerable knowledge concerning their activities. In certain conditions they put rocks in the bottom of a cave, built a fire on them, and then sat by them until they became very warm and perspired freely; then they ran out and jumped into cold water. Thus they practiced a rudimentary physiotherapy. The medicine men had considerable knowledge of the herbs, and drugs derived from them and their medicinal effect. These herbs were carefully selected and saved, and later brewed into forbidding concoctions.

In general, the morbid conditions that occur frequently and those that occur more rarely among the South-Western Indians than among average white Americans are as follows:

Frequent in Indians: Affections of the gastro-intestinal tract, affections of the respiratory organs, affections of the eyes, muscular and senile arthritis, smallpox, measles, malaria, dysentery.

Rare in Indians: Anemia, affection of breast, diseases of heart, arteries, and veins, asthma, affections of the liver, affections of the female sexual organs, many affections of the skin, dental caries, cancer, rachitis (high grade), insanity, nervous diseases (excepting epilepsy), scarlatina, bone fracture.

In every Indian tribe there were a number of persons, called medicine men by the whites, who were regarded as the possessors of supernatural powers which enabled them to recognize and cure disease. They were believed to have received their powers from some supernatural being, either as a direct gift, or as the result of instruction by some person who had received such powers.

The methods used to work cures varied with the nature of the disease and the customs of the medicine men. Diseases of unknown origin and those ascribed to witchcraft could only be treated by some one who could work a counter spell. Such diseases were usually eradicated by sucking a feather, small stone, blood, or some other object from the patient, singing and the shaking of a rattle being part of the performance.

Methods of opening veins for the purpose of blood-letting are known to many quite uncivilized tribes. Central Californian Indians used to open the veins of the right arm for diseases of the trunk, and of the left arm for diseases of the extremities. They have always had faith in the actual cautery, using red-hot needles, made of bone or flint or shell, for relieving rheumatic pains.

*   *   *

206

In evaluating the old time family doctor the human-interest factors must not be overlooked. The relations between doctor and patient were personal. He was sensible and kindly and was aware of the family tendencies and susceptibilities. The very limitations upon the doctor forced him to become the comforter and helper of those in distress and trouble. If he could not save the life of a child, he at least could comfort the bereaved parents. If he could not cure the aged man of his affliction, he could make life appear a little brighter and less forbidding.

The greatest accomplishment of American medicine is Anesthesia, which will be treated in Modern Medicine.

CHAPTER TWELVE

Medicine in the Nineteenth and Twentieth Centuries

(MODERN MEDICINE)

IN THE nineteenth century Robert Massengill Porter developed the medical department of the University of Nashville, which became the largest medical college in the south and the third largest in the nation. He became its first professor of anatomy and physiology and was recognized as one of America's most brilliant students of the form and function of the human body.

"There was genius in the new department, the compounded genius of John Berrien Lindsey, Paul Eve, John M. Watson, W. K. Bowling, A. H. Buchanan, C. K. Winston, and Robert Massengill Porter, as bright a group of luminaries as ever shed radiance upon an American medical campus."

Clinical medicine was evolved in the eighteenth century, after attention had been given to the importance of pathology and post-mortem examinations of diseases, and this work led to better diagnostic practices.

Modernization of medicine began in the nineteenth century with the extension of physics, chemistry and biology, all branches of medicine and surgery developed with rapid strides.

The nineteenth century was an era of almost incredible accomplishments, and we feel that it is ours, for there is a sense of proximity to the nineteenth century that is absent from our thought relationship to the preceding eighteen centuries.

Systems had seen their best day by this time and the first half of the nineteenth century was a period of transition, and there was a tendency to stabilize knowledge on the basis of facts. The early part of the nineteenth century was merely an appendage of the eighteenth; the last half of the nineteenth century, a period that we may justly characterize as the glitter time of medicine, leading onward into a more brilliant future. However, we must not make the error of thinking all was well during the wonderful nineteenth century, for we encounter several types of medical prostitution.

Mesmerism has already been mentioned under Quacks.

Francis Schlatter in 1893 left Denver, Colorado, and wandered as far as New Mexico, bareheaded and barefooted, over the mountains and plains, led, as he asserted, by divine inspiration. He returned to Denver as a faith healer, and his fame grew until he was visited by patients from all over the United States. Each day a line of four or five thousand people formed before his house, where he stood behind a picket fence to touch each sufferer that filed past him.

John Alxander Dowie was a faith healer, whose work has extended well into the twentieth century. For some years he was connected with the Divine Healing Association, but eventually he broke away from this organization and established the Christian Catholic Church which after 1901 was centered at Zion City, a suburb of Chicago. Dowie maintained that disease was the work of the devil and that prayer and the laying on of hands was a cure for it.

Phineas Quimby, of Maine, was an outstanding faith healer of the nineteenth century. His importance comes not so much from his own work as from the influence he exerted in the origin of New Thought and Christian Science. Quimby began faith healing with the use of hypnotism, which was then called animal magnetism.

During his early days as a practitioner of faith healing Quimby's method of treatment consisted in sitting beside his patient—usually a woman—putting his left hand on her bare abdomen, and with the other hand rubbing her head. He told the patient that in so doing animal magnetism flowed out of his body into hers and that the animal magnetism thus acquired would cure her.

Quimby's metaphysical conception of disease led directly to the founding of Christian Science. Its organizer, Mrs. Mary A. Morse Baker Glover Patterson Eddy, was born in Bow, New Hampshire, about 1821. As a child she was said to be neurotic and subject to fits of nervousness which interfered with her schooling. At the age of twenty-two she married George Washington Glover, a stone mason, who died six months later and before the birth of her only child. During ten years of widowhood she stayed with relatives and had long periods of illness of a hysterical character. In 1853 she married Daniel Patterson, an itinerant dentist, who deserted her in 1862 and from whom she subsequently obtained a divorce.

Her nervous disorders persisted in spite of—or because of—this unsatisfactory marriage, and she turned to Quimby for help. Under his ministrations her health improved, thus clearly showing the neurotic origin of her affliction. She studied Quimby's methods and, later, dates her discovery of the principle of Christian Science from the year of his death, 1866. Mary Eddy never quite succeeded in getting away from some of the ideas of animal magnetism which she had obtained from Quimby. Her cures had nothing to do directly with this belief, but she developed what would appear to be delusions of persecution and felt that malicious animal magnetism emanating from her enemies was producing many ills and had caused the death of her third husband, Asa Eddy.

To mention and describe the methods of the numerous faith healers, many of whom have reaped fortunes from the credulous, would require a large volume.

As offsets to the cults and quacks we have anesthesia, antisepsis and bacteriology as nineteenth century conquests, greater than which no other century has ever boasted.

SOME GREAT DOCTORS

A remarkable group of incisive thinkers and brilliant workers during the nineteenth century must be passed in review:

LEOPOLD AUENBRUGGER (1722-1809) laid the foundations of anatomical diagnosis. He was a pupil of van Swieten, and from 1751 to 1762 was first assistant physician and then physician at the Spanish hospital in Vienna. It was there he began his experiments in tapping, in percussion, doing so directly with the finger-tips of one hand.

After seven years' study and practice he made his discovery known to the world:

"I here present the Reader with a new sign which I have discovered for detecting diseases of the chest. This consists in the Percussion of the human thorax, whereby, according to the character of the particular sounds thence elicited, an opinion is formed of the internal state of that cavity. In making public my discoveries respecting this matter, I have been actuated neither by an itch for writing, nor a fondness for speculation, but by the desire of submitting to my brethren the fruits of seven years' observation and reflexion. In doing so, I have not been unconscious of the dangers I must encounter; since it has always been the fate of those who have illustrated or improved the arts and sciences by their discoveries to be beset by envy, malice, hatred, detraction and calumny."

A man who wishes to know whether a barrel is full or empty taps it. Auenbrugger was the son of an innkeeper, and must often have seen his father engaged in this simple operation.

Persons with "a good musical ear" learn percussion and auscultation far more speedily than those without musical gifts. Auenbrugger was an accomplished musician.

CLAUDE BERNARD (1813-1878), was a Burgundian, the son of a vine-grower. He was sent in early youth to Lyons as an apothecary's apprentice. There he began to write plays: a comedy, which had a fair success in a small theatre; and then a tragedy, with which he wanted to try his fortune in Paris. Certain art critics read his piece, and advised him to study medicine in preference to becoming a playwright. The up-shot was that the apothecary's apprentice became a student of medicine.

He was a professor of physiology at the University of Paris, where a chair for him had been especially established. Simul-taneously he was professor at the College de France as successor to his teacher Magendie.

Claude Bernard, working in a damp and gloomy hole, with apparatus constructed by himself, became the greatest experi-mental physiologist of his time.

Experiments on animals attracted the unfavourable atten-tion of the police. By ill-luck, one day, a dog with a silver cannula protruding from its belly-wall escaped from the lab-oratory. Bernard was prosecuted, and it transpired that the animal in question had belonged to the commissary of police and had been stolen from him! Then Bernard explained the circumstances, and secured a respectful hearing. Indeed, the commissary of police became his protector, and invited Bernard to remove the laboratory into his own district, where these im-portant physiological investigations could be carried on with-out molestation.

THEODOR BILLROTH (1829-1894) was the son of a pastor in the island of Rugen. He wanted to become a musi-cian. Since his relatives dissuaded him from adopting this profession as one at which it would be hard to make a liveli-hood, he qualified as a doctor. All the same, he remained an artist, was an instrumentalist throughout his life. He quali-fied in 1852, took post-graduate studies in Vienna and Paris,

213

and took up his residence as a practitioner in Berlin. In 1860 he accepted a call to Zurich, where he remained seven years.

In 1867, he became professor of surgery at Vienna, and remained at work in the Austrian capitol until shortly before his death at Abbazia in Istria on February 6, 1894. It was Billroth who worked out the methods of gastro-intestinal surgery. Above all his name will remain associated with the history of the surgery of the stomach. He was the first, in the year 1881, to prove successful in the excision of the pylorus in a female patient who was suffering from cancer of that part of the gastro-intestinal tract. Before this he had successfully extirpated a larynx, and these two operations of his attracted widespread attention.

Billroth was a cautious operator and wrote: "We are only entitled to operate when there are reasonable chances of success. To use the knife when these chances are lacking is to prostitute the splendid art and science of surgery, and to render it suspect among the laity and among one's colleagues. We have to ask ourselves, then, by what standard we can measure the chances of success. We shall learn them through the indefatigable study of our science, through shrewd criticism of our own and others' observations, through careful consideration of individual cases, and through the meticulous appraisement of our results."

JEAN NICOLAS CORVISART (1755-1821), a pupil of Desault, was the founder of modern clinical medicine in France.

Corvisart had originally been destined for the legal profession. At school he was not only diligent in his studies, but had distinguished himself by bodily vigor. His father was solicitor to the crown, and took the lad into his own office. Corvisart, however, found the copying of legal documents a tedious affair. Whenever he could, he escaped from this thraldom, made his way into the Latin Quarter, listened to one lecturer or another, visited the Hotel-Dieu (the largest hospital in Paris), and there gave ear to what Desault had to say. He found this fascinating.

At length he broke away from his father's profession, and became a medical student.

In 1807, Corvisart became physician-in-ordinary to Napoleon, and his new duties tended more and more to withdraw him from his work as a clinical teacher. His practice increased from day to day, and his social obligations became more comprehensive. Napoleon was a difficult and exacting patient, but Corvisart got on with him very well. It is recorded that the Emperor once said he had no faith in medicine, but he had faith in Corvisart.

After the fall of the Empire in 1815, Corvisart likewise vanished from the stage. He had been paralyzed by an apoplectic seizure, and retired to his country estate.

PAUL EHRLICH (1854-1915) studied in Breslau, Strasburg, Freiburg, and Leipzig. He was mainly interested in histology and chemistry. Histology gave him an insight into the minutest formative elements of the organism. Chemistry provided him with the means of recognizing the substance that lay beneath the form. Although Ehrlich, because of his seemingly haphazard "trial and error" methods, referred to his chemical researches as "play chemistry," he realized that his "chemical imagination" was his chief asset. This imagination made him the greatest bio-chemical philosopher of all times.

Ehrlich was not a good student, he was irregular in attendance, especially avoided the classes in chemistry, and after five years could not pass the required examinations. He remained another year, and was graduated to the great relief of the janitors. For Ehrlich was constantly playing with dye-stuffs, and never was a neat worker, he squirted color-spots everywhere.

A favorite story, that Robert Koch told very often, was to the effect that when he came to Breslau to demonstrate the anthrax bacillus, he was taken on a tour of inspection through the laboratory: they pointed out Ehrlich's table to him with the remark, "This here belongs to little Ehrlich, he is a very good dyer, but his examination he will never pass."

By following his lead August von Wasserman discovered the diagnostic test for syphilis. Ehrlich introduced the arsenical derivative—the six hundred and sixth of the series—for the sterilization of syphilis. As a therapeutic achievement, the production of salvarsan (606) and neosalvarsan (914) has never been surpassed.

EDWARD JENNER (1749-1823) was a native of Berkeley in Gloucestershire, England. His father was the vicar of Berkeley, and his mother was descended from an ancient family in Berkshire.

Round Berkeley, and elsewhere, the cows occasionally suffered from a malady in which pustules closely resembling those of smallpox appeared on the udders and the teats. Jenner called the illness "variolae vaccinae"—cowpox. This malady was transmissible to human beings. The cowherds and milkmaids became infected from time to time with similar pustules, which appeared on their hands and arms. The trouble, however, remained purely local, the attendant general symptoms being of trifling importance, and there being no tendency to the outbreak of a generalized crop of pustules.

He wrote to his master Hunter, telling him he thought that on this fact could be based an attempt to secure acquired immunity to smallpox on a large scale. Hunter replied with the famous bit of advice, "Do not think, try; be patient, be accurate." Jenner did try, he was accurate and he was patient, making observations from 1788 until May 14, 1796, when he performed his first vaccination on a boy, using pus from the arm of a dairymaid infected with cowpox. About two months later the boy was inoculated with smallpox virus and proved to be immune. Previously, no one had suspected that vaccination, as Jenner called his discovery, was anything more than a curiosity of medicine.

Thus inoculation with smallpox was replaced by inoculation with cowpox. "Vaccination" was substituted for variolation, and a means had been discovered by which smallpox became a preventible disease. During the latter half of the nineteenth century, vaccination was made compulsory in most civilized countries, with the result that smallpox is now extremely rare.

Jenner's introduction of preventive inoculation for smallpox furnished medicine with one of her greatest victories.

ROBERT KOCH (1843-1910) sprang from a miner's family and from early youth showed a strong inclination toward scientific research. Lister and Pasteur established the bacterial theory of disease, but it remained for another man to develop a systematic method of cultivating, grouping and classifying bacteria. This man was Robert Koch, whose efforts constituted what practically amounted to the birth of the science of infectious diseases. Koch, a native of Germany, took his medical degree at the University of Gottingen in 1866.

In 1876 Koch wrote to Ferdinand Cohn, who was then the leading authority on microscopic plants: "After many vain attempts, I have finally been successful in discovering the process of development of the anthrax bacillus. After many experiments, I believe to be able to state the results of these researches with sufficient certainty. Before, however, I bring this into the open, I respectfully appeal to you, esteemed Herr Professor, as the foremost authority on bacteria, to give me your judgment regarding this discovery."

Cohn asked leading investigators to examine his new methods, among them Cohnheim, the leading experimental pathologist of Europe, who told his assistants: "Drop everything and go at once to Koch. This man has made a splendid discovery which is all the more astonishing because Koch has had no scientific connections and has worked entirely on his own initiative and has produced something absolutely complete. There is nothing more to be done. I consider this the greatest discovery in the field of bacteriology and believe Koch will again astonish and shame us with still further discoveries."

217

Koch spent a considerable part of his life in travel. He could not hear of an epidemic anywhere without wanting to set forth and study it. Every nation owes an immeasurable debt to the man who gained victories over typhoid and rinderpest and sleeping sickness, uncovered the source of tuberculosis and cholera and Egyptian ophthalmia, and invaded continents to lead physicians in the warfare against pestilence and plague.

One malady, above all, interested Koch throughout his life. Again and again he returned to the problem of tuberculosis. Tuberculin is looked upon as the one folly of a great scientist. As a therapeutic agent, tuberculin has failed to fulfill the expectations which Koch prematurely raised, but as a diagnostic aid it has proved of great value.

When, on May 21, 1910, an end came to Robert Koch's laborious life, it was possible to look back upon unexpected advances which were due to him, to Pasteur, and to their pupils. The infectious disorders had lost many of their terrors. They were better known than they had ever been known before.

EMIL BEHRING (1854-1917) was a pupil of Koch and later his fellow-worker. The success of his serum treatment of diphtheria was amazing. Wherever the use of Behring's antitoxin was tried, there was an immediate and notable decline in mortality.

JAKOB HENLE (1809-1885), a rabbi's grandson and a pupil of Muller at Bonn, was the greatest anatomist of the nineteenth century. He later removed to Berlin with Muller.

Becoming suspect to the authorities as a member of the Burschenschaft, he was prosecuted, and was sentenced to six years' detention in a fortress, but was amnestied, and in 1840 went to Zurich as professor of anatomy.

"The life of Henle was a drama. None familiar with his career can forget his disastrous love-affair in boyhood, celebrated in a cycle of songs dedicated to the flames, but which

218

nevertheless survived; his duels, in one of which he was successful, only to pierce his foot when he put down his rapier in
triumph; his attempt to fling away his bachelorhood in three
cities, including a proposal to Felix Mendelssohn's sister, who
was already secretly betrothed; his romantic marriage to Elise
Egloff, the beautiful nurse-maid, who was really the illegitimate daughter of a well-to-do Swiss."

Henle did a great many pathological studies but primarily
he was an anatomist. He was the discoverer of epithelium,
was the founder of histology, the science of the minute structure of the tissues.

In 1844, Henle had a call to Heidelberg, and in 1852 he removed to Gottingen, where, until his death more than thirty
years later, he was busied in fruitful work as a teacher and
investigator.

RENE THEOPHILE HYACINTHE LAENNEC (1781-
1826), took his degree in Paris in 1804, filled many important
posts, and belonged to the faculty of the College de France.
He was a distinguished anatomist, a great clinician, and developed auscultation.

The Hippocratists had long ago pointed out that certain
sick people had strange noises going on in their chests. "It
bubbles like boiling vinegar," and "It creaks like a new leather
strap," they had said. Still, little use could be made of these
perfectly accurate observations until doctors began to think
anatomically.

"Laennec had under his care an exceedingly stout woman
suffering from heart disease. Listen as he might, he could not
hear the heart-sounds clearly. On his way to visit his patient,
Laennec was passing through the courtyard of the Louvre. A
heap of old timber was lying in one corner, and some children
were playing there. They had discovered a new game. One
of the pieces of wood was a long beam. A youngster had his
ear at one end of it, and another was signalling by tapping the

other end. This gave Laennec an idea. He quickened his steps, and, when he reached his patient asked for a quire of letter-paper. Having rolled this paper into a cylinder, he applied one end of it to the site of the cardiac impulse and listened at the other end. The result was marvelous. He could hear the heart-sounds much better, much more plainly, than with his ear on the chest. Moving his paper cylinder from place to place, he listened to the sounds that were forthcoming all over the heart. Then he listened to the breath-sounds. They were so loud that they startled him. The stethoscope had been discovered, the auditory tube which was to become symbolical of latter-day physicians as the urine-glass was of the medieval doctor. Indirect auscultation had replaced the direct method. A new process of physical examination had been revealed, a new means of access to the interior of the organism."

Like Auenbrugger, Laennec had musical gifts. He was an instrumentalist as well as an amateur, being, we are told, an excellent performer on the flute.

JOSEPH LISTER (1827-1912) sprang from a Quaker family. His father was a wine-merchant, but also a man well versed in mathematics and physics, and one who devoted his leisure to microscopical studies. Having qualified in London, young Lister went to Scotland, where in 1854 he became Syme's house-surgeon at the Edinburgh Hospital. After distinguishing himself by various anatomical, physiological, and pathological researches, he was in 1861 appointed professor of surgery in Glasgow. It was there that his decisive life-work began.

In 1869, Lister became professor of clinical surgery at Edinburgh. In 1877, he became professor at King's College, London, where he worked until his retirement in 1892. He laboured strenuously at the development of his method, and introduced the use of absorbable aseptic catgut for ligatures and sutures. He attained the age of eighty-five, and was able

to enjoy the satisfaction of seeing that his work had borne
magnificent fruit. He had made surgery safe for patients.
He had banished sepsis from hospital wards. The general belief was that contused wounds necessarily suppurated. In 1867
he showed that infection in wounds could be prevented by
antiseptics and by cleanliness. It has been said that there are
only two periods in the history of surgery—before Lister and
after Lister.

WILLIAM OSLER (1849-1919), a Canadian of Celtic
stock, the son of a minister of religion, was originally intended
to adopt his father's profession. Having early begun to take
an interest in natural science, he soon abandoned the idea of
becoming a clergyman, and devoted himself to medicine. He
studied the elements at the McGill University in Montreal, and
took his degree there in 1872. Then he went abroad for post-
graduate work.

Returning to Canada in 1874, Osler soon became professor
of medical institutions at McGill University. In 1884, he accepted a summons to become professor of clinical medicine in
the University of Pennsylvania. Five years later, he removed
to Baltimore, and began clinical work at Johns Hopkins
Hospital.

In 1905, Osler left Baltimore. He was suffering from
over-work, and therefore accepted a call to Oxford as professor of medicine—the highest distinction open to a British physician. But though he was absent in the flesh, in the spirit
he remained active in America.

At Oxford, his hospitable home was always open to American doctors. A heavy blow befell him in 1917 when his only
son was killed at Ypres. Two years later, when William Osler
was hard upon seventy, he also passed away. His library was
sent back to America, to the McGill University in Montreal,
where he had taken his medical degree.

LOUIS PASTEUR (1822-1895) was a chemist, not a physician. However, he did far more for the prevention of illness, did far more in this respect on behalf of human welfare in general, than many "great doctors" who lived before and after him. Few men of science have become so widely known as he.

Pasteur was a Burgundian. Born at Dole in the year 1822, the son of a tanner, he was destined for the scholastic profession. Having been sent to Paris to study, he showed from the outset noteworthy scientific talent. After spending several years engaged in teaching activities at Dijon and Strasburg, Pasteur removed to Lille as dean of the newly founded faculty of natural science there.

Coming as he did from a wine-growing district, Pasteur had often heard his compatriots complain that wine so readily "fell sick," just like living creatures. They did not know how to explain the process, and were therefore unable to ward it off and to avoid the losses it entailed. Now Pasteur's studies on fermentation showed him how wine was spoiled.

In the year 1865 the silk-growing industry of southern France was faced by a catastrophe. Everywhere the caterpillars were dying. Whole districts were being impoverished. Pasteur was sent for to study the malady. He had never before had a silkworm in his hand. He went to the region, examined the question without prejudice, made experiments, and after a few years, having had to cope with immense difficulties, he was able to elucidate the nature of the disease, to ascertain the method of infection, and to indicate a way of breeding healthy stock. The French silk industry was saved.

Pasteur's discoveries had benefited the wine industry, the silk industry and the animal and fowl industries, but his work was not yet complete, for he had before him the problems of applying his principles to the control of human diseases. For this effort he chose to study rabies, or hydrophobia.

Pasteur's first human patient was Joseph Meister, an Alsatian boy nine years of age. He had been bitten in fourteen places by a rabid dog. Pasteur hesitated to apply his immunizing vaccine for fear it would harm the boy, but finally he was persuaded to do so, since otherwise it was inevitable that the boy would die of rabies. Pasteur administered the new prophylaxis and rabies did not develop. Soon afterward a second case was brought to him. A shepherd boy of fourteen, named Berger Gupille, had struggled with a rabid dog to prevent it from biting some younger boys. He had himself been bitten. The vaccine of Pasteur saved him from rabies. In the yard of Pasteur Institute at Paris there is a statue of this shepherd boy showing him struggling with the rabid dog.

After these two successful cases people who had been bitten by rabid dogs came from all over Europe to receive the vaccine. The first Americans to receive treatment were four children from Newark, New Jersey. They were sent to Paris and treated there in December, 1885, six months after Pasteur had treated Joseph Meister. The following year a supply of the virus was sent to America.

Pasteur applied none of his discoveries to the treatment of disease. They were all directed to preventing disease. The recognition of the cause of infectious diseases made possible the development of preventive medicine. He was a man of genius, impulsive, intuitive, full of fruitful ideas. Medicine owes him much. His practical achievements and the knowledge he garnered where, in other hands, soon to produce even more important results.

Pasteur's and Koch's work resulted in the founding of bacteriology.

MAX PETTENKOFER (1818-1901) founded the science of experimental hygiene. He had not originally intended to devote himself to public health, having reached it by a circuitous route. The son of a peasant, he was destined by the family to become an apothecary, like his uncle. For a time he was refractory, and went on the stage. Then he resumed his studies, becoming in 1843 a qualified apothecary, and at the same time taking his degree as doctor of medicine.

At the age of eighty-three, Pettenkofer, his health being broken, sought a voluntary death. His work was left as his monument. Hygiene had taken an outstanding place in the system of medicine. Since then it has continued to develop, achieving new conquests year by year. To it belongs the future.

RUDOLF VIRCHOW (1821-1902), born at Schievelbein in Pomerania, a son of the town treasurer, went to Berlin in 1839 to become a pupil of the army medical school. Johannes Muller and Schonlein were his principal teachers. He took his degree in 1843.

For almost half a century, extending from 1856 to his death in 1902, Virchow lived in Berlin as professor of pathological anatomy and director of the Pathological Institute— the first independent institute of the kind. He had founded a school; he reigned as pope of German medicine, supreme though not without adversaries. Throughout his epoch, his researches were mainly concerned with anthropology.

Virchow was the founder of modern pathology, went a step further and opened up the new field of cellular pathology. There was practically no field of pathology that Virchow did not enrich.

CARL AUGUST WUNDERLICH (1815-1877) was the son of a physician. His mother belonged to a family of French refugees. Born at Sulz on the Neckar, he attended the high school in Stuttgart, and subsequently, from 1833 onwards, studied at the University of Tubingen.

Wunderlich did not discover the use of the clinical thermometer. We have already seen how, long ago, Santorio, with a primitive instrument, made measurements of bodily temperature. But it was Wunderlich who taught us to read and to understand the curves of fever. He showed that the course of fever is not determined by chance, but reflects the essential nature of the disease; that each of the specific infectious disorders is sharply characterized by the temperature chart. It was mainly through his instrumentality that the clinical thermometer was adopted for daily use by general practitioners, whereas up till then the instrument had been used only by hospitals. Nay more, it made its way into family life.

WILHELM CONRAD ROENTGEN OF WURZBURG, a man of fifty years of age, was working in his darkened laboratory on November 8, 1895. He was experimenting with the so-called cathode rays. When he noticed an unusual phenomenon, he began a thorough and patient investigation of it. In less than two months he was sufficiently certain of the results he had obtained to present a paper on "A New Kind of Ray" to the Physical Medical Society of Wurzburg. He admitted that he still did not know much about the nature of the rays, and therefore referred to them as X-rays. They penetrated with ease a surprising variety of objects, books and clothes, for example. They would affect a photographic plate, but could barely be seen by the human eye. They would pass through a human hand, yet show on a photographic plate the outline of the bones and of the flesh in very different densities.

Roentgen was a famous physicist before he ever discovered X-rays, but the discovery was of such general interest that his name became a household word within the space of weeks. Morality brigades were formed overnight to resist to the death the destruction of all decency and privacy. A London firm rose to the occasion, and made a small fortune from the sale of X-ray-proof underwear. New York was also in the van, with a determined attempt to obtain legislation against "the use of X-rays in opera-glasses in theatres." Slowly—and with some disappointment—the general public realized that an X-ray picture was not pornographic nor ever likely to be.

225

Roentgen was awarded a Nobel prize in 1901. The introduction of anesthesia and of X-rays are two great discoveries which have contributed to progress in the field of surgery and medicine.

MAX NITZE (1848-1906) was born in Dresden in 1848 and died in Berlin February 24th, 1906 from apoplexy. The idea and the plan of construction of the cystoscope originated with Nitze (1877). He made many advances in diagnostic procedure in cystoscopy, urethroscopy and rectoscopy. "He had a very large practice, his patients including members of reigning families and foreigners from every part of the world. He lived very plainly, having few interests beyond his professional work."

EPHRIAM McDOWELL (1771-1830) was born in Rockbridge County, Virginia, and came of that sturdy Scotch Presbyterian stock which has done so well by this land of ours. His father was Samuel McDowell, an important man in his place, lawyer, judge, and legislator. In 1755 he married a Miss McClung, also Scotch and Virginian. To them were born twelve children, of whom Ephriam was the ninth.

American surgery during the earliest pre-Listerian and pre-anesthetic days became famous through the work of Ephriam McDowell (1771-1830) who after studying in Edinburg, settled in the backwoods village of Danville, Kentucky, where he performed the first ovariotomy in 1809, when thirty-eight years old and fourteen years in practice. It had never been done before. For centuries surgeons had regarded it as impossible, but out of the American wilderness came the pioneer to show the way.

At that time Danville, in the very center of Kentucky, was a far-distant place, in a rude country, little cultivated, with forests and bridle paths and Indians. There, any day, you might have seen young McDowell riding through the woods to visit his patients. It was a fine figure of a man, rising six feet, broad shouldered, erect, a splendid horseman; ruddy, with keen, sparkling black eyes and a ready smile. He could ride all day and all night without a murmur, and take off your leg at the end of it without winking.

Jane Todd Crawford was enormously distended; although beyond term, she thought she was in labor, and two physicians requested McDowell's aid in delivering her. Upon vaginal examination, McDowell found the womb empty, and thus realized that the enlarged abdomen was not due to a fetus but to an ovarian tumor. McDowell explained that never had he seen so large a substance extracted, nor heard of an attempt; he informed her that the situation was dangerous, and the experiment uncertain, but he promised to perform it if she would come to his home in Danville.

Mrs. Crawford lived sixty miles away; mounting a horse, resting her tumor on the horn of the saddle, she arrived after a journey of a few days in McDowell's village. Without trained assistants, anesthetics or a precedent, McDowell placed her on a table and operated. "In five days I visited her, and much to my astonishment found her engaged in making up her bed. I gave her particular caution for the future; and in twenty-five days, she returned home as she came, in good health, which she continues to enjoy."

Jane Todd Crawford reached the age of seventy-eight, outliving for several years the man whom she made the "Father of Ovariotomy."

JAMES MARION SIMS (1813-1883), a young doctor in South Carolina, in 1835 tore the tin sign from his office-door, and dropped it in an abandoned well. His practice had consisted of two patients, both babies, and both had died. He settled in Alabama. So little did he know himself that ten years later he said: "If there is anything I hate, it is investigating the organs of the female pelvis." He invariably informed gynecological cases, "This is out of my line."

Entirely against his will, cases of vesico-vaginal fistula were sent to him. He refused to attend these young colored

227

mothers, saying over and over again that nothing could be done for them. Later, he built a little hospital for six of these slave-girls, and kept them for four years at his own expense. He found that when he placed a woman in the knee-chest position, the admission of air expanded the vagina. With a pewter spoon he originated the duckbill vaginal speculum: "Introducing the bent angle of the spoon I saw everything, as no man had ever seen it before." Walking from his house to the office, he picked up in his yard a piece of brass wire that was used in suspenders before the days of India rubber; this fine brass wire gave him the idea for his silver-wire suture. "From an onrush of air, a bent spoon and a torn suspender, Marion Sims learned how to revolutionize gynecology."

On account of ill health he decided to change his location. "I was always a little better in New York and Philadelphia than in any other place." In 1853 he left his Alabama home and settled in New York. After some preliminary skirmishes with the foremost physicians, Sims organized the Woman's Hospital. Long afterward he wrote: "The Woman's Hospital from the day it was opened had no friends among the leaders—among hospital men. I was called a quack and a humbug, and the hospital pronounced a fraud." The sweet-tempered Sims was unusually bitter about his early New York experiences; in time, he dominated the gynecological practice of the metropolis.

At the age of forty-eight, Sims arrived in Paris in 1861. The most hopeless cases were brought to him and his successes were marvelous. It was customary for Americans to come to Europe to study, but few had come to teach. Sims was urged to settle in London; he was decorated by the governments of France, Portugal, Spain, Belgium and Italy. No American breast had ever been covered with so many ribbons.

Sims attended the medical college of the State of South Carolina for one year and then went to Philadelphia where he matriculated in the Jefferson Medical School, from which he graduated. He translated himself from the status of a more

or less obscure Southern country practitioner into a world figure, and is regarded as one of the founders of modern gynecology.

WALTER REED (1851-1902) was a United States army
doctor holding the title of major.

Yellow fever had for generations been the greatest scourge
of tropical America. Typhoid and smallpox were easily controlled because the means of preventing them were known;
but yellow fever was still a mystery. In the year 1900, a special commission of army doctors was sent to Havana to study
the problem. Its chairman was Walter Reed, and his associates were James Carroll, Jesse W. Lazear and Aristides Agra-
monte. They had good reason to suspect that the disease
might be carried by mosquitoes.

The difficulty, however, was that the lower animals were
not then known to suffer from yellow fever, and experiments
had to be made with human beings. The commission decided
that a solution of the yellow fever mystery, and all that this
would mean in the saving of life, would justify experimenting
on human beings. The members of the commission agreed
that it was their duty to be the first ones to run these risks.

The first successful experiment was made with Dr. Carroll,
who allowed himself to be bitten by a mosquito which had previously bitten four yellow fever patients. For three days his
life hung in the balance. He finally recovered, but Lazear,
the second man to be bitten, died.

An experiment station called "Camp Lazear" in honor of
the first martyred member of the party, was established in the
open country near Havana. Volunteers were called for; and
in spite of the danger, there were always men ready and willing to serve in this cause. The first two volunteers after
Lazear's death were a private, John R. Kissinger, and a civilian
government clerk, John J. Moran. Reed explained to them
fully the danger and suffering involved. Then, seeing they
were determined, he stated that a definite money compensa-

tion would be made them. Both young men declined to accept it, making it, indeed, their sole stipulation that they should receive no pecuniary reward, whereupon Major Reed touched his cap, saying respectfully, "Gentlemen, I salute you." Reed's own words, in his published account of the experiment on Kissinger and Moran, are: "In my opinion, this exhibition of moral courage has never been surpassed in the annals of the Army of the United States." Both Kissinger and Moran had severe attacks of yellow fever after submitting to the bites of infected mosquitoes. Fortunately, they recovered, as did all the men who developed yellow fever later as a result of the experiments at Camp Lazear.

In 1900 Reed wrote his wife ten minutes before the close of the year in which this discovery was made, he said: "I thank God that this has been accomplished during the later days of the old century. May its cure be wrought out in the early days of the new."

ROBERT MASSENGILL PORTER

Alexander James Porter, a Scotch-Irish Presbyterian, arrived in America from Ireland in 1793. His brother James was a distinguished Presbyterian preacher in Ireland, where his frankness cost him his life by court martial procedure in the Irish troubles of 1798. He was hanged in front of the church in which he had preached the offending sermon.

In 1796 Alexander James Porter set out on horseback from Delaware to Nashville, Tennessee, to establish a wholesale linen business, mostly Irish linens. It was a long and arduous trip, to add to the vicissitudes of which he developed typhoid fever en route. And thereby hangs a tale, a tale portraying vividly the sturdiness, the sympathy, and the romance of pioneer life. He didn't know he had typhoid. He thought he was just tired. He came presently to a home and asked for water. A girl took a bucket and ran to the spring. He was weaker than he thought and when she came with the water he lay on the ground in a faint, his horse nibbling at roadside grass. The girl

was Susan Massengill. They bore the young stranger into the
house. He lay ill for five weeks. Then for two weeks he
gathered his strength for the remainder of the trip to Nashville. When he left the Massengill home, Nashville bound, he
did not go alone, for that day he and Susan Massengill had
married.

The third child of this union was Robert Massengill Porter
who entered the University of Nashville in 1832 and was
awarded a Bachelor of Arts degree in 1836.

Dr. Porter continued his studies and graduated in law at
Harvard in 1838. He returned to Nashville and married Mary
Wharton Williams, a daughter of one of the city's most re-
nowned pioneers. Mrs. Porter survived that marriage by three

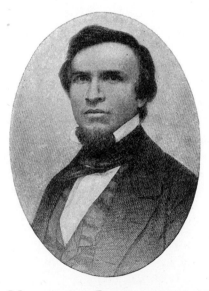

DR. ROBERT MASSENGILL PORTER (1818-1856) OF THE
MEDICAL DEPARTMENT OF THE UNIVERSITY
OF NASHVILLE

months. "His hopes of domestic happiness being thus rudely
interrupted, he was inclined to seek retirement from the

231

world." In June, 1840, he matriculated in the Theological Department of Princeton, and was graduated in 1843. He never preached.

In the fall he entered the University of Pennsylvania to study medicine and was graduated in the class of 1845. And so he came late to the choice his father had made for him early. He arrived in Paris, May 24, 1845, for a graduate course in anatomy. After finishing his course in Paris, he visited hospitals in Italy, Germany, England, Ireland, and Scotland. In 1848 he returned to Nashville and began the practice of medicine and was soon offered the chair of anatomy and physiology in the medical department of the University of Nashville. He threw all of his training, all of his character, and all of his engaging personality into the development of the university's new department, making it the largest medical college in the South, the third largest in the nation, acknowledging only the superiority of the University of Pennsylvania.

In 1852 he married Mrs. Felicia Grundy Eakin, a woman of great culture, the youngest child of Felix Grundy, lawyer of distinction, a United States senator, and a member of President Van Buren's cabinet.

The dissecting room of a college of medicine today is a vast improvement over one in 1856. How much of our improvement has risen out of tragic ashes! Men have died that other men might learn not to die. Martyrdom is not an infrequent phase of progress. On May 27, 1856, Dr. Porter took a cadaver, newly secured by the college, and made it the subject of an anatomical demonstration during a period of two hours. A peculiar infection developed within twenty-four hours, mild at first, then gathering in gravity.

Robert Massengill Porter died of blood-poisoning. His death caused much comment in the country's dissecting room circles and, more than comment, much preventive effort. Such tragedies are not heard of today. And so Robert Massengill Porter served by dying. But at the age of 38 he met death too young.

The esteem in which he was held is attested by the fact that
when he died there were standing at his bed-side his own Presbyterian pastor, a Catholic priest, and a Jewish rabbi. The
largest crowd that had ever assembled at a funeral in Nashville
followed his remains to Mt. Olivet cemetery.

DR. JOHN DAVID MASSENGILL (1844-1919)

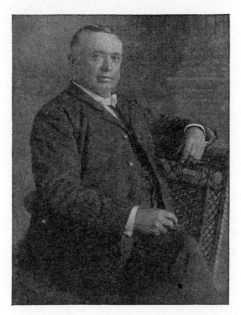

John David Massengill, father of Samuel Evans Massengill,
at the age of 16 years volunteered as a soldier in the Confederate States Army and rode four years under those great cavalry leaders, Generals Forrest and Wheeler. After the close of
the war he took up the broken thread of his education and life
and began the study of medicine. In 1874 he received his degree of M. D. from the Baltimore College of Physicians and
Surgeons. He began practice during the days of Reconstruc-
tion in the South, and on account of the poverty of that period
his practice was largely charitable, and remained so during his

entire life. During the early years of his practice it was the custom for the country doctors to extract teeth. S. E. Massengill's first connection with medicine was holding the heads of patients who came to have their teeth extracted.

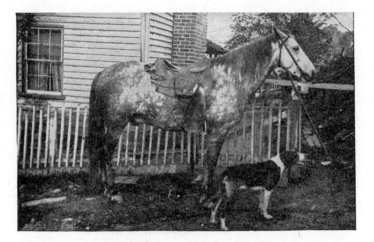

ONE OF DR. JOHN D. MASSENGILL'S SADDLE HORSES, EQUIPPED WITH THE SADDLE-BAGS AND SLICKER THAT WERE GENERALLY USED BY COUNTRY DOCTORS BEFORE THE ERA OF GOOD ROADS

Dr. Massengill, as was generally the case during his period, was also a farmer. He was a great lover of the chase and always kept a pack of fine fox hounds. Also, he was enthusiastic about fine horses and brought much of the best blood of Kentucky to his section. At one fair his trotters, pacers and show horses took seventeen first premiums.

CHRISTOPHER WREN, the architect, developed the hollow hypodermic needle in 1852.

The author has heard his father, Dr. John D. Massengill, tell of giving his first hypodermic injection. He was called in great haste to see Billy Leonard who had an attack of acute

234

indigestion and was in great agony. His prize possessions, and about all he did possess, was a team of jennets. He told father if he would relieve him he would give him his jennets. Father said that never thereafter did he see a hypodermic of morphine act so beautifully. The patient was soon completely at ease. When father started to leave he jokingly told his patient to have the boys bring the jennets from the stable and he would take them home with him. The patient was still grateful but insisted that he should be allowed to settle upon some other basis.

SENOR MANUEL GARCIA, who created the laryngoscope, was a singing-master who wanted to see how his larynx worked. The idea came to him out of a very blue sky. With two mirrors it is possible to see round a corner, and the larynx is so far round a corner as to be normally invisible. Garcia bought his two mirrors, a little dental mirror with a long handle, which cost 6 francs, and a hand mirror. The dental mirror he placed firmly against his uvula, and what appeared there he saw in the hand mirror, which reflected a ray of light on to the dental mirror.

By the time Garcia died in 1906, at the ripe age of 102, a distinct department of the surgical art had been firmly based upon the laryngoscope he invented. Again, we find a valuable discovery made in medicine by some one outside the profession.

In the first half of the nineteenth century, English physicians gave their names to various diseased conditions: Addison's, Bell's, Bright's, Hodgson's, Parkinson's. Many surgical operations were first performed in the nineteenth century.

Many instruments were invented that were invaluable in the practice of medicine: The hypodermic syringe by Pravaz, 1851; the ophthalmoscope by Helmholtz, 1850; the stethoscope by Laénnec, 1819; the cystoscope in 1877; the laryngoscope by Garcia, 1854.

235

Holmes says: "Medicine appropriates everything from every source that can be of the slightest use to anybody who is ailing in any way, or likely to be ailing from any cause. It learned from a monk how to use antimony, from a Jesuit how to cure ague, from a friar how to cut for stone, from a soldier how to treat gout, from a sailor how to keep off scurvy, from a postmaster how to sound the Eustachian tube, from a dairy maid how to prevent smallpox, and from an old market woman how to catch the itch insect. It borrowed acupuncture and the moxa from the Japanese heathen, and was taught the use of lobelia by the American savage."

Diphtheria antitoxin was placed in the hands of the medical profession in 1895, and in its dying years the nineteenth century bequeathed to the twentieth three important discoveries, the X-ray by Wilhelm Konrad Roentgen, the Finsen lamp by Niels Finsen, which gave us phototherapy, and radium by Pierre and Marie Curie.

Researches continued without pause! A whole generation of investigators devoted themselves to the campaign against pestilences. Each year brought fresh discoveries. In 1882, Loffler discovered the glanders bacillus; Bollinger and Harz discovered the actinomyces bovis, which is the cause of actinomycosis. Next year, Fehleisen discovered the exciting cause of erysipelas. The year 1884 was exceptionally fruitful, for in this came the discovery of the diphtheria bacillus by Loffler, of the tetanus bacillus by Nikolaier, and of the pneumonia bacillus by Fraenkel. In 1887, Weichselbaum discovered the exciting cause of epidemic cerebrospinal meningitis; in 1894, Kitasato and Yersin discovered the bacillus of bubonic plague; and in 1897, Kruse and Shiga discovered the exciting cause of dysentery. In 1901 came the discovery by Forde, Dutton, and Bruce of the exciting cause of sleeping-sickness; and 1905 was marked by Schaudinn's discovery of the spirochaeta pallida, the exciting cause of syphilis.

236

The perspective is not sufficient to fully evaluate the accomplishments of the twentieth century. The following are some of the outstanding ones:

The use of liver extract in the treatment of pernicious anemia.

Sulfanilamide and other sulfa drugs for infectious diseases.

The application of electricity to diagnosis and new techniques in surgery.

The discovery of insulin, the anti-diabetic hormone, discovered at the University of Toronto in 1922 by Dr. F. G. Banting.

The great advance in parenteral therapy, especially the use of arsenical preparations for the treatment of syphilis.

The development of the glandular products that have become popular in the treatment of disease.

The knowledge gained of anaphylaxis.

The use of preventive medicine and the reduction of mortality as a result of the growing control of the infectious and contagious diseases and the development of hygiene and sanitation.

The most important dietetic discovery of the twentieth century is that with regard to the vitamins.

A few of the outstanding American doctors of the nineteenth and twentieth centuries, not heretofore mentioned, are: Austin Flint, Joseph O'Dwyer, Lawson Tait, Thomas Addis Emmet, Howard A. Kelly, John B. Murphy, Victor Horsley, S. Weir Mitchell and the Mayo brothers.

During the latter part of the nineteenth century and the twentieth century the large scale manufacture of elegant pharmaceutical products was developed into a large industry.

Perhaps our age will live in the history of medicine chiefly as a time when men learned more and more about the physical and chemical reactions which go on in the human body. New chemical and physical tests, the X-ray, various electrical devices, are all helping to make medicine a more exact science. The sciences of chemistry and medicine, working together, have made possible much of the safety in daily living which we now enjoy.

ANESTHESIA

The greatest triumph achieved in any department of medicine, and worthy, perhaps, to be described as almost, if not quite, the most beneficent discovery in the world's history, is that of the successful employment of anesthetics. This great glory belongs to the nineteenth century—Ether, 1842; nitrous oxide, 1844; chloroform, 1847.

From the dawn of civilization attempts had been made to control or at least deaden pain. Incantations were used for a thousand years to render patients less conscious of the pain of an operation, and deities were invoked on their behalf. For another thousand years the victim was tied down with ropes and instructed to commend himself to God and bear his sufferings beneath the surgeon's knife with such fortitude as he could command.

The deep sleep of Adam was anesthesia.

Lyman suggests that it was mandragora wine mixed with myrrh that was offered to Christ on the Cross, as it was commonly given to those who suffered death by crucifixion to allay in some degree their terrible agonies. Another suggestion is that the anesthesia may have been vinegar and hyssop.

The deadening of pain by soporific potions was known even to some primitive peoples as well as those of the earliest civilizations. Helen cast "nepenthe" into the wine of Ulysees, and the Talmud of the Jews speaks of a narcotic called "samme de shinta;" there is the "bhang" of the Arabian Nights and the "drowsy syrups" of Shakespeare's time. Opium and Indian hemp, "hashish," were probably known to the Egyptians and Greeks, and the mandrake to the Babylonians and Hebrews.

238

This mandrake is the European plant, not the May apple, or mandrake, of America.

Mandrake was the most popular substitute for an anesthetic during the Middle Ages. It held its vogue up to the sixteenth century. It was an inefficient anesthetic and ceased to be employed.

In the teachings of the school at Salerno were revived the "surgical sleeping draughts" mentioned by the Church fathers Hilary and Origen, and previously referred to under the name of the "soporific sponge." One of these was composed of opium, henbane, mulberry juice, lettuce, hemlock, mandragora, conium and ivy. This was inhaled from a sponge by the patient, who was later revived by fennel juice applied to the nostrils. The plants were dried in the sun, dipped in warm water when required and applied to the patients' nostrils. A recent experimenter has found that these medieval narcotics "do not make even a guinea pig nod."

DR. CRAWFORD W. LONG

Crawford W. Long, M. D., discovered the use of sulphuric ether as an anesthetic in surgery on March 30, 1842, at Jefferson, Jackson County, Georgia. Dr. Long was born at Danielsville, Georgia, Nov. 1, 1815, and died at Athens, Georgia, June 16, 1878.

The statue of Dr. Crawford W. Long is in the Hall of Fame under the dome of the National Capitol in Washington. This honor is in recognition of Long's great discovery of the use of sulphuric ether as an anesthetic. Also of unusual interest is the fact that Georgia's other representative in the Hall of Fame is Alexander H. Stephens, Vice-President of the Confederate States of America, a classmate and roommate of Dr. Long at the University of Georgia.

He attended the academy in his native town, and at the age of 14 entered Franklin College, now the University of

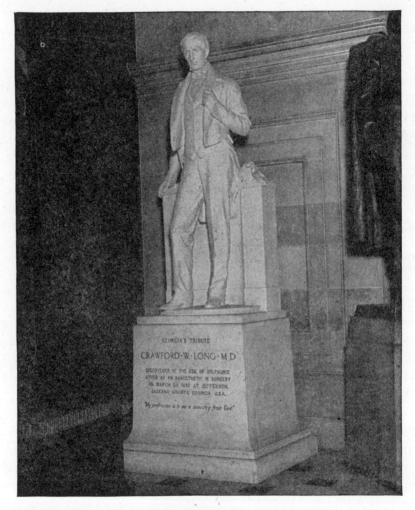

DR. CRAWFORD W. LONG (1815-1878)

Georgia, where he took the degree of master of arts, in 1835, at the age of 19, being considered "studious and wise" beyond his years, and called "The Baby" at college on account of his youth. He stood second in the graduating class.

He took a one-year course at Lexington, Kentucky, and in 1837 he entered the medical department of the University of Pennsylvania, where he received the degree of M. D. in 1839. After his graduation he went to New York and spent eighteen months with leading teachers. Specializing in surgery, he was impressed by the terrific suffering as a result.

At twenty-six he returned to Jefferson, Jackson County, Georgia, and began the practice of medicine. Later, he practiced in Atlanta for a year and, finally, located at Athens, Georgia, where he resided till his death, after practicing medicine for nearly forty years.

Long made the discovery of surgical anesthesia because he was looking for it, and because he was a keen observer and a courageous man. His experience in the New York hospitals, where he witnessed the pain of women in childbirth, convinced him of the need of an anesthetic agent, and he determined to find one if possible.

Dr. Long was the first man known to have used an anesthetic. In 1842 he gave ether to a patient and performed an operation on him. The bill for that operation still exists—$2 for the operation and 25 cents for the ether. Dr. Long placed his patient, a certain Mr. James Venables, profoundly under the influence of ether and removed a tumor from his neck painlessly. During the next twelve months, Long successfully repeated the use of ether several times.

The use of anesthetics to alleviate the pain of surgical operations and of childbirth was unknown before the discovery of Dr. Long. No greater boon has ever come to mankind than the power thus granted to induce a temporary but complete insensibility to pain.

It has been said that Dr. Long was in many respects in advance of his day. He treated and cured consumption by food and fresh air, and he treated typhoid fever practically as we do now. He operated several times very successfully for cancer of the breast, always clearing the ribs and removing the auxiliary glands. He cured several cases of lockjaw, and was especially skilled in the use of obstetrical forceps.

Those who knew Dr. Long declared him a man of exceptional qualities of mind and soul. Dignified in manner, his whole appearance betokened culture and high character. It is said he possessed no eccentricities, very unusual in a celebrity. He was sensitive, refined, and considerate of others; free from envy, malice, and uncharitableness. He maintained a slight reserve, except among intimates and congenial people. Cheerful in the sick room, he inspired his patients with confidence. He was fond of Shakespeare and good music; tall and slender, dressed in conventional black, always with frock coat; in short, a high-bred, scholarly Christian gentleman.

"My profession is to be a ministry from God."

Two years later, in 1844, Horace Wells, a dentist in Hartford, Connecticut, began to experiment with nitrous oxide, the anesthetic properties of which had been suggested by Sir Humphrey Davy in 1799. During the experiments, the sudden death of one of Wells' patients so upset him that he withdrew from practice, and four years later committed suicide.

William Thomas Green Morton of Massachusetts had been a partner of Wells and was naturally interested in the subject of anesthesia. On taking up the study of medicine, Morton came under the preceptorship of the chemist, Professor Charles T. Jackson of the Harvard Medical School. Jackson suggested to his pupil the possibilities of ether as an anesthetic. Morton began intensively to study the question with the result that on October 16, 1846, he administered ether successfully to a patient. Morton, maintaining secrecy as to its identity, tried to patent the new drug under the name of "letheon," had a quarrel with Jackson regarding their respective legal rights, but finally in 1847 published a paper announcing the new agent as sulphuric ether. Morton died of an apoplexy in 1868.

Wells claimed to be the sole discoverer of the principle of anesthesia; his mind unhinged by failing where Morton succeeded, he was caught throwing vitriol at the Broadway prostitutes, and committed to prison; Jackson insisted that he had told Morton everything, and he wrote to Humboldt of America's ingratitude; Morton quarreled over his patent-rights, and said he would sue every physician who used ether without his permission.

The other general volatile anesthetic, chloroform, was discovered independently in 1831 by the American Dr. Samuel Guthrie of Sacketts Harbor, New York, and the Frenchman Eugene Soubeiran. It was introduced as an anesthetic by Sir James Young Simpson of Edinburgh in 1847. His striking personality, dominating character and unquestioned fame served him in good stead in his stubborn fight to make a place for chloroform, as an aid to childbirth. Rigidly Presbyterian Scotland was inclined to construe the pains of labor as presented by the Holy Writ, and anything aimed at lessening them, as heretical, contravening the precept, "In sorrow shalt thou bring forth children."

Dr. Simpson bore the brunt of the opposition to the use of anesthesia. He weathered the storm of that opposition, and what is still more unusual, he lived to see the general acceptance of the cause he championed.

While Simpson was waging his battles in Edinburgh, a less picturesque struggle was going on in America. Dr. Channing of Boston was the champion of anesthesia in this country. The opposition he encountered was not based on a religious ground, but on one which would seem totally absurd and ridiculous if it were not for the fact that the same argument was raised again as late as 1921. The argument against ether for mothers was the sophistry that the suffering involved is one of the strongest elements in the love which the mother bears for her child. As one clergyman expressed it, "chloroform is a decoy of Satan, apparently offering itself to bless women; but in the end it will harden society and rob God of the deep, earnest cries which arise in time of trouble for help."

In the middle of April, 1853, an event occurred which exerted a greater influence on popular acceptance of anesthesia at childbirth, not only in Great Britain, but in America as well, than all the efforts of Simpson. Queen Victoria accepted chloroform for the delivery of her seventh child, Prince Leopold. Again in 1857 the Queen accepted chloroform for her confinement. Formal opposition ceased in Great Britain thereafter, and to a large extent in America also.

So surgical anesthesia became a demonstrated reality. Anesthesia? That word wasn't even known then, for the condition was new and there were no words in the language to describe it. The men concerned turned to our great physician and scholar and author, Oliver Wendell Holmes, and asked him for a name, and he gave us anesthesia, anesthetic, and anesthetist.

DR. JOHN GORRIE

Physician, scientist, inventor of the ice machine and mechanical refrigeration. His statue was the first to represent Florida, the state of his adoption, in the National Hall of Fame, Washington.

Dr. Gorrie was born on the island of St. Nevis in the West Indies, arrived at Charleston, South Carolina, where he was reared, on his first birthday. His mother was Spanish, probably of royal lineage.

There seems to be some doubt about where Dr. Gorrie received his medical education. On April 10, 1942, Vernon W. Lippard, M. D., Assistant Dean of Columbia University, College of Physicians and Surgeons, wrote as follows:

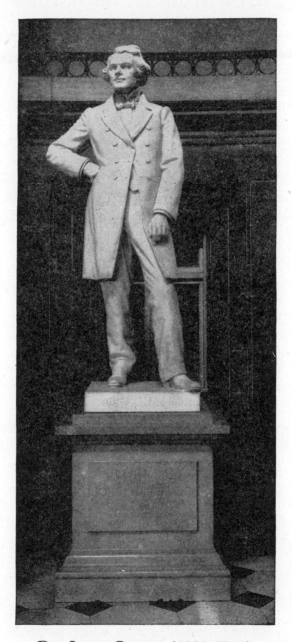

Dr. John Gorrie (1803-1855)

"During the past few years we have had a number of inquiries about Dr. Gorrie but repeated search of our records has failed to reveal any mention of his name among our graduates. I have recently received a communication from a biographer who states that Dr. Gorrie was a graduate of the Fairfield Medical College, located in Herkimer County, New York. Dr. Gorrie is said to have graduated in 1827 and the last session of the school was 1839-40."

After his medical education was completed he left Charleston and located for a time in Abbeville, South Carolina, where he was closely associated with the famous Calhoun family.

Traveling over the South, he came in 1833 to Apalachicola, Florida, and located there.

He made friends rapidly and was soon as popular socially as he was successful professionally. Between 1835 and 1839, while he was still in his middle thirties, he served first as a member and then as chairman of the city council, as treasurer of the city, postmaster and mayor. He had a part in establishing a Masonic lodge of which he was the first secretary, and he was a vestryman in the Episcopal Church which he helped to build and which still stands.

Dr. Gorrie published many articles on sanitation and related subjects and advocated sanitary measures, which mark him as a pioneer in public health work in the South.

The records of the United States Patent Office show that on May 6, 1851, he was granted letters patent No. 8080 for a period of fourteen years on a machine for the manufacture of artificial ice based on a process which was the precursor of the compressed-air ice-making machine used almost universally half a century later.

Although he apparently made ice as early as 1844, it was not until 1850 that Dr. Gorrie completed the first practical working model of his machine with which he produced blocks of ice little larger than ordinary building bricks, but in which

he saw a means of controlling fevers by conditioning the air of
sick rooms in the South during the heated term.

This achievement was merely incidental and secondary to
the primary objective which lured him more and more from
the routine of general practice to the fascinating field of research. Dr. Gorrie had concluded that in pulmonary consumption the disease might be modified and perhaps arrested
by confining the patient to a uniform temperature. This and
the humanitarian purpose of controlling temperature as a
therapeutic measure in treating fevers was what led to his discovery of the ice-making machine. Sub-tropical fevers created
a major problem for the practitioners of that day.

In 1850, Monsieur Rosan, French Consul at the Port of
Apalachicola, celebrated Bastille Day at the Mansion House.
The supply of stored ice was exhausted and the sailing vessel
from New England which now and again brought ice, a luxury
not to be spurned at from fifty cents to a dollar a pound, failed
to arrive with ice to cool the champagne.

In the company of guests were two physicians of Apalachicola, Dr. John Gorrie, the guest of honor, and his intimate
friend, Dr. A. W. Chapman, the South's distinguished botanist.
Dr. Gorrie offered the first toast.

"To our sister republic! My friends, we drink to France
in warm, red wine!" And so they drank.

Then Dr. Chapman, lifting high his glass, proposed a second toast.

"Now, our own country we toast in sparkling cold champagne, chilled by the genius of an American!"

Springing to his feet, their host exclaimed:

"We commemorate the day when France began giving her
people what they want. Gentlemen, if you, my guests, want
ice, you shall have it, even though your fellow countryman
and our honored guest worked a miracle to produce it."

247

As he spoke, from each of the four corners of the spacious dining room a waiter advanced bearing high a silver salver on which rested a cube of ice.

After dinner, Dr. Gorrie demonstrated his invention. Assisted by Monsieur Rosan, he explained the intricacies of his ice-making machine to the other guests. Dr. Chapman then told how his colleague had confided to him but a few weeks before the success of his experiment, conducted secretly for ten years.

Detecting a gleam of excitement beneath his usual reserve as Dr. Gorrie joined him behind the prescription counter in his drug store one warm June day, Dr. Chapman had inquired:

"Have you found a way to freeze all of your patients?"

With a glimmer of his infrequent smile, Dr. Gorrie had replied:

"Not exactly." Then, quietly, "I have made ice."

"The hell you have!"

"No," in quick response. "This has nothing to do with hell. But with continued success, I may even lower the temperature of that torrid clime!"

Commenting editorially on June 15, 1844, on his claim that he had manufactured artificial ice in the South in the summer time and that it could be manufactured at any time and in any place by his method, the Apalachicola ADVERTISER wisely declared: "The discovery and the invention of our correspondent, if true, are calculated to alter and extend the face of civilization." Less wisely, at a later time, a New York daily commented: "There is a crank down in Apalachicola, Florida, a Dr. John Gorrie, who claims that he can make ice as good as God Almighty!"

Dr. Gorrie became the father of modern air-conditioning when he conceived the idea of conditioning air as a therapeutic measure in the control of fevers. So intent was he upon his efforts to control temperature that he planned a room to compensate for the excessive heat of summer nights by assuring a definitely cool temperature for sleeping.

Pledging all that he possessed to secure capital for commercializing his invention, he sought additional funds, first in New Orleans and then in the East. The New York and New England newspapers so ridiculed his machine and decried its utility that he was unable to secure adequate financial backing. The Boston financier who at length agreed to furnish the necessary funds in return for a half interest in the undertaking, died before the project could be developed. Dejected, brooding over failure, stung by the ridicule of the world he sought to serve, he returned to Apalachicola. Broken in spirit, he was soon broken in body and died, some say, of a broken heart, thwarted in the development of his contribution to the science of mechanical refrigeration and unaware that he had planted the first milestone in the science of air-conditioning for a world that spurned his gifts because he lived three-quarters of a century too soon.

THE SOUTHERN MEDICAL ASSOCIATION

The forerunner of The Southern Medical Association was the Tri-State Society of Alabama, Tennessee and Georgia, consisting of two hundred members. This association was founded by Dr. J. B. Cowan, of Tullahoma, Tennessee, who was Surgeon on the Staff of General Robert E. Lee from 1861 to 1865.

Dr. Giles C. Savage, President of the Tennessee State Medical Association, was named chairman of a committee to communicate with the presidents of the state associations of Louisiana, Mississippi, Alabama, Georgia and Florida, and to ask them to send delegates to meet with the Tri-State Society of Alabama, Tennessee and Georgia at its October meeting in Chattanooga in 1906.

In compliance with the above invitation, delegates from the six Southern states mentioned met in Chattanooga on October

2, 1906, one day prior to the date of the annual meeting of the Tri-State Society.

Dr. H. H. Martin, Savannah, President of the Georgia State Society; Dr. Walter W. Crawford, Hattiesburg, President of the Mississippi State Society, and Dr. Jere L. Crook, of Jackson, Tennessee, acting for Dr. Savage, were named as a committee to form a tentative constitution and by-laws for a new organization, and it was finally decided that the new organization should eventually embrace all the sixteen Southern states and the District of Columbia.

As Chairman of the Committee it became Dr. Crook's duty to present the tentative constitution to the meeting and attempt to induce that small but loyal group composing the Tri-State Medical Association to dissolve, "thaw and resolve themselves into a dew," to die in order that the baby Southern Medical Association could be born. The chief obstacle to the plan was the well-known opposition of the founder of the Tri-State, Dr. J. B. Cowan, of Tullahoma, who very naturally was loath to destroy his own brain child.

"His plea was ably and enthusiastically buttressed by Dr. Crawford and Dr. Martin, and when the presentation was completed Dr. Cowan arose and under the stress of visible emotion stated his determination, when he first learned of the plan, to fight any move to kill his own brain child. He spoke of the fine record of the Tri-State Association and of the love and loyalty of its membership for their Society. 'But,' said he, 'Mr. President, after listening to the plea of these ambitious young doctors, who have come here today asking for a chance to try their wings over all of Dixie Land, I move that we adopt this tentative constitution as a whole, without changing one jot or one tittle.' The motion was carried unanimously, and thus was born the Southern Medical Association."

CHAPTER THIRTEEN

Medicine in the Bible

"Lo, and it was given unto men to know—
And to heal the sick—
But vouchsafed only unto the chosen."

—BIBLICAL

TO SOME extent the habits and practices of the Israelites were based on those of the Egyptians. The Mishnah, the book of Jewish legends, which forms part of the Talmud, mentions a treatise on medicines believed to have been compiled by Solomon. The Talmud also cites a treatise on pharmacology called Megillat-Sammanin, but neither of these works has been preserved. In the Talmud an infusion of onions in wine is mentioned as a means of healing an issue of blood. It was necessary at the same time for someone to say to the patient, "Be healed of thine issue of blood."

To them, health and success depended on the favor and protection of their Lord God Jehovah; and defeat in war, famine and pestilence come because Jehovah was angry with them. Disease was not to them the badgering of mankind by a host of malign demons, but the just expression of Jehovah's wrath. To avert this wrath, the people may pray and make sacrifice, but they were forbidden to resort to the magic and charms which their ancestors saw used in Egypt. The whole conception of disease, under the early Christian religion, can be summed up in the words of St. Augustine in the fifth century: "All diseases of Christians are to be ascribed to demons, chiefly do they torment the fresh baptized, yea, even the guiltless new-born infant."

There were, to be sure, physicians and pharmacists in Jerusalem. Simple surgery was practised and wounds were dressed with oils, wines, and balsams, but curing a sick person was largely a matter of appealing to Jehovah, who could both inflict sickness and bestow health.

In the prevention of disease, however, the ancient Hebrews made real progress. The teachings of Moses, as embodied in the Priestly Code of the Old Testament, contain two clear conceptions of modern sanitation—the importance of cleanliness and the possibility of controlling epidemic disease by isolation and quarantine.

The Papyrus Ebers was supposed by its discoverer to have been compiled about the time when Moses was living in Egypt, a century before the Exodus. It is not certain that in the whole of the Bible there is any distinct reference to a medicine for internal administration. Poisons are mentioned several times but in all cases in an allegorical sense. It is assumed that Rachel wanted the mandrakes which Reuben found to make a remedy for sterility, but that is not definitely stated. Nor is it certain that the Hebrew word Dudaim, translated mandrakes, meant the shrub we know by that name. The European plant is not the May apple, or mandrake, of America. Besides having narcotic properties, mandrake was said to have the power of arousing the sexual passions; Rachel sought mandrakes of Leah (Gen. XXX:14-16), but it is uncertain for which purpose she used them.

Violets, lilies, jasmin, truffles, mushrooms, citrons, melons, and other fruits have been proposed by various critics. There are three passages in Jeremiah where Balm of Gilead is mentioned in a way which may have meant that it was to be used as an internal remedy.

Among all the ancient Eastern nations olive oil was one of the most precious of products. It was used lavishly by the Egyptians for their hair and the skin, as well as in all sorts of ceremonies.

To the Israelites in the Desert the anticipation of the "corn and wine and oil" of Canaan was always present, and throughout their history there are abundant evidences of how they prized it.

The prescription for the "holy anointing oil" given in Exodus, xxx, 23, is very remarkable. It was to be compounded of the following ingredients:

Flowing myrrh	500 shekels.
Sweet cinnamon	250 "
Sweet calamus	250 "
Cassia (or costus)	500 "
Olive oil	One hin.

A hin was a measure equivalent to about 5½ of our quarts. The shekel was nearly 15 lbs., and some of the Rabbis insist that the "shekel of the sanctuary" was twice the weight of the ordinary shekel.

The manna of the wilderness provided for the children of Israel on their journey towards Canaan has no claim to be regarded as a drug, except that a drug has in modern times usurped its name.

Among the drugs named in the Bible are: Bdellium, aloe wood, myrrh, wormwood, hyssop, juniper, jonah's gourd, the wild gourds, the horse leech, nitre, mustard seeds, vinegar, anethon, saffron, pomegranates, the poultice of figs, spikenard and eastern imagery.

No case of poisoning either suicidal, murderous, or accidental, is alluded to in the Bible, unless we regard the story of the wild gourds (2 Kings, ch. iv, v. 39), as coming within the last description.

Between the time of the opening of the Christian Era and the period of Galen's activity, medicine and pharmacy had deteriorated very much. Great numbers of specialists had arisen, most of whom were charlatans claiming super-natural powers (a distinct retrogression). Many of these specialists (the CIRCUMFORANEI), traveled from place to place like the itinerant Indian herb doctors and their like of today.

Among the Great Physicians in early Christian times are Aetius, Alexander of Thralles, Paul of Aegina, Theophilus, George (Dschordschis) and Alkindus.

CHAPTER FOURTEEN

Surgeons and Surgery

IT APPEARS that surgery was born of demonology. By far the most important phase of prehistoric surgery was the operation known as trepanation—the removal of part of the skull vault. The chief indications for trepanation were infantile convulsions, relief of cerebral tension, cranial injuries, headaches, epilepsy and blindness. The object of the perforation was to give the confined demon an opportunity to escape.

Some Stone Age skulls show that this painful operation had been performed five or six times on the same patient. The prevalence of that operation is shown by the fact that the bones of one hundred and twenty persons found in a mound in France yielded forty trephined skulls. This would seem to indicate that thirty-three per cent of the people in that locality had undergone the operation.

The following gives an account of a substitute for trephining that occurred in the thirteenth century:

"Albert of Hapsburg was a hard, cold man, with all of his father's will and energy, yet without his moderation and shrewdness. He was haughty and repellent in his manner, and from first to last made no friends. He was one-eyed, on account of a singular cure which had been practiced upon him. Having become very ill, his physicians suspected that he was poisoned; they therefore hung him up by the heels and took one eye out of its socket, so that the poison might escape from his head."

It was Elliot Smith who showed that the operation of circumcision was practiced about 4000 B. C. He actually found a number of pictures of the operation which were carved at least 2,000 years before the time of Rameses II, and other evidence proving that it had been employed over a thousand years earlier. The first written record of the operation was made about 800 B. C. and is in the seventeenth chapter of Genesis.

Circumcision is the only operation the Bible mentions apart from Adam's rib excision.

The earliest known pictures of surgical operations are engraved on the stones over a tomb near Memphis, Egypt. These engravings were made 2,500 years before Christ; their age is more than twice that of the Christian era. The pictures show the operation of circumcision and operations on the legs and arms, and these operations, with the addition of castration, included all the surgical procedures performed by the Egyptians.

Ophthalmology is one of the oldest specialties. Hammurabi, laying down his code in 2250 B. C., legislated specifically for operations on the eye—ten shekels for a successful operation, amputation of both the surgeon's hands in the event of failure.

Accidents during sport must have been common, and that is why the surgery of fractures and dislocations was well developed in Hippocratic times, with the result that many a page of these early surgical treatises has a modern ring. Even major operations were performed, although with considerable hesitation. Scrupulous cleanliness was impressed upon the surgeon, and this provided, in some measure, for asepsis.

Surgery was by no means overlooked by our savage brothers. They performed the operations of circumcision, infibulation, tatooing, and tooth extraction; they had instruments for opening abscesses. Hot and cool applications were used. Arrow wounds were thoroughly sucked out. Fractured bones were splinted with stiffened mud bandages, or with wooden splints made of tree branches; dislocations were reduced, and amputations were done, mostly, it is true, as punishment for crime. Litters and hanging mats were used for transportation and trusses were devised for hernia. Urethrotomy and cystotomy were performed for stone. In certain primitive races, the so-called "Mica" operation was done; this consisted in making a permanent urethral fistula in male subjects. Trepanation was common and cataractous lenses were removed.

Old China never had any real system of surgery, nor had Japan. Of the Babylonians we know little except that they practised surgery in a fairly advanced form and that to them must be given credit for freeing surgery from the trammels of religion, at least for a time. Surgery in Egypt, and to an even greater extent in India, reached heights which only the Greeks equalled, and only our own civilization has bettered.

In the Middle Ages, under the influence of the church, the practice of surgery in Europe was relegated to barbers, bath-house keepers, sow-gelders, executioners, and any strolling vagabond who cared to try his hand at the art. Surgeons were looked upon as menials. Surgery was considered beneath the dignity of the physician, ecclesiastical opposition, strictly prohibited dissection and popular prejudices were antagonistic to all things medical. Surgery fell into the hands of the so-called "barber-surgeons" who matched their technic with the tempo of their time.

In England there were hospitals, there were physicians, and there were apothecaries. Surgeons had yet to appear, but the barbers, who understood what surgery there was, were quietly creating a guild to protect their own interests, a guild which was to have a considerable influence upon the rise of surgery in England.

The following shows the attitude toward surgeons during the Middle Ages:

Surgery was regarded an unfit occupation for a gentleman and scholar, and was largely relegated to barbers. There was once a time, about four hundred years ago, when, if you needed your hair cut and your face shaved, you inquired the way to the nearest surgeon. In those days the town barber and the leading surgeon of the community were one and the same person. "If possible, the surgeon should avoid a bad reputation, because the people, since ancient times, consider all surgeons to be thieves, man-killers, and the worst kind of frauds."

During the early part of the Middle Ages there were no trained surgeons in Europe. The only men with any medical education were the Jews; they studied in Arabia. Even as late as the eleventh century the armies had no surgeons. The pay of the English army surgeons was good; a first-class surgeon in the fifteenth century received two hundred dollars a year and twelve cents a day for expenses. The wage for a laboring-man at that time was about five dollars a year. The attitude toward men practicing surgery in the Middle Ages and Renaissance was such that the surgeons were continually in jeopardy of life.

Surgeons, as distinct from both barbers and "barbers exercising the faculty of surgery," belonged originally to a small Guild of Surgeons within the City of London, which was officially recognized in A. D. 1368 by the appointment of Master Surgeons, who were given authority over their brethren of the craft.

Surgery was becoming more and more widely separated from medicine, and the belief that it was an inferior art was held almost everywhere. Debarred from university education and with their art regarded generally as more of a trade than a profession, surgeons in London, in Paris, and a few other great centers banded together to protect themselves and their profession, and evolved an educational system of their own.

The first Act regulating the practice of surgery in England was passed in A. D. 1421. No woman was to practice.

In 1210 a guild of surgeons was instituted at Paris in which the members were divided into two classes. The "surgeons of the long robe" were the clerical barber-surgeons, who possessed some educational attainments. The "barbers of the short robe" were the lay barbers or surgeons. The word barber comes from *barbatonsorium*, or beard cutter. The lay barbers were later restricted to blood-letting and the treatment of ordinary wounds.

Formerly in England the patient, while undergoing vene-section, was wont to grasp a pole in order to make the blood flow more freely, and as the pole was likely to be stained, it was painted red. When it was not in use, the barber would hang it up on the outside of the door, with white linen swathing-bands twisted round it. The red and white pole of the present day, so conspicuous in front of barber shops, has resulted by evolution from this custom. It is worthy of note that, since the Revolution, a blue stripe is frequently added, making the patriotic combination of the "red, white, and blue."

Hippocrates had taught that in inflammatory disease, the patient should be bled freely from a vein near the site of the lesion and on the same side of the body—so-called revulsive bleeding. The later Greeks, and their followers the Arabians, taught that at the outset of inflammatory disease, the blood should be taken slowly, drop by drop, at a site far removed from the lesion, and on the opposite side of the body—so-called derivative bleeding. The Hippocratic method of revulsive bleeding had for centuries, been in disrepute as a most dangerous procedure, until Pierre Brissot (1478-1522) in the early sixteenth century, reintroduced it.

The supposed value of phlebotomy in the Middle Ages is stated as follows:

"Phlebotomy is the beginning of health. It strengthens the mind and memory, purges the bladder, dries out the brain, warms the spinal cord, clears the hearing, restrains tears, relieves anorexia, purifies the stomach, invites digestion, induces sleep, is believed to favor longer life, and drives away disease. Phlebotomy should be done with caution, and the amount of blood withdrawn is large or small according to the strength and age of the patient, the time of year, and the state of his bodily heat. If the blood runs black at first, bleed until it becomes red; if thick or greasy, bleed until it has the consistency of water; but the bleeding should not be allowed to run until the patient is overtaken by lassitude or weakness of the stomach."

The barbers had been growing into an increasingly important civic body. A grant of arms in A. D. 1452 merely crowned their achievement of A. D. 1450, when the Mayor and Aldermen of London sanctioned a code of laws they had drawn up for the protection and government of their craft. In it they again insisted on their right to practice surgery.

From the point of view of numbers and in the superiority of their position and power, thanks to Edward IV's charter, the barbers had the advantage of the surgeons. But on the other hand the surgeons had a better social standing and much higher professional attainments. As a result each body was able complacently to point to certain advantages it had over the other, and they lived in comparative amity from that point onwards. So much improved were the relations of the two bodies that in A. D. 1493 they entered into an agreement whereby all the chartered privileges of the barbers were conceded also to the surgeons, with the sole exception of admission to the freedom of the Barbers' Company.

In 1515, the surgeons were finally admitted as a department of the university, and the barber-surgeons were also admitted to the lectures on anatomy and surgery. From now on, surgery began to look up. In 1686 the royal surgeon Félix cured Louis XIV of fistula-in-ano, and was knighted as a reward. This incident marks the final step in the complete elevation of surgery. However, the barber-surgeon crudely plied his trade in England until 1745, when an act declared, "That the business of trade of a barber is foreign to and independent of the practice of surgery."

GUY DE CHAULIAC, who lived in the fourteenth century, was the greatest authority on surgery in Europe at that time, and is called the Father of Modern Surgery. He accomplished the best of his work some five centuries before surgery in our modern sense of the term is supposed to have developed.

It is usually considered that he was born some time during the last decade of the thirteenth century, probably toward the end of it, and that he died about 1370. He was born Guido de Chauliac, the son of an Auvergne peasant. His early education must have been reasonably efficient, since it gave him a good working knowledge of Latin. He was educated in a little town of the south of France, made his medical studies at Montpellier, and then went to Italy, in order to make his post-graduate studies. Italy occupied the place in science at that time that Germany has taken during the nineteenth century.

Even his post-graduate experience in Italy did not satisfy Chauliac, however, for, after having studied several years with the most distinguished Italian teachers of anatomy and surgery, he spent some time in Paris.

One of Chauliac's most important contributions to major surgery was in rescuing the treatment of rupture from the hands of quacks. Just as there were many quack cutters for stone, so there were quacks who specialized in the treatment of ruptures. They would apply a cautery, which did little harm but less good, or, worse still, make some flourishing incision, which was more likely to cut across the intestine than to cure the rupture. He described an operation for the radical cure of hernia, or rupture, and made it clear that the treatment of this condition should not be left to itinerant quacks and peddlers. His comprehensive text-book of surgery appeared about A. D. 1363.

A few of his criticisms evidence that his pen was as sharp as his scalpel: "There is a sect composed of military men,

German chevaliers and others following the army, who with conjurations and potions, oil, wool, and cabbage leaves, dress all wounds, basing their practice on the maxim that God has given his virtue to herbs and to stones." "Another sect consists of women and of many fools who treat all diseases by referring them to the saints." After receiving John of Gaddesden's Angelic Rose of Medicine, Chauliac thus reviewed it: "They have sent me this insipid rose; I thought I might find some fragrance in it, but discovered only vapidness."

The black death ravaged Avignon in 1348. In many of the European cities the physicians joined the fugitives, and the ailing were left to care for themselves. With a few notable exceptions, this was the case at Avignon, but Chauliac was among those who remained faithful to his duty and took on himself the self-sacrificing labor of caring for the sick, doubly harassing because so many of his brother physicians were absent. He denounces their conduct as shameful, yet does not boast of his own courage, but on the contrary says that he was in constant fear of the disease. Toward the end of the epidemic he was attacked by the plague and for a time his life was despaired of. Fortunately he recovered and, later, wrote a very clear account of the epidemic, which leaves no doubt that it was true bubonic plague.

In the Introduction chapter of his CHIRURGIA MAGNA he said:

"The surgeon should be learned, skilled, ingenious, and of good morals. Be bold in things that are sure, cautious in dangers; avoid evil cures and practices; be gracious to the sick, obliging to his colleagues, wise in his predictions. Be chaste, sober, pitiful, and merciful; not covetous nor extortionate of money; but let the recompense be moderate, according to the work, the means of the sick, the character of the issue or event, and its dignity."

ROGER FRUGARDI, a surgeon of school of Salerno, was one of the founders of modern surgery. He introduced the use of the seton, a method of stitching a bundle of linen threads through a fold of skin and leaving them to act as a counter-irritant. He was also the first to suggest that torn intestines, which had always presented difficulties to contemporary surgeons, might be sutured more easily over a hollow tube of elderwood. Roger ligatured blood-vessels which had been ruptured, if cauterization and styptics failed to check the bleeding; and, like Albucasis, he refractured and set again bones which had been broken and had united in bad position.

However, Roger erred greatly in one particular. He did not believe that clean healing, by first intention, was possible. This theory was opposed by Hugo of Lucca and his son Theodoric of Cervia: "For it is not necessary, as Roger and Roland have written, as many of their disciples teach, and as all modern surgeons profess, that pus should be generated in wounds. No error can be greater than this. Such a practice is indeed to hinder nature, to prolong the disease, and to prevent the conglutination and consolidation of the wound."

In the Middle Ages Roger and Roland and Jehan Yperman used ligatures, and so did many lesser surgeons. But despite the fact that ligatures were known, surgeons were never enthusiastic about undertaking the larger amputations. They had good reason for avoiding these operations. Whether ligatures were used or forgotten, the results of amputation was uniformly disastrous. This was simply because the battered stump of the limb was always smothered in scalding oil or roasted with a red-hot iron, or else favorite styptics of rabbit's fur and aloe and the like were applied.

It might have been thought at Paré's death in 1590 that his carefully recorded experiences and his undoubted authority would have ended forever the controversy as to whether gunshot wounds were or were not poisoned. Actually, the debate continued.

BRANCA OF SICILY, regarded as the first surgeon of the world, 1442, established a reputation of building up noses from the skin of the face.

Some other great surgeons of the Middle Ages were: Roland, a pupil of Roger; Bruno; Theodoric and his father, Hugo of Lucca; William of Salicet; Lanfranco; Henri de Mondeville; Yperman and John Ardern.

In 1308 a human body was publicly dissected for the first time in many hundreds of years in Venice. At first there was an outcry against the sacriligious immorality of such a proceeding. In the course of years, however, the practice became accepted and remarkably elaborated.

Had it not been for the lawyers of Bologna demanding an autopsy in cases of suspicious deaths, pigs might have continued to be used for anatomical studies. Thus, dissection was brought to the cadaver! In 1315, Mundinus, University of Bologna, obtained two female cadavers which he dissected for his students.

Frankish surgery during the Middle Ages and later was an accepted barbarity. A Saracen surgeon relates the following experiences:

He had been shown first a man with an abscess of the leg. To this he applied poultices, and the patient seemed to be making satisfactory progress until a Frankish surgeon intervened. He denounced the poultices as useless and asked the man whether he would prefer to die with two legs or live with one. The patient said he would rather live. The Frankish surgeon assured him of the wisdom of his choice, and summoned a man-at-arms who bore a huge battle-axe. Calmly, the surgeon instructed the soldier to chop off the offending leg at one blow. The axe fell, but the leg was not completely severed. The surgeon directed his stalwart assistant to try again, higher up. At the second blow the patient died.

Another patient was a consumptive woman, whom the physician was treating with the appropriate drugs and diet. In a second uncalled-for consultation the Frankish surgeon diagnosed positively the presence of a devil within the woman's head. The physician's diagnosis of consumption was laughed at, and the surgeon ordered all the woman's hair to be shaved off and restored her to a dietary of garlic and oil. When she rapidly grew worse he embarked on more active treatment. He made a deep cross-incision through her scalp right down to the bone, and rubbed salt violently into the cruciform wound.

Up to 1616 the physicians and the Barber-Surgeons had been at peace, if not in amity. In that year, since the apothecaries had been created in a separate company, the College of Physicians approached James I and received from him a new charter. This conferred several new privileges, notably that of being able to take proceedings against anyone who administered "inward medicines" and was not a member of the College.

Surgery was advancing in every country in Europe. Almost to the end of the sixteenth century Ambroise Paré was the doyen of French surgeons. Germany had two surgeons at this time who rose far above the barbers who let blood, set broken bones, and treated almost everything.

ABMROISE PARÉ (1510-1590), a French military surgeon, was born in Brittany. He was not born a gentleman. He studied under a Paris barber and was such an apt student that he was taken in by the barber-surgeons of the Hotel Dieu. He made the discovery that gunshot wounds are not poisonous. During his first campaign he followed the usual method of treatment—he poured scalding oil into the wounds. When the boiling oil gave out, the inexperienced surgeon could do nothing better than apply a simple dressing. He passed a most uneasy night, fully expecting that when he looked at his non-cauterized patients the next morning, they would be dead. He arose earlier than usual, and was astonished to find that those whom he had treated according to authority with the scorching oil were in great agony, suffering with severe inflammation at the edges of the wounds, while the others were quite comfortable, and had neither pain nor swelling. "See," says he, "how I learned to treat gunshot wounds; not by books."

This experience taught him to no longer place faith in the Hippocratic aphorism, "Diseases which are not cured by medicines are cured by iron; those which are not cured by iron are cured by fire; those not cured by fire are incurable."

There is practically no chapter in surgery that Paré did not embellish. He simplified wound dressings, invented an ingenious armamentarium of useful surgical instruments, discarded the common practice of castration in the operation for hernia, popularized the use of the hernia truss, described fracture of the femoral neck, introduced the operation for cleft palate, and a simplified operation of trephining, and was the first to perform direct excision of loose cartilage of the knee joint. Yet, he opposed Caesarean section, and his opinion checked its further advance for more than a century; in its stead he suggested podalic version.

The fact that he was allowed to preside at the deaths of three kings in succession, and still live, attests to Paré's sterling character and to his worth. It is even said that he was a Huguenot, and the only one spared by royal edict on the night of the great massacre.

At one time Paré was obliged to defend himself against the whole faculty of the University of Paris because he taught that neither ground up mummies nor unicorn horns possessed therapeutic value. His modesty regarding his accomplishments in wound healing is refreshing. "I dressed him and God cured him," he said in explaining the cure of an important officer.

Paré, reviewing his life-work, wrote: "God is my witness, and men are not ignorant of it, that I have labored more than forty years to throw light on the art of surgery and to bring it to perfection. And in this labor I have striven so hard to obtain my end, that the ancients have naught wherein to excel us, save the discovery of first principles: and posterity will not be able to surpass us (be it said without malice or offense) save by some additions, such as are easily made to things already discovered."

266

One rather striking feature of the seventeenth century is the failure of practical medicine to react to the stimulating ferment of this period; and likewise the failure of surgery to progress despite the fact that the work of Paré seemed to promise an enthusiastic development of this specialty. As a matter of fact surgery had to wage a stubborn battle for recognition, and the fruit of battle was not won to a satisfying degree until much more than a century after Paré.

During this transition period, Medicine and Surgery became separate and distinct; for the clergy, forbidden by the church to shed blood, abandoned the practice of surgery to barbers who were employed to shave and leech the priests. These barbers, for many years the only surgeons, were for the most part ignorant artificers or adventurers, and they degraded surgery into a vulgar trade of butchery and charlatanry. They travelled about, remaining at a center as long as patients and public confidence warranted. Some barbers confined themselves to a limited repertoire of operations, the formulae of which were handed down from barber-father to barber-son as a family heritage; others were more versatile and obliging. The story is told of one of these itinerant surgeons, who in order to relieve a corpulent nobleman of his paunch, "ripped up his belly" so that he died on the spot. These were the men who in later days were known as the barber-surgeons of the short robe in contradistinction to the surgeons of the long robe who practiced general surgery after training in schools. In hands so unskilful, surgery became an alternative more dreaded than the disease itself.

In Virginia in the seventeenth century the early records in regard to surgery are concerned chiefly with the treatment of wounds, burns, frostbite, fractures, dislocations and ulcers. The York County records show several surgeons at work. Dr. Haddon's treatment of an amputation was to give two cordials on the day of the operation and a purge four days later, with frequent ointments and external applications. After two months it became necessary to bleed the patient. Sores of the

267

feet and legs are frequently mentioned and were probably due to the custom of going barefooted.

The seventeenth century was notable for improved instruments, yet the surgical achievements are indeed disappointing. The gulf between physician and surgeon was not yet bridged: the physician scorned to think surgically, and the surgeon feared to trespass on medicine.

During the seventeenth century, surgery was excluded from the curriculum at the University of Paris and witchcraft wrote a bloody chapter for the history of the world. Surgery was still not only questionable but exceedingly dangerous and advanced no further than Paré.

RICHARD WISEMAN was the leading English surgeon of the period.

WILLIAM CHESELDEN was the most outstanding figure in English surgery during the first half of the eighteenth century.

JOHN HUNTER (1728-1793) was the outstanding English surgeon of the eighteenth century. Modern surgery was founded by him.

Throughout the eighteenth century German surgery was a crime. A barber's apprentice, who sought to evade the humiliations inflicted upon him, was hunted like an escaped animal; the regimental surgeon was compelled to shave the army officers; the oculist, the bone-setter, the stone-cutter, the rupture-specialist, preyed upon the credulity of the people; the Prussian executioner, experienced in the disarticulation of joints and the breaking of bones, was granted permission to treat wounds and ulcers and to set fractures. Frederick the Great replied to the complaints of the Berlin surgeons: "If you are as skillful as you pretend to be, every one will trust themselves to you rather than go to an executioner; but if you are ignoramuses, the public must not suffer, and rather than remain lame and crippled, let them go to the executioner."

The nineteenth century opened with surgery nearly as crude and barbarous and as limited in its scope as it had been in the earliest civilizations, and is now among the most primitive peoples. Guillaume Dupuytren was a brilliant but eccentric surgeon (1777-1835) who died refusing surgical aid, preferring, as he said, "to die at the hands of God rather than those of man." The nineteenth century closed with modern surgery well developed. In the early part of the nineteenth century, the distinction between surgeons and physicians was broken down and both were required to obtain the degree of doctor of medicine.

Medicine developed much more slowly than surgery, or, rather, lagged behind it, as it seems nearly always prone to do. Surgical problems are simple, and their solution belongs to a great extent to a handicraft. That is, after all, what chirurgy, the old form of our word surgery, means.

It has been said that there are only two periods in the history of surgery—before Lister and after Lister. Joseph Lister, later Lord Lister (1827-1912), made surgery safe for patients. A recital of the accomplishments of surgery, after the general acceptance of antisepsis, would appear to be out of place in a sketch of this scope.

CHAPTER FIFTEEN

Women and Medicine
WOMEN DOCTORS

WOMEN have been prominent as physicians since the remotest times. In many of the early social settlements, women physicians greatly outnumbered the men. Throughout the ages there have been medicine women of exceptional ability who have been as shrewd, rational, and as capable as any of the medicine men. At all times the midwife and nurse rendered first aid to the sick, and tended cases, until the greater skill of a medicine man became necessary.

The first woman doctor to receive historical notice is mentioned in the Ebers papyrus. She was the goddess Tefnut, and she compounded a medicine for the Great God Ra. It gave him a headache, but the goddess Isis cured this by another medicine which contained Berry-of-the-Poppy-Plant. This is one of the very early records of the use of opium to relieve pain.

The practice of obstetrics in the early dawn days of the race was almost exclusively left to women. But when men became more advanced in medicine, they began to resent the competition of women and that resentment has continued. The history of the struggles of women doctors has therefore been a long recital of oppression. Yet in all ages there have been strong-minded women who have braved exclusion from the medical societies and schools and have ignored the adverse legislative enactments regarding their practice. There are numerous examples of Egyptian, Greek, and Roman women physicians who have won renown.

Among the women doctors of the Empiric School, the name of Cleopatra, Queen of Egypt, is widest known. Her early books dealt with cosmetics and perfumes, later books dealt with the diseases of women. These appear to have been such excellent books that some critics have doubted whether Cleopatra was the actual author, although during her lifetime that question was not raised.

Trotula, a woman, was a teacher at Salerno in the middle of the eleventh century. An interesting chapter in the history of the medical school at Salerno is to be found in the opportunities provided for the medical education of women and the surrender to them of a whole department in the medical school, that of Women's Diseases. After Trotula we have a number of women physicians of Salerno whose names have come down to us.

The organization of the department of women's diseases at Salerno, under the care of women professors, and the granting of licenses to women to practice medicine, is not so surprising in the light of this tradition among Greeks and Romans, taken up with some enthusiasm by the Christians.

Laura Bassi was professor of experimental physics at the University of Bologna which was founded in the twelfth century.

When it was announced that Miss Blackwell, the first American woman physician, had received the degree of M. D. at Geneva Medical College, a correspondent of the Boston Medical and Surgical Journal wrote as follows:

"It is to be regretted that she has been induced to depart from the appropriate sphere of her own sex, and led to aspire honors and duties, which, by the order of nature, and the common consent of the world, devolve alone upon men; and I am

272

sorry that Geneva Medical College should be the first to commence the nefarious process of amalgamation."

Among the American Indians there were instances of unusual medical knowledge being attributed to old women. Under the primitive conditions existing in the early years in Virginia, doctors' widows occasionally dispensed medical advice. As late as 1700 we find Mrs. Mary Seal, former wife of Dr. Power, winning a suit for four pounds seven shillings "for phisicall means, etc., by her administered in the time of Richard Dunbar's sickness."

Reverend John Clayton, writing to the Royal Society in 1688 of his observations in Virginia, reports that "A Gentlewoman, that was a notable female Doctress, told me, that a Neighbour being bit by a Rattlesnake swelled excessively; some Days afterwards she was sent for, who found him swelled beyond what she thought it had been possible for a skin to contain, and very thirsty. She gave him oriental Bezoar shaved, with a strong Decoction of the aforesaid Dittany, whereby she recovered the Person."

In Virginia the modern Trotula had to wait a long time for recognition. It was 1910 before women physicians were admitted to membership in the Richmond Academy of Medicine.

There were few medical schools in 1847 when Elizabeth Blackwell applied at a dozen of them in different university centers for admission to the lectures. Those were days when, as Oliver Wendell Holmes said, a professor filled a whole settee in a medical college.

Elizabeth's brother described the ceremony of her graduation as follows: "She wore a black brocaded silk gown, invisible green gloves, and black silk stockings. The dress must have been long and voluminous, well-fitted over the spreading hoop skirt and the inevitable bustle, but he does not mention that. He adds that all the ladies of Geneva turned out *en masse* to see a lady receive a medical diploma. The ceremony took place at 10 A.M., and the procession of graduates was headed by a band, the Bishop of New York, the Dean, Dr. Hale, the curators, faculty, etc. Elizabeth refused to march with them lest it should not seem lady-like. The church galleries were crowded with ladies but gentlemen sat in the aisles. Elizabeth was called up to receive her diploma after all the rest, and in a flattering speech she was addressed as DOMINA. She bowed her thanks properly and on the impulse of the moment she turned again to the speaker saying, 'Sir, I thank you; by the help of the Most High it shall be the effort of my life to shed honor upon your diploma.' There was great applause and all the faculty smiled approvingly to one another, and the function was ended."

After her graduation she soon sailed for Europe, where she studied for two years in England and France. She had a very distinguished career in medical pioneering both in America and in England—founding dispensaries, hospitals, medical schools, and lecturing and writing.

Women were not generally accepted in medicine at that period and in Paris in 1859 a French author expressed his opinion in this amusing manner: "A doctress imported from America, Miss Elizabeth Blackwell, has come to shine among us. She is the personification, not of American bloomerism but of therapeutics in crinoline. She has already founded a college for women in the United States. Today more than two hundred beautiful Yankees are making medical efforts like the men for whom hitherto the practice of medicine has been reserved."

Five years after Elizabeth Blackwell graduated, her sister Emily Blackwell (1826-1910) graduated in 1854 at the medical school of Western Reserve University. Then, like her sister, she went to Europe for a two years' course of study. Her career was not as spectacular as that of her sister Elizabeth's, but she had quite a distinguished career in medicine.

There were many noted midwives in New England in early times. The third wife and widow of Samuel Fuller (1580-

1633) of Providence, came to Boston in 1623 and was urged by the citizens of Rehoboth, Mass., in 1663, to accept a regular salary and move to their town where the services of a midwife were urgently needed. She refused because of her age and died in 1664. There was also Mrs. Ann Eliot, wife of the Apostle to the Indians, whose tomb, erected by the town of Roxbury in 1687, bears the legend, "She was thus honored for the great service she hath done this town." Old Mrs. Wiat, who died in Dorchester in 1705 at the age of 94, was given a laudatory epitaph, an excerpt from which tells us, "She assisted at ye births of one thousand and one hundred and odd children." Of Mrs. Thomas Whitmore, of Marlboro, Vt., the historian said, "She officiated at more than two thousand births and never lost a patient." Mrs. Elizabeth Phillips, a well-trained English midwife living in Charlestown, near Boston, "had by the blessing of God brought into the world upward of 3,000 children." She died in 1761. Mrs. Janet Alexander, of Edinburgh, settled in Boston in 1818 to practice midwifery. At one time she was offered a good salary if she would move to New York, but the women of Boston quickly raised the sum of $1,200 to induce her to stay with them. When she died, in 1845, it was said, "She was universally mourned for her great worth and eminent usefulness."

There had been at least four men who taught obstetrics in the Colonies, James Lloyd, in Boston (1728-1810), Dr. William Hunter of Providence, R. I. (1729-1777), a cousin of the famous Hunters of London, William Shippen (1736-1808), and Charles D. Meigs (1792-1869), both of Philadelphia, and teachers in its medical schools.

There was a school for women midwives in Boston as early as 1846.

The Female Medical College of Philadelphia, the first medical college in the world for women, began its work in 1850. The moving spirit was Ann Preston, who had been refused admittance by the four regular Philadelphia medical schools. She was graduated in 1852 and in 1856 became professor of physiology.

A few years later a somewhat eclectic school called Penn College admitted several women who got their start within its walls.

Harriot Hunt (1805-1875) applied twice, in 1847 and 1849, for admission to the medical school of Harvard College, and finally she was almost admitted because of the promise of a gift of ten thousand dollars to the College by Miss Hovey of Boston, on condition of the admission of women students, but as a negro man applied at the same time both applications were refused.

To the world of men in general movements for the education of women were preposterous for, as Sarah Grimké said, to them "woman was merely a lapse of nature" and not an independent entity.

Between 1849, when Elizabeth Blackwell was graduated from a man's medical school, and 1877, five medical colleges for women were opened in the United States and one in England. The Women's Medical College of Pennsylvania is the only one solely for women still in existence in America.

The medical colleges about the middle of the nineteenth century were commonly spoken of as "regular" and "irregular," the latter being the Central Medical College of Syracuse, eclectic, the Cleveland Medical College, also eclectic, the Western College of Homeopathic Medicine, and the Female Medical College of Philadelphia. Between January 23, 1849, when Elizabeth Blackwell received her diploma at Geneva, N. Y., and March 3, 1852, when Nancy Clark received hers at Cleveland, there were twenty women graduates from four "irregular" schools.

At this period the reaction from the mineral drugs like calomel and arsenic was so strong that when herbs came into fashion the propaganda for their use was loudly advertised and widely accepted. Probably homeopathy was gained in popularity for the same reasons, and each system in its way led to more rational prescribing than heretofore among the adherents of the "old school," who needed more than one lesson as to the cause and effect and scientific use of drugs and the quantities to be administered.

Those were the days of heroic medication. We read that Dr. Frederick Dorsey of Hagerstown, Md., treated himself for cholera. He took 200 grains of calomel in 24 hours and survived.

In 1869 the University of Michigan Medical School opened its doors to women medical students. Dr. Ruth Gerry was active in accomplishing this.

The second woman, in point of time, to be graduated from an American medical college, or from any medical college in the nineteenth century, was Lydia Folger-Fowler (1822-1879).

The third woman in the United States to receive a diploma from a medical school was Sarah Adamson-Dolley (1829-1909).

The fourth medical pioneer appears to have been Rachel Brooks-Gleason (1820-1905), who was also graduated at Rochester in 1851, a few months after Dr. Dolley.

The story of the Homeopathic schools begins with the graduation of Dr. Helen Cook, whose diploma was dated 1852 from the new sectarian school in Cleveland. Her graduation scarcely antedated that of the first medical class of 1852 at the new school for women in Philadelphia where Ann Preston and Hannah Longshore of Philadelphia, and Martha A. Sawin of Boston, were among the graduates in January of that year. It is, therefore, impossible to say which was the fifth woman to graduate in medicine in the United States, but Helen Cook must have been the first in homeopathy, and among her immediate successors were Myra K. Merrick, 1852, and Clemence Sophia Lozier, '53.

A great pioneer surgeon in America was Emmeline Horton Cleveland (1829-1878), of the Philadelphia Woman's Medical

College (M. D. 1855), who was the first woman ovariotomist in America, trained in Philadelphia and in Europe.

Among the pioneer medical women in America was Marie Zakrzewska (1829-1902), a Polish woman of noble birth who received her medical diploma from the Western Reserve University in 1856. Connected with Dr. Zakrzewska was Sophia Jex Blake (1840-1912), the second English woman to study medicine. Also, Mary Putnam-Jacobi who belonged to a well-known New York family of publishers. Though born in England, in 1842, she was brought up in America and studied pharmacy in New York, and medicine at the Philadelphia school, where she was graduated in 1864.

Dr. Emma L. Call, one of Dr. Zakrzewska's students, was graduated from the University of Michigan in 1873 with the highest honors. She was at the head of the class of the ninety-six members among whom were twelve women. Dr. Call was the first woman to be admitted to the Massachusetts Medical Society, in 1884.

Mary Harris Thompson (1829-1895) founded the Women's Medical School of Chicago. Dr. Zakrzewska said: "Dr. Thompson was the first woman surgeon who performed capital operations entirely on her own responsibility."

Elizabeth M. Cushier (1837-1932), was a graduate of the College of the New York Infirmary, in the year 1872. She spent much time studying in Europe and was closely associated in her travels and study with Dr. Elizabeth Blackwell. Dr. Cushier is said to have been the leading woman surgeon of her time and also an eminently successful practitioner.

The women surgeons, Dr. Croasdale and Dr. Bromall of Philadelphia, and Dr. Cushier of New York, were praised by such noted men surgeons as Marion Sims, Horatio Storer and Thomas Addis Emmet, as equal in operative results and technique to any surgeons in the world.

Clara Barton (1821-1912), who undertook hospital service during the Civil War and later established hospitals in the

Franco-German War, and formed the Red Cross Society in 1881 of which she was president until 1904.

The Medical Women's National Association was founded in 1915 by Dr. Bertha Van Hoosen, who became its president. Dr. Van Hoosen is a distinguished teacher and writer, a professor of obstetrics, and has entered foreign field to help medical missionaries with their work.

Women doctors have been of outstanding value in the foreign missionary field. Dr. Rosetta Sherwood-Hall, a graduate of the Women's Medical College of Pennsylvania, is an example of the women doctors who, as missionaries, have shown their ability as well as character in medical emergencies.

Dr. Hall began her foreign work in Korea and continued for 45 years. She established four women's hospitals and educational work for the blind and deaf.

One of the institutions that she founded was the Women's Medical College of Korea. This work started out with five girls. Today it is as large as many schools in this country and as modern as any American foundation.

Dr. Hall is still living and is a distinguished resident of Liberty, New York.

The story of the discovery of radium has taken its place as one of the episodes of man's age-long struggle to gain supremacy over nature. Marie Sklodowska, the daughter of a Polish college professor, went from her native Warsaw to study at the Sorbonne and to become one of the world's greatest scientists. She met and married Pierre Curie. Radium is the Curies' gift to humanity.

DOCTORS' WIVES

The doctor's wife is really an important personage and a great auxiliary in the practice of medicine. The life of a prominent physician in active practice is unlike that of an ordinary business man. He is called upon at all times of the night and day to meet all manner of emergencies. Unless he is aided in his home, half of the effectiveness of his work will be lost.

How many people ever stop to consider the influence the doctor's wife must bear upon the doctor's character for good or evil—and how that influence must react upon the community which trusts its life into the doctor's keeping?

Every man is master of his home except the doctor. Day or night, at any hour, any one is free to ring his bell and ask for help. When the doctor is away, the rearranging of visits to patients, business schedules, consulting work, and innumerable other disordered events, all these duties often fall upon the doctor's wife. Upon her administrative and diplomatic abilities in these times her husband's success largely turns. She can make a practice successful or otherwise.

One author has written of the requirements of a successful physician's wife:

"Tact, discretion and a particularly large bump of curiosity are essential in a successful physician's wife. Her husband is sure to be deficient in powers of observation. He will often appear to be absent-minded. Her abnormally developed curiosity must be used to balance that defect. She must observe closely so as to be always well-informed, and her discretion must be used even in that. She must not know about the doctor's cases; but she must know much about his other experiences, if she is to be able to guide him wisely. Yet she must not ask him for information; but cause him voluntarily to impart it to her. She must gain his complete confidence without ever indicating that she wants it."

NURSES

The training of women in the art of "helping the patient to live," which is the office of the nurse, began in the nineteenth century. Prior to that time there were nurses in hospitals, but they were untrained. In Roman Catholic institutions the nursing was done by nuns, but in all other hospitals

280

the sick were cared for by the worst type of women conceivable for the service.

A note in the London Times for April 15, 1857, described the servant nurses of the large hospitals in these words: "They were sworn at by surgeons, bullied by dressers, grumbled at and abused by patients, insulted if old and ill-favored, talked flippantly to if middle-aged and good-humored, and tempted and seduced if young and well-looking." In short they were the worst type of women conceivable for the work of nursing. The hospitals under their care were filthy and vermin-ridden, and the wards were scenes of repulsive squalor. Nor did the physicians in charge pay much attention to any need for cleanliness. Here is an extract from the regulations of one of these hospitals; it is in reference to the linen of the patients. It says: "Their sheets shall be shifted once a fortnight; their shirts once in four days; their nightcaps, drawers, and stockings once a week." The windows of the hospital were kept tightly closed against fresh air. The wards were inconceivably horrible.

In Europe the seventeenth century was the dark age of nursing, and the care of the sick sank as low as the hospitals in which it was practiced. Conditions were little changed two hundred years later, when Dickens immortalized Sairey Gamp. She, with her pawky umbrella and talk of the hypothetical Mrs. Harris, was a type of the "pudgy, slatternly, dowdy looking female, of drunken and dubious habits" who was the nurse of that day.

FLORENCE NIGHTINGALE

Florence Nightingale did not found nursing, for nursing is one of the oldest occupations of women. What Florence Nightingale did was to make nursing a dignified profession and a branch of medicine. She instituted also the modern methods of training nurses.

Florence Nightingale was born in 1820, the daughter of a well-to-do country gentleman. She grew up to be an intelligent and popular young woman. Yet she was wholly un-satisfied with what her apparently fortunate life seemed to offer. She longed to do something useful and was deeply moved by sympathy for the sick and suffering. At the age of 24, her longings began to crystalize about the thought of be-coming a nurse. This idea was bitterly opposed by her family. Eighty years ago nursing (except that done by the religious orders) was looked upon as an occupation for the lowest type of woman.

At last, however, her growing conviction of her mission in life proved strong enough to overcome the power of conven-tion. She studied nursing in Germany and France, and at the age of 34, she was ready for the call of her country in its time of need.

Two seemingly fortuitous events seemed to favor her—the Crimean war and the condition of nursing in hospitals, par-ticularly in those of England, in the first half of the nineteenth century. This period was one in which all social relations were marked by extreme prudery—so much so, in fact, that this at-titude had affected even the Sisters of Charity. A series of ab-surd restrictions were imposed upon them by their religious or-ders. They were forbidden to perform all sorts of necessary practical bits of nursing on the grounds of impropriety. Con-sequently, while they retained their serenity and gentleness, they had lost their practical usefulness. The Sisters watched the sick, maintained discipline and system in the hospital, and shed an atmosphere of refinement over the wards. All the actual care of the sick was performed by lay attendants.

Theodor Fliedner (1800-1864), a Lutheran clergyman, settled in Kaiserswerth, Germany; was urged by his wife Friederike to establish a home for deaconesses to visit the sick and poor of the church parishes. These good people already supported a home of reclamation for discharged women crim-inals and in 1836 they opened the deaconesses' home. Eliza-beth Fry, the British prison reformer, visited the Fliedners in

1840 and adopted their system in England. Other countries gradually followed.

Florence Nightingale applied the idea to the British Army medical department when the Crimean war started in 1854, and in the following year, Pirogoff introduced nurses into the Russian Army.

The picture of Florence Nightingale going through the dim wards at night with a lantern led Longfellow to write one of his best-known poems called "The Lady with the Lamp."

In 1856 the Crimean war came to an end and Miss Nightingale returned to England. She decided to select the best of her nurses and secure positions for them in hospitals. But, like all pioneers, she met with opposition from the medical profession. She succeeded in having a fund subscribed to establish the Nightingale School for Nurses at St. Thomas' Hospital in London. The school was opened on June 15, 1860, with fifteen students. This was the first institution of its kind and it has continued to lead the world in nursing progress.

The Nightingale Hospital nursing movement astonished the world. It was so different from anything before experienced, and it proved so successful that other countries rapidly followed in establishing nursing schools.

The leadership of Miss Nightingale—her social rank, her position as a national heroine, her vision and her dauntless courage—changed the whole conception of nursing, first in England, then throughout the world. Today, we see at some of our leading universities, schools of nursing standing on an independent basis alongside of the schools of medicine and law.

Miss Nightingale has been pictured as a saintly, self-sacrificing, delicate woman who threw aside a life of pleasure to help the afflicted. But this picture is not a true one. She was a strong-minded, determined woman with a gift of caustic sarcasm. Her one great interest in life was to establish the independence of women and to elevate nursing to a dignified profession.

VIRGINIA NURSES

We encounter nurses early in Virginia history. In 1612 the hospital at Henricopolis was supplied with "keepers" to attend the sick and wounded. These were probably male nurses. During the rest of the century we find references to both male and female nurses, although male ones were apparently more common. Nursing was at that time indeed a task for men, entailing physical labor that would horrify the modern nurse.

The records of Surry County in 1663 show that Ralph Creed presented a bill for his wife's attendance on a patient "with the comfortablest things a Man in his Condition could expect" and for the "entertainment of those that came to bury him with 3 vollys of shott & diging his grave wth the trouble of his funeral included."

The duties of the seventeenth century nurse in Virginia were not to take the temperature, record the pulse, give daily baths, or follow elaborate orders from physicians; but to prepare food, give the "draughts regularly," wash the linen, watch by the bedside, and when death came (as it usually appeared to do when the patient was ill enough to warrant a nurse) to shroud the body and to furnish the entertainment of those who came to the funeral.

There is nothing to show that nursing in Virginia during the eighteenth century surpassed it in the preceding century. It was not a profession at all and did not achieve that distinction for more than a hundred years. It was still the business of slovenly old women. Florence Nightingale once observed that "at one time or another every woman is a nurse." We can be sure that on the women of Virginia homes rested the chief responsibility for the care of the sick—a duty that even the advent of specialized nursing has not entirely lifted.

A new figure did appear during this period—the negro nurse. She was the natural outgrowth of slavery and of the economic and social life of the South. As mammy, midwife, wet nurse or nurse-maid she became a figure of increasing importance. Mammies had large responsibilities in the nursery and often took entire charge of the dosing of the children. Out on the plantation negro nurses had even more responsibility, especially in the larger establishments where they presided over the infirmary and where the care of the small slave children was almost completely committed to them.

CHAPTER SIXTEEN

Midwifery

WOMEN and priests were the first obstetricians. The Greeks called the men who assisted women in labor Maeutai or "men-grandmothers." Hippocrates speaks of their customs. Peter Chamberlen, the inventor of the modern forceps about 1632 A. D., was called a man-midwife, and his descendant, Hugh Chamberlen, bore a similar title. Obstetrics, or the art of aiding human birth, is consequently one of the oldest and most important of the medical specialties.

The position of woman in any civilization is an index of the advancement of that civilization; the position of woman is gauged best by the care given her at the birth of her child.

Among most primitive peoples the mother bathed in cold water when the child was born, and either returned immediately to take her tasks or waited for some time until she had undergone a period of isolation and sacramental purification.

Most primitive peoples have held the belief, which has persisted even among some civilized peoples almost to the present time, that labor was a voluntary act upon the part of the child, due to its desire to escape from its confined quarters. The woman who assisted at the birth did all she was able to coax out the child by promises of food, and resorted to threats if the child was obdurate. The expectant mother was even starved during the last week of her pregnancy in order that the child might be more willing to emerge and obtain the milk that awaited it.

If the labor of the primitive mother was difficult, assistance of the straightforward type might be called into play. She was picked up by the feet and shaken, head down, or rolled and bounced on a blanket, or possibly laid on the open plain in order that a horseman might ride at her with the apparent intention of treading on her, only to veer aside at the last moment, and by the fear thus inspired aid in the expulsion of the child. Again, she might be laid on her back to have her abdomen trod upon, or else be hung to a tree by a strap passed under her arms, while those assisting her bore down on a strap over her abdomen. Such practices as these last were known in Europe four hundred years ago.

In the most primitive stages of man's development, as in the animal world, the mother aided her own parturition. But as soon as attention was given to medicine, friends and specialists helped in the simplest manipulations. Thus arose the midwife, at first a blessing and a comfort, but later the greatest impediment to the advance of the obstetrical art.

Child-bearing among primitive peoples is today what child-bearing was to our ancestors twenty-five centuries ago, and little different from what it was three centuries ago, except that some of the hazards were greater at the later period than at the earlier. The woman of native or primitive peoples was not in horror of the devastation of childbed fever. Nor did she take her place in the filthy bed of a hospital of the seventeenth, eighteenth and even early nineteenth centuries.

Susruta, the Hindu Hippocrates, wrote a book containing the ancient system of midwifery formerly handed down by word of mouth. It states: "That a woman should be delivered by four aged and knowing women whose *nails were well trimmed*. The law regarding midwives, as it appeared in Athens, states that the midwives must be women themselves past the age of child-bearing, but who have had a child."

The Alexandrian doctors appear to have attained the greatest skill in obstetrical practice. Demetrius and Herophilus lectured on the dangers of foot presentments. Celsus tells us about the means for foot-version.

Soranus wrote a special textbook for midwives in which he collected all the knowledge of the medical schools. Like Celsus, he devoted many of his monographs to foot-presentments, and if version failed, he suggested resorting to embryotomy.

There was little about the female genitalia that Soranus did not know, and after his description of the anatomy of the womb, there was no longer any excuse for confusing the vagina and the uterus. He popularized the vaginal speculum, and his obstetric chair or labor-stool was the parent of numerous offspring. Instead of hastening the expulsion of the fetus by manhandling the mother in the traditional manner—shaking her, rolling her, making her run up and down stairs, or jolting her on a ladder—he instituted gentleness in the lying-in chamber. He knew that conception can be prevented by closing the mouth of the womb with cotton or ointments, that the os uteri opens during coitus and menstruation, that the woman conceives most readily following the menstrual period, and that sterility occurs in men as well as women.

Soranus' fame rests upon his textbook of midwifery and gynecology. He is usually esteemed the ablest gynecologist of classical times. As to gynecology, there must have been noted gynecologists in ancient days, both before and after Soranus, but unhappily, their writings have vanished.

In ancient Athens, we are told, there were as yet no midwives, since women were forbidden by law to practice any sort of healing activity. However, a noble-hearted woman, Agnodice by name, eager to help her sisters in the pangs of childbirth, dressed herself up as a man and, in this disguise, studied under Herophilus. It need hardly be said that, as a matter of fact, midwives had practiced in Athens long before the days of Herophilus.

The divinities of child-bearing gave a Roman bride little privacy and little credit for her share in bringing a child into the world. Altogether there were nineteen deities who attended her from the time of her courtship, through all the intimate acts pertaining to procreation, and till the child was taught to cry and suckle. The Fates hovered about, and if anything went wrong, they still had additional recourse for, Opigena, the divine midwife, was invoked.

The cynical Juvenal spoke as follows about pregnant women:

"These poor women, however, endure the perils of childbirth, and all the troubles of nursing to which their lot condemns them; but how often does a gilded bed contain a woman that is lying in? So great is the skill, so powerful the drugs, of the abortionist, paid to murder mankind within the womb. Rejoice, poor wretch; give her the stuff to drink whatever it be, with your own hand: for were she willing to get big and trouble her womb with bouncing babies, you might perhaps find yourself the father of an Ethiopian; and some day a colored heir, whom you would rather not meet by daylight, would fill all the places in your will."

Trotula, a woman of noble family who was a teacher at Salerno in the middle of the eleventh century wrote a series of works known as the Trotula. The procedure recommended for the treatment of difficult labour:

"When there is difficult labour with a dead child, place the patient in a sheet held at the corners by four strong men, with her head somewhat elevated. Have them shake the sheet vigorously by pulling on the opposite corners, and with God's aid she will give birth."

The Middle Ages were the most unfortunate period in the history of womankind. Complete ignorance prevailed, without the intuitive skill of the primitive period and without the knowledge of previous civilizations. Women were deprived of the aid, however poor, of the male physician, and at the same time the penalties of urban civilization were making childbirth more and more hazardous.

In the fifteenth century cradles were merely boxes with detachable rockers; sometimes they were hooded. The baby at birth was bathed; then it was salted all over and its head bandaged to shape it. Next it was bound tightly in swaddling bandages until it was unable to move. This swaddling was continued for several months, the bandages being taken off for a few minutes each day. About half the children so treated died during the first year of life.

About the year 1500, the wife of a sow-gelder, Jacob Nufer of Sigershaufen, went into labour. For some reason or other she could not deliver herself of her child. Jacob himself knew nothing about midwifery, but had been engaged in sow-gelding for some years. Feeling that he could be no more unsuccessful than the midwives and the lithotomists, Jacob took up a razor and did the obvious things with it. The end results of his impromptu performance have never been bettered. His wife recovered completely. It was over a hundred years later, in 1637, that the first book on Caesarean section appeared, and from that time onward the operation was attempted more often.

The surgical branch of pure midwifery had no real existence, however, till antisepsis changed Caesarean section from a last-minute attempt to extract a live child from a dying mother to an operation which would almost always save the lives of both mother and child.

In 1580 a law was passed in Germany to prevent shepherds and herdsmen from attending obstetrical cases—an indication both of the advance of civilization and what it had advanced from.

Dr. Wertt of Hamburg, in the sixteenth century, realized that he could only study the process of birth at an actual labour, and knew well that as a man he would never under any circumstances be admitted to a lying-in room. He did the only thing possible—dressed himself as a woman and went boldly in to the next confinement in the district. For a brief while all went well, then somehow or other one of the mid-wives realized that he was a man, masquerading in a woman's garments. The mere idea of a male being present at a con-finement raised a storm of protest. Punishment was swift and salutary. Wertt was burned to death in 1522. Other physicians watched him die and realized then, if they had not done so before, that midwifery was a woman's art protected by every possible taboo. The only men who dared even dis-cuss the subject were cloistered and celibate clerics, for their motives only could be deemed pure.

Of all the branches of practical medicine, obstetrics was at the lowest ebb during the sixteenth century. The result was that the mortality rate in normal labor was 50 per cent and in complicated labor was appalling. Two great advances were made during this century, however. Eucharius Roeslin made a special study of obstetrics, as taught from the time of Hippocrates down, and as early as 1513 he described the ad-vantages of podalic version, a procedure that was popularized and firmly established, some forty years later by Paré. The other great step forward was the development of the operation of Caesarean section.

Greek medicine as developed at Rome culminated in the ancient practice of midwifery as told in the writings of Soranus of Ephesus, second century after Christ. His teachings brought the child-bearing woman a kindness of treatment she had never before received. He disapproved of the reckless employment of medicines for hastening labor or applying force to the woman for this purpose. He reintroduced podalic version. This procedure of turning and extracting the child, instead of employing instruments to destroy it, marks the peaks of an-cient midwifery. Its revival in the sixteenth century after Christ marks the point where medieval midwifery was finally raised to a par with that of the ancients.

William Chamberlen, a Huguenot refugee, came to South-ampton from France in 1569. He had two sons, Peter the

Elder, and Peter the Younger, both members of the Barber-Surgeons' Company. It was probably the elder brother who invented midwifery forceps for the extraction of a live child in the course of a difficult confinement. Unfortunately, the Chamberlens kept their invention as a family secret.

For thirteen centuries the physicians of Europe were not allowed to attend normal cases of delivery, but in the seventeenth century they began to participate to some extent. Except among royalty they met with amazing prudery and were often forced to carry out their manipulations under a sheet in order to spare the blushes of their modest patients.

In Colonial days in America obstetrics did not receive the attention in this country that it did abroad. Child birth in those early days of American civilization was considered a simple physiological function, to be carried out in secrecy with a friend or a midwife. The wife of Dr. Samuel Fuller, who landed from the Mayflower, was the first midwife of the Colony. The next was Mrs. Hutchinson of Boston, who was banished for her political heresy. She was succeeded by Ruth Barnaby, who lived to be one hundred and one. The first person to be executed in the Colony of Massachusetts Bay was Margaret Jones, female physician; she was accused of witchcraft. In 1716 the professional ability of anyone and everyone in this country to officiate at childbirth was still, nearly a hundred years after the landing of the Mayflower, taken for granted.

Dr. John Moultrie of Charleston, South Carolina, began practice in 1733 and was the first regular obstetrician in the state or in the South. He died in 1775, after having gained great popularity, both as an obstetrician and as a physician.

The prejudice in favor of women midwives was still very strong, and newspaper advertising was expected to influence public sentiment in favor of the physicians. Evidence of the changing attitude toward the medical care of pregnancy may be found all through contemporary Virginia records. In 1766 one William Coakley appeared from the West Indies, settled in Norfolk and announced that his practice would include "every branch of surgery, midwifery, and physic." In 1769 Andrew Anderson advertised himself as "surgeon and man midwife" in Williamsburg.

Midwives did not give up their place in the community without a fight. There appeared on the first page of the Virginia Gazette in 1772 an article denouncing the fashion of having man-midwives, attributing the large number of adulteries to the practice and declaring that women midwives were safer because they trusted to nature rather than to forceps.

The eighteenth century was notable in obstetrics for the popularization of the forceps and the return of the man-midwife. In fact, one of the most remarkable changes witnessed during the century was the altered attitude of the profession and the laity toward the medical care of pregnancy. A certain obstetrician told Joseph II that "the Viennese women were too modest to have men as midwives." The technique of the lying-in room was an example of the ridiculous and obstructive prudery of the times—the physician working under cover of a large sheet with one end tied around his neck and the other similarly attached to the patient.

Obstetrics was not a man's profession in America until the middle of the nineteenth century. The first lectures on midwifery were given by Shippen in 1765. Before this midwives were women, whose training was acquired in a crude apprenticeship or through unaided personal experience.

In the eighteenth century in Virginia an ordinance was passed providing against fraud in obstetrics, making it unlawful to misrepresent a child's father, to be party to a false delivery or to conceal births, especially the births of bastards. Midwives were pledged to expose infanticide, to summon other midwives in suspicious cases, and not to induce abortion or charge exorbitantly.

The records show not a few bastard births. Moral obliquity of this nature was not readily hidden in the small communities of colonial Virginia. The unfortunate woman, usually of the servant class, if not forced to wear the scarlet letter was commonly punished publicly with stripes or prolonged servitude. Dr. Daniel Parke's servant, Elizabeth Holloway, in 1662 was ordered to receive ten stripes on her bare back for her misconduct, and a servant of William Townsend in 1672 had to serve him two years longer, besides receiving twenty-nine lashes, for a similar offense.

Chloroform was not used to relieve the pains of childbirth until 1847, and the Biblical injunction "in sorrow thou shalt bring forth children" was not lightened until that time.

One of the greatest boons conferred by gynecologists upon women in labor was the introduction of anesthesia into obstetrical practice. The glory of bestowing this is enjoyed by Sir James Young Simpson (1811-1870), the professor of obstetrics in Edinburgh University. This great authority made this great innovation in a Scotch hospital early in 1847 when, in a difficult case, he employed chloroform successfully.

There was violent opposition to the use of chloroform in labor. Dr. Simpson waged his battle in Edinburgh and concluded a paper on anesthesia with a bit of irrefutable logic. He takes the weapons of his opponents from their own hands. He shows that the first surgical operation ever recorded was carried out under anesthesia. The deep sleep of Adam was anesthesia! The controversy was at an end so far as the Scotch clergy were concerned.

Dr. Channing, of Boston, was the champion of anesthesia in this country. In April of 1853, there occurred an event that had a more profound influence on the general acceptance of anesthesia than the work of both Simpson and Channing. Queen Victoria accepted chloroform at the birth of her seventh son, Leopold. And such was the influence of the example of royalty that formal opposition to anesthesia ceased altogether in Great Britain thereafter, and to a large extent in America also.

Modern science has intervened in obstetrics and is able to compensate, and more than compensate, for the handicap of civilization. It can now save lives that would have been lost even under the most natural conditions. It can do more, for it can minimize for women the effects that child-bearing might have upon length of life, a consideration that did not affect the short-lived primitive peoples.

The interesting history of the evolution of obstetrical practices has been briefly outlined. Today the practitioner is furnished with the instruments, drugs and skill to meet any conditions which might arise with assurance.

CHAPTER SEVENTEEN

Dentistry

DENTISTRY was well known to the ancients. Considerable progress had been made in it 4,000 years ago. The mouths of Egyptian mummies with their filled, pivoted and artificial teeth bear silent witness to the proficiency of the dentists of the Pharoahs. It was a long time before Europe made similar progress.

In the post-Roman era, to the great calamity of the human race, dental knowledge decayed. If Albucasis is not the restorer, at least he is the conservator of dentistry in the Arabian period. Histories of dentistry are always embellished with illustrations of his instruments for shaking, loosening and removing teeth, the earliest type of turn key for extraction, dental saw and file, set of fifteen dental scrapers, small axe for resection of irregular teeth, elevators and forceps for extraction of roots, vulsella for removal of portions of the jaw, and the gold and silver wire with which he bound a loose tooth to a sound one. He realized that irregular or projecting teeth are particularly displeasing in women, and described the operation for their correction.

In the absence of a dental chair, his method of holding a patient during extraction, was sensible: "The head of the patient should be taken between the knees of the operator, in order to keep it steady." He was a pioneer in discussing oral deformities, dental arches, formation of tartar, replanting teeth, and artificial teeth: "The space left by missing teeth can be filled up with artificial ones made of ox-bone; such teeth can be anchored with a suitable gold wire to the firm teeth; they will be found of esthetic and functional value."

The "Royal Book of Medicine" of early Arabia, directed that in pulling a back tooth the gums be incised so as to loosen them around the roots, and then the tooth itself may be drawn with a special forceps which is called a molar forceps.

Ernest Renan, during an exploring expedition in Phenicia, found in the old necropolis at Sidon a set of teeth wired together, two of which were artificial. It was a striking example of bridgework, very well done, and may now be seen in the Louvre.

The old Etruscans, who inhabited the Italian hill country, have left in their tombs some fine examples of bridgework. In one specimen, which is especially notable, two incisor teeth are replaced by a single tooth from a calf. This was grooved in such a way as to make it seem like two separate teeth. Guerini suggests a very interesting and quite unexpected source for this. While examining the specimen he wondered where the old Etruscan dentist had obtained a calf's tooth without a trace of wear on it. He came to the conclusion that he must have cut into the gums of a young calf before the permanent tooth was erupted in order to get this structure absolutely unworn for his purpose.

At the end of the Republican times at Rome and the beginning of the Empire there appear to have been many forms of dental appliances. Martial says that the reason why one lady's teeth—whose name he does not conceal—are white and another's—name also given—were dark, was that the first one bought hers and the second still had her own. In another satiric poem he describes an elderly woman as so much frightened that when she ran away her teeth fell out, while her friends lost their false hair. Fillings of many kinds were used, dentrifices of nearly every kind were invented, and dentistry evidently reached a high stage of development, though we have nowhere a special name for dentist, and the work seems to have been done by physicians, who took this as a specialty.

In the Middle Ages there was, owing to conditions, a loss of much of this knowledge of antiquity with regard to dentistry, or an obscuration of it, it never disappeared completely, and whenever men have written seriously about medicine, above all about surgery in relation to the face and the mouth, the teeth have come in for their share of scientific and practical consideration.

When the great revival in surgery came in the twelfth and thirteenth centuries it is not surprising that there should also have been an important renewal of interest in dentistry. The great surgeon, Guy de Chauliac, in the middle of the fourteenth century, wrote about dentistry in connection with surgery, and exposed many dental fallacies.

Four hundred years ago you would not have consulted a dentist for any reason except the toothache. You had a wide choice to select from. You could apply to the state executioner, who conducted dentistry as a sideline. If not engaged in his major occupation he would gladly lay aside his rope and axe and gouge out the aching molar for you, with only a small fee in recompense for his services. The keeper of the public bathhouse was also an amateur in extraction. But for really expert treatment you would have applied to the mountebank who had his booth on a raised platform at the street corner. These vagabonds practiced dentistry as a sideline to roguery.

The barber-surgeon of four hundred years ago would, if you request it, do more than merely relieve the pain of toothache by extraction; he would repair the blemish to your appearance by filling in the gap in your teeth. He could whittle out an ivory peg and tie it in place with gold wire. If you ask him what causes decay he will probably tell you that it results from worms that eat away the substance of the tooth just as they eat away the flesh of an apple. If you ask him how to prevent toothache he may hand on to you the ancient treatment recorded by Pliny, which was to eat a whole mouse twice a month.

An advertisement appearing in the British Journal for 1724 suggesting the idea that toothache is due to worms in the roots of the teeth is very ancient. An old method designed to remove them consisted of heating onion seeds in a small funnel, the stem of which was held against the aching tooth. Tiny worms, presumably from the tooth, but in reality driven out of the onion seeds, were found in the funnel after it had cooled.

Pierre Fauchard's method has been cited as an example of the dentistry of two hundred years ago. Carefully and skillfully he extracts the tooth. Then he puts it back, driving its roots into their former socket. He ties the tooth in place with thread, and fills its cavity with lead. The lady will soon have an abscess in her jaw-bone; perhaps rheumatism will follow, and her stiffened fingers will lose their skill. But in the meantime she will retain her beauty—at least until she has married.

When Fauchard filled the cavity in the tooth he had no dental engine with which to drill; he used a file instead. John Greenwood, dentist to George Washington, is said to have devised one in connection with a spinning-wheel, but it was not until 1870 that a practical form of the dental engine came into use.

Fauchard's next patient is an aged courtier whose only remaining teeth are those in the front of his jaws; even these teeth Fauchard finds have become so loose that they must be pulled. Fauchard makes false teeth, which he carves from ivory and fastens the pair together with springs. They resemble the famous set that George Washington used and which were repaired for him by Paul Revere, for Paul Revere was not only a silversmith and patriot, but also a dentist. Fauchard will, if you wish, insert a pivot tooth; to do so he suspends the carved ivory crown on a wooden peg driven into the old fang. These ivory teeth were horribly insanitary, for they absorbed fluids from the mouth and could not be kept clean; they also decayed. It was not until the nineteenth century that really satisfactory porcelain teeth were successfully manufactured.

Dentistry has always been afflicted with quacks, just as other branches of medicine. The methods of one of the best known ones in London in the eighteenth century was a little man with a long grey beard, who every morning rode solemnly up and down Rotten Row on a white pony painted with purple spots. This was Mr. Martin Van Butchell, who made "Real or Artificial Teeth from one to an Entire Set, with Superlative Gold Pivots or Springs, also Gums, Sockets, and Palate fitted, finished and fixed without drawing stumps or causing pain."

Butchell had a magnificent house in Mayfair, which attracted even more attention than the Gold Pivots or the purple-spotted pony. Butchell's wife died, in January, 1775, and he had her body embalmed. The embalming was done by packing the abdominal cavity with camphor, and injecting into the blood-vessels a preservative made of oil of turpentine and camphorated spirit of wine. A more than lifelike reality was finally achieved by two glass eyes and the injection of a carmine solution into the vessels of the head and neck, so that the lips were bright red and the cheeks rosily flushed. This greatly improved edition of Mrs. Van Butchell was arrayed in fine linen and lace, placed in a glass-lidded case, and kept in the sitting-room. The lady was formally introduced to each and every visitor as the "dear departed", and not unnaturally the visitors were many. Mrs. Van Butchell the first remained in the sitting-room and proved a good advertisement till she was displaced permanently by Mrs. Van Butchell the second.

Up to the sixteenth century dentistry was a part of medicine, but during that and the succeeding centuries dental practice was almost exclusively in the hands of the barber-surgeons. Real progress was not made before the eighteenth century, when dentistry first became a separate art. The dental operations practiced by Fauchard in his forty years' experience and enumerated by him in 1728 included cleaning, straightening, shortening, scraping, cauterizing, filling with lead, fastening, removing, replacing, transplanting and artificially constructing teeth. This is an excellent summary of the state of dental knowledge at that time. Fauchard had exposed the common belief that toothache was caused by worms and that cupping was a remedy.

In America dentistry languished until 1776, and the few dentists known to have practiced were confined to the northern states. James Mills, 1785, and Robert Woofendale, 1766, in New York, and John Baker, 1767, and Paul Revere, 1768, in Boston, enjoyed local reputations. Better known was John Greenwood, who served in the Revolutionary army and was highly regarded by Washington, for whom he made at least two sets of false teeth. One set was buried in Washington's mouth and the other is now in the Museum of the Baltimore College of Dental Surgery.

EARLY DENTISTRY IN VIRGINIA

In colonial Virginia of the seventeenth century the doctors and chirurgeons practiced what dentistry there was. Their work was limited to extraction and the treatment of toothache.

Dental troubles are added to the chronicle of ailments given by Francis Taylor in his long and illuminating diary. For treatment he relied upon home remedies, or in extreme cases upon his brother Charles, who was a physician:

Jan. 23, 1787: "Had the toothache violently."

Feb. 3, "My face swelled with sore tooth and Gum boil."

Mar. 9, 1791: "Heard that Chas. Porter died yesterday —his death was caused by drawing a tooth which turned to a mortification."

Jan. 1, 1794: "I had the toothache last night violently in one of my fore teeth."

302

Aug. 27, 1797: "Walked to C. Taylor's—he drew a tooth for me it was the farthest in my jaw and some bone came with the tooth."

Aug. 1, 1798: "I went to C. Taylor's, got him to draw the roots of two of my jaw teeth, one of them hard to extract."

May 10, 1799: "I went to C. Taylor's—he drew the only remains of four of my upper fore teeth, which makes my mouth very sore."

William Byrd's account of pulling his own tooth shows the ingenuity of one Virginia gentleman:

"I had an impertinent Tooth in my upper Jaw, that had been loose for some time, and made me chew with great Caution. Particularly I cou'd not grind a Biscuit but with much deliberation and presence of mind. Tooth-Drawers we had none amongst us, nor any of the Instruments they make use of. However, Invention supply'd this want very happily, and I contriv'd to get rid of this troublesome Companion by cutting a Caper. I caused a Twine to be fasten'd round the Root of my tooth, about a Fathom in Length, and then ty'd the other End to the Snag of a Log that lay upon the Ground, in such a Manner that I cou'd just stand upright. Having adjusted my String in this Manner, I bent my Knees enough to enable me to spring vigorously off the Ground, as perpendicularly as I cou'd. The force of the Leap drew out the Tooth with so much ease that I felt nothing of it, nor should have believ'd it was come away, unless I had seen it dangling at the End of the String. This new way of Tooth-drawing, being so silently and deliberately perform'd, both surprized and delighted all that were present."

According to Samuel Mordecai, in Richmond in the late eighteenth century "one Tooth-drawer, who probably never heard the word dentist, did all the work and all the mischief in the dental line." He goes on to describe this unique person:

"Peter Hawkins was a tall, raw-boned, very black negro, who rode a raw-boned, black horse, for his practice was too extensive to be managed on foot, and he carried all his instruments, consisting of two or three pullikins, in his pocket. His dexterity was such, that he has been known to be stopped in the street by one of his distressed brethren, (for he was of the church,) and to relieve him of the offending tooth, gratuitously without dismounting from his horse. His strength of wrist was such, that he would almost infallibly extract, or break a tooth, whether the right or the wrong one. I speak from sad experience, for he extracted two for me, a sound and an aching one, with one wrench of his instrument.

"On Sundays he mounted the pulpit instead of black barebones, and as a preacher he drew the fangs of Satan with his spiritual pullikins. Peter's surgical, but not his clerical mantle, fell on his son, who depletes the veins and pockets of his patients, and when he has exhausted the latter, the former are respited."

The dentists of the eighteenth century in Virginia were for the most part itinerant practitioners who heralded their arrival in a community with a conspicuous newspaper advertisement notifying the public of their ability to extract and fill, supply false or natural teeth, treat pyorrhoea, furnish dentrifices to preserve the teeth and sweeten the breath, in fact to perform any dental operation "hitherto performed in Europe." They often took pains to explain that their former patients had been among the nobility, and that they hailed from no less a city than London. They warned the public that, due to the press of business, their stay in the community would be short.

Previous to 1839 there were still no schools of dentistry; the students learned their trade by apprenticeship to older dentists. Soon after 1839, schools of dentistry were opened and the technical aspects of the profession progressed amazingly. In the decade following 1880, mechanical dentistry reached its culmination in the vogue for ingenious and expensive crown and bridgework.

The American Journal of Dental Science, the first journal pertaining to dentistry, was founded in 1839, in New York City.

CHAPTER EIGHTEEN

Advice to Physicians

THE PHYSICIANS of the Middle Ages seem to have had a deep understanding of human nature.

Henri de Mondeville made the following suggestions:

"Keep up your patient's spirits by music of viols and ten-stringed psaltery, or by forged letters describing the death of his enemies; if he is a canon, inform him that his bishop has just died and he has been elected in his place."

Also: "Never dine with a patient who is in your debt, but get your dinner at an inn, otherwise he will deduct his hospitality from your fee." "If you have operated conscientiously on the rich for a proper fee, and on the poor for charity, you need not play the monk, nor make pilgrimages for your soul."

One very interesting contribution to medical literature that comes to us from Salerno bears the title, "The Coming of a Physician to His Patient, or An Instruction for the Physician Himself."

The instruction for the immediate coming of the physician to his patient runs as follows: "When the doctor enters the dwelling of his patient, he should not appear haughty, nor covetous, but should greet with kindly, modest demeanor those who are present, and then seating himself near the sick man accept the drink which is offered him (*sic*) and praise in a few words the beauty of the neighborhood, the situation of the house, and the well-known generosity of the family,—if it

307

should seem to him suitable to do so. The patient should be put at his ease before the examination begins and the pulse should be felt deliberately and carefully. The fingers should be kept on the pulse at least until the hundredth beat in order to judge its kind and character; the friends standing round will be all the more impressed because of the delay and the physician's words will be received with just that much more attention."

John of Arderne was in distinguished company when he wrote "Of ye manere of ye Leche" in one of his works. Since the days of Hippocrates surgeons—and physicians—had been writing on this theme, but John amplified their exhortations. "Consider not over openly the lady or the daughters or other fair women in great men's houses, nor proffer to kiss them, nor touch their breasts privately or openly" and more to the same effect. Like everyone else, John advised that the estimated time of cure for any condition should always be increased for the benefit of the patient and his friends, even going so far as to advise doubling it.

The following passage is taken from a work of general guidance as to medical conduct written about A. D. 1100 by one Archimathaeus:

"When you are called to a patient, may the name of God be your help, and may the angel who walked with Tobias be the companion of your mind and body. At your entrance inquire of him who greets you from what disease the sick man suffers and how his illness progresses; this is advisable in order that when you come to him you may not seem entirely uninformed as to the illness. Again when you reach the house and before you see him, ask if he has seen his confessor, and if he has not done this, arrange for him to do so, or have him promise to do so, for if the sick man hears talk on this subject after he has been examined and the signs of his illness studied, he will begin to despair of his safety, because he will think that you despair of it. Entering the sick-room you should have neither proud nor greedy countenance; you should repeat the greeting of those who rise as you enter, and with a gesture seat yourself when they sit down. Next you may resume the conversation with a few remarks in which you praise the neighbourhood, commend the arrangements of the house, if it seems appropriate, or compliment the liberality of the family.

"Then turning to the patient you may ask how it goes with him, and have him put out his arm. At first there may be differences between your own state and that of the patient, either because he is excited at your arrival, or because he is worried about the size of your fee, so that you find the pulse rather confusing; therefore you should consider the pulse only after the patient has become steadier. Take care that he does not lie upon his side nor has his finger over-extended or flexed against his palm. Support his arm with your left hand and observe the pulse for at least 100 beats in order to feel all its variations, and thus you will be able to satisfy the expectant bystanders with words which they are glad to hear.

"Next have the urine brought to you, that the sick man may see you study his illness not only from the pulse but from the urine. When examining the urine you should observe its color, substance, quantity, and content; after which you may promise the patient that with the help of God you will cure him. As you go away, however, you should say to his servants that he is in a very bad way, because if he recovers you will receive great credit and praise, and if he dies, they will remember that you despaired of his health from the beginning. Meanwhile I urge you not to turn a lingering eye upon his wife, his daughter, or his maid-servant, for this sort of thing blinds the eye of the doctor, averts the favor of God, and makes the doctor abhorrent to the patient and less confident in himself. Be therefore careful in speech, respectable in conduct, attentively seeking Divine aid. If the people of the house invite you to a meal, as often happens, do not seem too much gratified, and do not seek the first place at the table, although it is the custom to give this to the priest or the doctor. Do not criticize the food or drink, and when in the country do not show distaste for country food, for example millet bread, even though you can scarcely control your stomach.

"While you eat you may inquire as to the condition of the patient from any one who is present, for in this way the sick man will confide in you all the more, since he sees that you do not forget him while seeking your own comfort. When you rise from the table you may mention that you have been well looked after; this too will give pleasure to the patient."

CHAPTER NINETEEN

Poisons

POISONS, those subtle and silent weapons capable of destroying life mysteriously, secretly and without violence, have ever had a peculiar fascination for mankind.

They have played so large a part in history at various periods, also in romance as well as crime, that the subject must be regarded as one of great human interest.

The word poison, which appears to have been originally employed for a potion or draught prepared with a deadly or deleterious drug or ingredient, is used in that sense in English literature as early as 1230. The words venym, venum or bane, though no doubt originally applied to the poison of serpents, appear to have also been used for any poisonous or noxious substance which had the effect of a poison and was capable of destroying life.

The sketch that will be found in the following pages does not pretend to be a complete history of poisons, but has been confined mostly to those that have been employed for criminal purposes.

Our knowledge of the use of poisons by primitive man is chiefly derived from archaelogical research which shows that from the earliest times, in every age and in every inhabited part of the globe, he has endeavoured by some means or other, to make the weapons he employed more deadly to his enemies or his prey.

That he observed the poisonous effects of plants and herbs on animal life is evident from the names given to them in early times. Instances of these are perpetuated in cowbane (the water hemlock), which often has a fatal effect on cattle; sowbane, so called, says Parkinson in his Herbal, as it was observed to kill swine; wolf's bane, leopard's bane, henbane, and many others which might be mentioned.

It is remarkable that certain animals and birds can consume plants and substances that are poisonous to man, with impunity. Thus storks and quails can feed on hemlock and aconite. Water hemlock can be eaten by oxen, goats, horses and sheep without apparent ill effects.

In human beings the state of health and disease have considerable influence over the action of poisons. Climate also has its effect and it is well known that natives of southern countries, especially those with warm climates, are more susceptible to narcotics and other vegetable poisons, than those who live in more northern and colder latitudes.

Almost every savage tribe and people throughout the world have been found to have their own particular poison for making the wound caused by their weapons more deadly, and this method has been practiced from a period of great antiquity.

The earliest known deity associated with poisons is Gula, whose name was revered by the Sumerians about 4500 B. C. She was known as "The Mistress of Charms and Spells," the "Terrible Goddess," "Controller of noxious poisons," and was the deified form of the sorceress.

Leaving the period of tradition there is evidence from ancient records that the Assyrians possessed a considerable knowledge of poisonous substances, both of mineral and vegetable origin, at least three thousand years ago. From these records inscribed in cuneiform on clay tablets, we know that they employed such mineral poisons as orpiment, the yellow trisulphide of arsenic, antimony oxide, copper acetate, lead, litharge, mercury and verdigris, and among the vegetable poisonous plants mentioned are poppy, aconite, mandragora, henbane and hemp.

Coming to times of early culture in Greece, we find the knowledge of poisonous substances had considerably increased. The ancient Greeks knew of arsenic in the form of realgar and orpiment, also antimony, mercury, gold, silver, copper and lead and probably had a knowledge of their properties, as they recommended hot oil as an antidote in a case of poisoning and mention other means to promote vomiting and preventing poison being absorbed into the system.

The Greeks looked upon suicide under certain conditions as a noble act, and sanctioned the use of the poison-cup by those who desired to terminate their existence on earth.

A curious custom prevailed among the ancient inhabitants of the island of Ceos in which poison played a part. When the old men found they were no longer of service to the State and began to feel life a burden, they assembled at a banquet of death and, with their heads crowned with chaplets, cheerfully drained the poison-cup.

Of the vegetable poisons known and used by the Greeks, hemlock appears to have been chiefly employed. From all accounts the poison draught does not appear to have been either very powerful or rapid in its action, as a second dose was often required before it proved fatal.

The circumstances attending the death of Socrates, who was poisoned with hemlock, which happened in the year 402 B. C., are thus recounted by Plato:

"When the fatal cup was brought, he asked what it was necessary for him to do. 'Nothing more,' replied the servant of the judges, 'then as soon as you have drunk of the draught, to walk about until you find your legs become weary and afterwards lie down upon your bed.'

"He took the cup without any emotion or change in his countenance and, looking at him in a steady and assured manner:

" 'Well!' said he, 'what say you of this drink?'

" 'May a libation be made out of it?'

"Upon being told that there was only enough for one dose, 'At least,' said he, 'we may pray to the gods as is our duty and implore them to make our exit from this world and our last stage happy, which is what I most ardently beg of them.'

"Having spoken these words he remained silent for some time and then drank off the whole draught.

"After reproving his friends for indulging in loud lamentations, he continued to walk about as he had been directed until he found his legs grow weary. Then he lay down upon his back and the person who had administered the poison went up to him and examined for a little time his feet and legs, and then squeezing his foot strongly, asked whether he felt him? Socrates replied that he did not. He then did the same to his legs, and proceeding upwards in this way, showed us that he was cold and stiff, and he afterwards approached him and said to us that when the effect of the poison reached the heart Socrates would depart. And now the lower parts of his body were cold, when he uncovered himself and said, which were his last words: 'Crito, we owe Æsculapius a cock. Pay the debt and do not forget it.'

" 'It shall be done,' replied Crito. 'But consider whether you have anything else to say.'

"Socrates answered in the negative, but was in a short time convulsed. The man then uncovered him; his eyes were fixed and when Crito observed this, he closed his eyelids and his mouth."

The poisonous plants enumerated by Dioscorides include the poppy, black and white hellebore, henbane, mandragora, hemlock, elaterium, the juices of a species of euphorbia and apocynae. The black and white hellebore were known to the

Romans and used by them as an insecticide, and Pliny states that the Gauls used a preparation of veratrum to poison their arrows.

Dioscorides throws a further light on the poisons of antiquity in his work on Materia Medica, which for fifteen centuries or more remained the chief authority on that subject. He mentions cantharides, and copper, mercury, lead and arsenic among the mineral substances.

In the early ages the knowledge of poisonous substances appears to have been more general among Eastern races than among nations in the West.

The Persians in ancient times are said to have studied with care the art of poisoning. The Carthaginians were apparently also skilled in the art of poisons, and it is related that they killed Regulus, the Roman general, by this means.

In India and the Far East, poisons have been used from very early times, not only for the destruction of human life, but also for destroying animals. Arsenic, aconite, opium and many other poisonous mineral and vegetable substances were employed for this purpose.

In India, when powdered glass is employed for lethal purposes, it is generally given with sherbet or some kind of food. It acts as a powerful irritant to the coats of the stomach or intestines and produces gastro-enteritis. Both powdered glass and diamond dust have for centuries had the reputation of acting as powerful irritants.

The Hindus have many curious traditions concerning poisons, and like the Western nations, attribute to some the property of causing a lingering death which can be controlled by the will of the poisoner. The knowledge of the substances employed is guarded with great secrecy and even now are not fully known.

Both the Chinese and Japanese, from early times down to the present day, have studied the action of poisons. The Chinese are said to have employed gold leaf for suicidal purposes

315

from a time of great antiquity and until recent times, when a high official put an end to his life, it was officially announced that he had "taken gold-leaf."

Judging from the earliest laws on record, criminal poisoning does not appear to have been common amongst the ancient Egyptians or Hebrews. The first law against criminal poisoning was passed by Sulla in Rome in the year 82 B. C. and it continued in force until the fall of the Empire. The penalty was confiscation of property and exile or exposure to wild beasts.

There have been certain periods in the world's history when every eminent personage, king, prince, minister of favorite, was deemed in danger of poison, and when not a particle of food was swallowed by them until it had first been tasted.

"Tasters" were often employed in the castles of nobles and houses of the wealthy to taste the wine before it was handed to their masters, and dishes made of electron, which were believed to become tarnished if poisonous food was placed upon them, were frequently used at table. Beakers of Venetian glass which were warranted to fly into atoms if poisoned wine was placed in them, were also among the detectors used in the sixteenth century, when the dread of poison was greater than the assassin's dagger.

The strict precautions taken by Royal personages against attempts at poisoning, are evidenced in the orders made by Henry VII for protecting the infant Prince of Wales. It was laid down by command that: "No person of whatsoever rank, except the regular attendants in the nursery should approach the cradle except with an order from the King's hand. The food given to the child was to be largely 'assayed' and his clothes were to be washed by his own servants and no other hand might touch them. The material was to be subject to all tests. The Chamberlain and Vice-Chamberlain must be present morning and evening when the Prince was washed and dressed and nothing of any kind bought for the use of the nursery might be introduced until it was washed and perfumed."

During the Middle Ages a strange dread of wholesale poisoning spread throughout Europe and caused numerous panics. Some of these rumors may probably have been circulated by unscrupulous traders who had articles to sell, or some business interests to forward, but of this disturbing fear, authentic record still exists that it affected whole communities.

Wholesale poisoning appears to have been frequent in Eastern countries, especially in India and Persia. The wells or other water sources were usually chosen as the media for disseminating the poison, and in this way whole villages have often been destroyed by some miscreant.

The priests of Notre-Dame became appalled at the number of self-accusations of murder by poison made to them in the confessional, and conveyed an intimation of the fact without names to Colbert and Louvois, then Ministers of State. A judicial commission was appointed by Louis XIV, by which strict justice was to be done, without distinction of person, condition or sex. It sat for three years, and was known as the *Chambre Ardente*, or Chamber of Poisons, and was established at the Arsenal near the Bastille.

The stir and mystery made by the examinations of this Court apparently drew more attention to poisons than before, and many began to learn how to employ them, with the object of succeeding to heritages or of ridding themselves of persons they disliked.

Among those arrested and brought before the Court were members of some of the noblest families of France, together with magistrates, priests and a number of women, who had practiced as witches, fortune-tellers, *sages-femmes* and poisoners. Confessions, which were extracted from these people by torture showed that systematic poisoning had for some time been carried out by the ladies of the Court of the *Grand Monarque*.

In 1662 it was thought necessary to devise some more drastic method of dealing with the secret sale of poisons, and a decree was issued by Louis XIV, forbidding apothecaries to sell arsenic, sublimate, or any drug reputed to be a poison except to persons known to them. It further required that the purchaser should sign a register declaring the purpose for which he was buying the poison. A similar condition had been imposed by the local authorities in Montpellier about twenty years previously, but Louis applied it to the whole of France.

In early times there is little doubt that many people died from the effects of poison without suspicion.

The death of Niccolo Macchiavelli, whose abbreviated Christian name according to Macaulay, was the origin of the term "Old Nick" commonly applied to the universal enemy of mankind, is said to have been due to a magic potion.

In the eighteenth century, there is evidence that poisons were sometimes secretly administered by means of a clyster, the use of which was very common at the time. Arsenic, corrosive sublimate, cantharides and opium are said to have been given in this way.

POISONS IN CHRISTIAN ERA

The study of poisons was forbidden in the early Christian era, and Galen mentions the fact that only a few philosophers dared treat the subject in their works.

Theophrastus states that the poison of most subtle operation of his time was extracted from wolf's bane (aconite); no antidote had been discovered to this poison and it was a capital crime to have in one's possession the plant from which it was extracted.

Nicander's particular remedies were such drugs as birthwort, alkanet, and Theriaca of vipers, which was prepared with a great many aromatic roots and fruits, including ginger, cinnamon, myrrh, iris and gentian.

In his work he mentions twenty-two poisonous substances including aconite (wolf's bane), litharge (lead oxide), buprestis (a beetle resembling cantharides), ceruse (white lead), conium (hemlock), cantharides, hyoscyamus (henbane), ixias (probably a species of chameleon), coagulated milk, sea-hare, poppy (opium), pharicum (probably a composition of agaric), the red toad and marsh frog, the salamander, bull's blood, taxus (yew), and toxicum (an unknown poison). As general antidotes he recommends warm oil, warm water and mallow or linseed tea to excite vomiting.

From this list we have some idea of the knowledge of poisons in the second century before the Christian era. Most of the substances enumerated are of vegetable or animal origin, few of the soluble mineral poisons being known at that time.

POISONS IN MEDIEVAL TIMES

Many poisons revealed by modern chemical research were unknown to the chemists of the Middle Ages, and it is equally certain that the latter knew of few poisonous bodies that are not familiar to chemists of the present day.

Our knowledge of the substances regarded as poisons from the ninth to the fifteenth century is derived from manuscripts that have come down to us from those periods, although few are devoted especially to the subject.

Arsenic, red oxide of mercury, corrosive sublimate, nitric and hydrochloric acids were known to the Arabs in the ninth century and in the twelfth century, Albertus Magnus described the preparation of the acetates of copper and lead.

Several of the vegetable drugs he describes as poisonous we know to be innocuous, but among the more potent venoms he includes aconite napellus, mandrake, opium, hellebore, and muscus (fungi).

Another manuscript in which we have a fuller list, is "The Book of Venoms" written by Magister Santes de Ardoynis in 1424. He describes three kinds of arsenic, viz., arsenic sub-

319

limate, yellow and red. He also includes silver, turpeth mineral among his mineral poisons; aconite, hellebore, laurel, opium, briony, mandrake and agaricus among the vegetable, and cantharides, buprestis, sea-hare, leopard's gall, cat's brains, menstrual blood as animal poisons.

Still later, Maister Peter of Abano wrote a treatise on poisons which was first printed in 1470. How far the knowledge of these substances had increased by the end of the fifteenth century is evidenced from the fact that he enumerates seventy drugs that were then regarded as venoms. Among the more powerful are sublimated arsenic, litharge, the juices of water-hemlock, poppy, mandrake, mezereon, hellebore, and briony. He also mentions opium and nux vomica, poisonous fungi, cantharides, scorpions, bull's blood, brain of a cat, sea-hare, menstrual blood and the venom of serpents.

The hallucinations of the witches which we read about in the Middle Ages, may be compared with those of the medicine-men of many savage tribes today. In all probability these effects were produced by the action of various drugs which they knew were capable of causing hallucinations and temporary insanity. Weak-minded women, who probably formed the greater part of the class known as witches, made use of an unguent with which they anointed themselves in preparation for the so-called "witches' Sabbath." Johannes Wierius, who was a witness of such a gathering, recorded in 1566 the composition of the witches' ointment and states it contained such powerful narcotic poisons as mandrake, belladonna, henbane and stramonium. The absorption of this unguent was followed by unconsciousness and sleep, and on being awakened the person so anointed was fully assured that she had visited the "Sabbath."

POISONS TRIED ON MAN

From an early period science has been gradually built up by experimental methods and even the ancients were cognizant of the fact that the remedial properties of a substance could only be proved by actual experiment. Not only animals but human beings were utilized for this purpose by many famous physicians in the Middle Ages. Criminals who had been condemned to death were generally selected when available.

It is recorded that Cosimo de Medici, Grand Duke of Tuscany, on one occasion ordered the magistrates of Pisa to hand over two men to Fallopius, "in order that he may put them to death in whatever way he pleases, and then anatomize them." Fallopius, however, seeing the men were condemned to death, seems to have acted with both dignity and humanity. He gave them opium; one died and the other recovered. Cosimo pardoned him, but, if we may believe contemporary records, Fallopius did not: he gave the man eight grains more, and this time he died.

At Bologna, poisons were habitually administered to criminals without their knowledge to obviate the perturbing influence of fear upon natural toxic effects. Arsenic was employed in the same way at Mantua and Florence.

On the ethics of such experiments some diversity of opinion may exist, but only when the subjects voluntarily submit themselves, as was recently done in connection with the researches on yellow fever, can such a course be in any way justified.

ANCIENT VEGETABLE POISONS

Aconite, belladonna, digitalis, hellebore, hemlock, hyoscyamus, mandrake, nux vomica, opium, stramonium.

ACONITE

Among other poisonous plants known to the ancients, aconite may rightly be claimed to be one of the most important. It has been called the "Queen Mother of Poisons" and has been a matter of comment and note by early historians for over two thousand years. It is also said to have been derived from the Greek word for javelin or arrow, because "some barbarous nations employed the juice to poison their arrows and spears."

It was used by the Chinese in ancient times and is still employed by the less civilized of the hill tribes of India as an arrow poison. It is said also to have been used for the same purpose by the aborigines of ancient Gaul.

BELLADONNA

Among the poisonous plants with powerful narcotic properties is belladonna (*atropa belladonna*) or deadly night-shade which is a native of Southern Europe but is often found growing wild in several of the Southern counties of England.

It cannot be identified with certainty earlier than the sixteenth century, where it is mentioned in the GRAND HERBIER, printed in Paris about 1504. In 1542, Leonard Fuchs included it in his HISTORIA STIRPIUM and recognized its poisonous properties.

Matthiolus who noticed it a few years later, calls the plant *Solatrum majus* and says it is commonly called by the Venetians *Herba Bella donne*, because the Italian women use a distilled water of the plant as a cosmetic. Whether this is true or not, it was certainly used by women in several European countries on account of its property of enlarging the pupils of the eyes which they thought added to their beauty.

It began to be used in medicine about the middle of the last century.

In 1833, Mein prepared from the root, and Geiger and Hesse isolated from the leaves, the alkaloid called atropine, a powerful poison of which they contain a large proportion.

DIGITALIS

Another plant of a highly poisonous nature which is commonly seen growing in our woods and gardens is the foxglove (*digitalis purpurea*) with its handsome spikes of purple or white flowers, but probably it has not been used for criminal purposes.

The name digitalis, from digitale, a thimble or finger stall, was given to the plant by Fuchs in 1542 who figured it in his "Herbal." The Germans called it *fingerhut*, while to the French it was known as gantelée.

In folk-lore it was regarded as the special flower of the fairies and its little bells were supposed to afford the tiny elves a safe retreat and hiding place. In Ireland it was called the "fairy cup" and in Wales it was known as "goblin's gloves."

The flower is also said to have been held in high favor by the witches who decorated their fingers with the largest bells and it was thus known in some parts of England as "witches bells" or "fairy folks glove."

Foxglove was used as an external remedy by the physicians of Wales as early as the thirteenth century. It became known as a remedial agent in the seventeenth century and was first included in the London Pharmacopoeia in 1650.

Its value in reducing the heart's action was recognized by Dr. Withering of England in 1785, who also used it with advantage in cases of dropsy.

Its active principles are digitalin, digitalein and digitoxin, the latter being discovered by Schmiedeberg in 1874.

HELLEBORE

Hellebore or Melampus root, like Hemlock, has been associated with mystery and evil throughout the ages. The poet Campbell thus refers to its reputation:

"By the witches' tower,
　Where Hellebore and Hemlock seem to weave
Round its dark vaults a melancholy bower
For spirits of the dead at night's enchanted hour."

It is supposed to have taken its name from Melampus, a traditionary physician who is said to have cured the daughters

323

of Proetus, King of Argus, of mental derangement and leprosy, by administering the root.

On the other hand, Pliny states that the daughters of Proetus were restored to their senses by drinking the milk of goats that had fed on hellebore. Melampus is reputed to have flourished at Pylus about 1530 B. C., and after his time the plant was generally known as Melampus root and later as Christmas Rose.

The root of the black hellebore was used by the ancients to hallow their dwellings and they believed that by strewing it about it would drive away evil spirits. The ceremony of laying it was performed with great devotion and accompanied with the chanting of solemn hymns. Cattle were also blessed with hellebore in the same manner, to keep them free from the spells of the wicked. For these purposes it was dug up with solemn religious ceremonies.

HEMLOCK

Hemlock or cicuta was a classical poison well-known in ancient times and has had an evil reputation from an early period. References are made to it in Greek literature from the fourth century before the Christian era.

Dioscorides describes it as "a very evil, dangerous, hurtful and poisonous herb, insomuch that whosoever taketh it into his body dieth remediless, except the party drink some wine before the venom hath taken the heart." Pliny declares that even serpents flee from its leaves.

It was used in Anglo-Saxon medicine and is mentioned in the Vocabulary of Alfric as early as the tenth century, the name hemlock being derived from the Anglo-Saxon words "hem," border or shore and "leac."

Its chief active principle, conine, is a colorless oily liquid which resembles nicotine in its action.

Judging from all accounts, and the evidence afforded by the description of its action, there seems little doubt that the Greek State Poison consisted of hemlock, probably in the form of the concentrated juice expressed from the leaves, to which a proportion of poppy juice was added to render its action more certain.

HYOSCYAMUS

Hyoscyamus, commonly called henbane, is an herb which has been employed in medicine from early times. Over three thousand years ago it was used by the Babylonians to relieve toothache.

Gerard writing in the sixteenth century says, "the seed was used by quack-doctors to cause worms to come forth of the teeth by burning them in a chafing dish of coles, the party holding his mouth over the fume thereof, persuading the patient that those small creepers come out of his mouth."

There is an old tradition that once in the refectory of an ancient monastery, the monks were served in error by the cook with henbane instead of some harmless vegetable. After partaking of the dish they were seized with the most extraordinary hallucinations. At midnight one monk sounded the bell for matins, while others walked in the chapel and opened their books, but could not read. Others sang roystering drinking songs and performed mountebank antics, which convulsed the others with uncontrollable laughter, and the pious monastery for the nonce was turned into a lunatic asylum.

MANDRAKE

There is probably no plant around which clusters more legendary lore and superstition than the mandrake (*mandragora officinalis*). Sufficient has been recorded about it to fill volumes, and between the years 1510 and 1850 no less than twenty-two treatises are known to have been written on the subject.

It was known to the Babylonians over 3,000 years ago, and their women carried a mandrake root as a charm against sterility.

The Greeks believed that when dragged from the earth the root gave a dreadful shriek and struck dead the person who had the presumption to pull it up. They therefore adopted the following ingenious method of obtaining it: A dog was allowed to fast, and was then brought near the plant round which a cord was fastened. The end was then tied to the tail of the dog. The gatherer would then place some food within a few feet of the hungry animal, who in his struggles to reach it would uproot the plant and be immediately killed by the evil spirit. At the moment of uprooting the gatherer generally sounded a horn, in order to drown the shriek of the demon that dwelt in the plant.

Many of the traditions and superstitions connected with the plant appear to have arisen from the curious natural shape of the root, which often bears a strong resemblance to the human form. Beyond the effects attributed to it by tradition, the mandrake has undoubted powerful narcotic properties. Its active principle, mandragorine was discovered by Ahrens, and is said to be a mixture of bases of which hyoscyamine is the chief, mixed with scopolamine.

The ancients attributed powerful aphrodisiacal virtues to the plant and claimed that it could produce a condition of sexual excitement which was often attributed to natural and magical powers, and for this reason included it in the composition of their love-philters. It was among the more important narcotic drugs employed for producing anaesthesia, and Dioscorides gives the formula for a wine made by infusing the root in Cyprus wine, which was directed to be administered before amputation of a limb or before the application of a hot cautery.

Shakespeare alludes to the mandragora and its properties in several of his plays. Thus we have Cleopatra asking for the drug that she may "sleep out this great gap of time" while her Anthony is away.

Iago, whilst the poison begins to work in the mind of Othello, exclaims:

326

"Not poppy, nor mandragora
    Nor all the drowsy syrups of this world
    Shall ever medicine thee to that sweet sleep."

Both in Germany and France the mandrake was said to spring up where the presence of a criminal had polluted the ground. It was sure to be found near a gallows, and so was popularly called in Germany *Galgemannlein*.

In some parts of England the Mandrake is said to be still carried by women to prevent sterility, and the same superstition survives in Greece, where pieces of the root are worn by young people as love-charms. Mandrake roots are also carried by women in Syria and Turkey to promote fecundity and may still be bought in the drug shops.

NUX VOMICA

Nux vomica from which strychnine is chiefly obtained was not known to the ancients. It was first used in England about 1640 for poisoning dogs and birds.

The chief active principles, strychnine and brucine, both of which are highly poisonous, were isolated by Pelletier and Caventou from St. Ignatius bean in 1818-19. These alkaloids are obtained from both sources.

OPIUM

There are few drugs used today with a more interesting history than opium. It figures not only in history but also in romance and crime. It has been associated with the acquisition of wealth and prosperity and with the most terrible degradation. Opium has been the cause of war, of bitter feeling and punishments. Whilst it has enslaved many with the most pleasurable hallucinations and relieved the most agonizing pains, it is capable of reducing human beings to the level of the beasts.

It is mentioned in the Papyrus Ebers, one of the earliest records of medicine, as having been known and used by the

Egyptians about 1550 years B. C. It is described by Theophrastus as having been used by the Greeks 300 years B. C. and is supposed to have formed the chief ingredient in the potion known as "Nepenthe" which Helen of Troy gave to the guests of Menelaus to drive away their care.

It was well known to the Arabs, who transmitted their knowledge of its properties first to the Persians and then to other nations of the East. In India its introduction would appear to be connected with the spread of Mohammedanism.

It is believed that opium was introduced by the Arabs into both India and China.

Opium smoking does not appear to have been practiced in China until the latter part of the seventeenth century, but within a hundred years it spread like the tentacles of an octopus over the entire empire.

Paracelsus is generally credited with being the originator of the word laudanum, the name by which tincture of opium is commonly known.

STRAMONIUM

The stramonium (*datura stramonium*) or thornapple, which contains the highly poisonous alkaloids, atropine and hyoscyamine, appears to have spread itself about the middle of the fifteenth century from the regions near the Caspian Sea. We know from Gerard, that it was cultivated in London near the close of the sixteenth century. He tells us that he received the seed from Constantinople. When dried, the leaves were smoked to relieve asthma and were so used by the Nubians for other chest troubles. Both the leaves and seeds contain daturine which was discovered by Geiger and Hesse in 1833, and who considered it to have the same composition as atropine, although the latter is double as poisonous as the former.

DRUG INTOXICANTS and DELERIENTS

The best known drug intoxicants and delerients are hashish and mescal.

HASHISH

Hashish or Bhang, is the Indian name applied to the dried flowering tops of the Indian hemp, from which the resin has not been removed.

It is cultivated largely in India, and is now considered to be the same, botanically, as the *Cannabis sativa* of European cultivation. There is however great difference in their medicinal activity, that growing in India being much more powerful. The method of using it in India is chiefly for smoking in combination with tobacco.

The Chinese herbal, *Rh-va*, which dates from about the fifth century B. C., mentions the fact that the hemp plant is of two kinds, the one producing seeds and the other flowers only. The drug is said to have been used in China to produce insensibility when performing operations as early as the year 220. In 1803 Visey, a French scientist, published a memoir on hashish, and attempted to prove that it was the Nepenthe of Homer; there is little doubt, however, that the use of the drug was known to Galen.

Silvestin de Lacy contends that the word assassin is derived from "hashishin," a name given to a wild sect of Mohammedans who committed murder under its influence.

The following is a description of one of the curious and interesting effects of hashish:

"The Orientalist, when he indulges in hashish retires into the depth of his harem; no one is then admitted who cannot contribute to his enjoyment. He surrounds himself with his dancing girls, who perform their graceful evolutions before him to the sound of music; gradually a new condition of the brain allows a series of illusions, arising from the external senses, to present themselves. The mind becomes overpowered by the brilliancy of gorgeous visions; discrimination, comparison, reason, yield up their throne to dreams and phantoms which exhilarate and delight. The mind tries to understand what is the cause of the new delight, but it is in vain.   It seems to know there is no reality."

MESCAL BUTTONS

The Kiowa and other Mexican Indians use the fruit of the *Anhelonium Lewinii*, known as "mescal buttons" to produce a species of intoxication and stimulation during certain of their religious ceremonies. They treat this cactus with great veneration, gathering it with uncovered heads and amid clouds of incense.

The effects of mescal, like Indian hemp, varies considerably in different individuals.   The effect has been described as follows:

The eating of the fruit first results in a state of strange excitement and great exuberance of spirits, accompanied by volubility in speech.   This is shortly followed by a stage of intoxication in which the sight is affected in a very extraordinary manner, consisting of a kaleidoscopic play of colors ever in motion, of every possible shade and tint, and these constantly changing.   The pupils of the eyes are widely dilated, cutaneous sensation is blunted and thoughts seem to flash through the brain with extraordinary rapidity.   The color visions are generally only seen with closed eyes, but the coloring of all external objects is exaggerated.   Sometimes there is also an indescribable sensation of dual existence.

The Mexicans also make a drink from the mescal, popularly known as peyote, which is distilled from the juice of the plant, and during their social entertainments swallow it in copious draughts.   The intoxication produced by it is manifested by prolonged visual hallucinations, often followed by vertigo, headache, nausea and confusion of thought.

The properties of mescal are due to an alkaloid called mescaline, and while not a dangerous drug, mescal is undoubtedly habit-forming and is eventually harmful both mentally and physically.   According to the reports of authorities 90 per

330

cent of the crimes perpetrated in the ranches and villages are
due to this drug.

POISONOUS FUNGI

Manuscripts dealing with poisons written in the Middle
Ages show that certain fungi "those evil fermentations of the
earth that spring up in a night no man knows whither," played
a more important part in criminal poisoning than is generally
supposed.

The two outstanding examples of poisonous fungi are
mushrooms and ergot.

MUSHROOMS

There are at least twenty-five poisonous varieties of mushrooms, but the most deadly of all which accounts for more
than ninety per cent of the deaths from fungi, is the *amanita
phalloides.*

The toxic properties of several varieties were known in the
early Christian era and mention is made of them directly or indirectly in works on medicine from the fourteenth to the sixteenth century. The facts that they could so easily be obtained and when carefully dried and powdered could be mixed
with food or wine no doubt led to their frequent use as secret
poisons.

The fungi are collected in the hottest months and dried in
the air. They are sometimes rolled up and swallowed without
chewing or they are eaten fresh in soups and sauces, but in this
way they lose much of their intoxicating properties.

One writer observes that external indications that death
has been caused by poisonous fungi, are numerous violet colored spots which afterward appear on the skin over the whole
body.

331

ERGOT

The story of another poisonous fungus now known as ergot, is one of historic interest and forms a page in the romance of science.

Ergot is a peculiar form of the fungus *Claviceps purpurea* which is developed in the ovaries of certain kinds of grasses but is now chiefly found in rye. It develops gradually in the ear of the rye and by the summer appears as a long, black, triangular "horn," some eight or ten often being found in one ear.

As early as the eleventh century it was observed by Sigebert de Gremblour, who remarked that an epidemic followed the consumption of damaged crops, but it was not until the end of the seventeenth century, that it was recognized as the cause of a terrible disease which had decimated mankind for centuries.

About the sixteenth century it began to be noticed that these epidemics occurred at particular seasons of the year, and that certain sections were more frequently visited than others.

The first suggestion that a fungus might be the cause of the disease, resulted from an investigation made by the Medical Faculty of Marburg following an outbreak in Hesse in 1597. Their conclusions led to the belief that the epidemic had been caused by the use of "spurred rye."

By the end of the eighteenth century it was generally concluded that the eating of rye contaminated with ergot was the cause of the gangrenous disease which came to be called ergotism.

Ergot is now only employed in medicine, and thus through scientific investigation and research, what was once the cause of terrible suffering and death has been transformed into a medicinal agent of great value to the human race.

A mysterious poison, kept as a secret by some of the gipsy tribes which wander Europe is said to be composed of a certain poisonous fungus. When mixed with food it causes death in from two to three weeks after administration. The symptoms produced are said to resemble those of typhoid fever.

THE POISON LORE OF SPIDERS, SALAMANDER AND TOADS

Certain species of spider possess poisonous properties, notably the *Chiracanthium nutrix* and the *Epeira diadema*. The bite of the female of the former is distinctly venomous, and one milligramme of the juice of the latter variety injected into a cat resulted in death.

The secretion of the skin glands of the salamander (*salamandra maculosa*) contains a strong poison called salamandrine.

TOADS

From early times the toad has had an unenviable reputation for evil and has been suspected of poisonous properties. Some of the early historians attribute the death of King John of England to a friar who squeezed the secretion of a toad into his cup of wine. The story is probably fictitious, but there is some ground for the evil reputation that has so long been associated with this unlovely reptile. The venom of some toads is believed to possess poisonous properties in certain countries throughout the world, and some species are said to be particularly virulent. A few years ago, Phisalix and Bertrand undertook an investigation to ascertain if there was any truth in the story of the poisonous properties attributed to toads. They succeeded in extracting two powerful principles from the parotid gland and skin of the common toad. One of these, phrynine, was found to act on the heart in a similar manner to digitalis, and the other known as bufotenine, exercised a powerful paralyzing action on the nerve centers.

The toad was an ingredient in the witches' hell-broth in "Macbeth." When dropped into the wine-cup it was believed to act with deadly effect on those who drank its contents.

Although the toad under certain conditions was credited with poisonous properties, during the Middle Ages it was esteemed a valuable remedy for the plague and was employed for that purpose in Austria as late as the year 1712.

The country people of Brazil believe the milky secretion of the common toad possesses wonderful curative properties and use it externally as a cure for shingles. In these cases living toads are generally applied to the part affected.

SOME CLASSICAL MINERAL POISONS

The most commonly used mineral poisons are antimony, arsenic and mercury.

ANTIMONY

Antimony has played an important part, both in medicine and chemistry, from a very early period. Known to the ancients as "stibium" or "stimmi," the native sulphide was used by women in Egypt and in the East for darkening the eyebrows and eyelids over three thousand years ago. Arab women still use it in the form of "kohl," finely ground, for making lines between the eyelids, which they regard as an aid to beauty. It was a favorite metal with the alchemists, who hoped to obtain from it a remedy for all ills. They soon discovered how readily it formed alloys with other metals, and found it a simple matter to make salts of the metal.

In the seventeenth century it was probably one of the most popular remedies in France for ague, dropsy, smallpox, syphilis and other diseases. Louis XV bought the formula for its preparation from La Ligerie for a considerable sum in 1720.

In the sixteenth and seventeenth centuries cups were made of an alloy of antimony and tin, called "antimony cups" (*pocula emetica*). A cup, when filled with wine, was allowed to stand for some little time and become slightly impregnated with tartar emetic, and the liquid when drunk caused vomiting. These cups are said to have been frequently kept in

334

monasteries, so that the monks who took too much wine could be punished by having to drink from the *poculum emeticum*.

In the seventeenth century Basil Valentine published a work entitled the "Triumphal Chariot of Antimony," in which he describes its virtues as a remedy, and the manner in which it could be prescribed. It was translated into English and published in London in 1678.

One of the peculiarities of antimony when given in large doses is its property of preserving the tissues of the body after death. In one case, the body of a victim who had been poisoned with antimony was exhumed after five years, and was found to be completely mummified and as well preserved as if it had only been buried a few days.

ARSENIC

Arsenic appears to have had an extraordinary fascination for the poisoner for centuries past and has, perhaps, been more frequently used for criminal purposes than any other poison. Through its history runs a vein of mystery and romance which has continued until the present day.

Arsenic has ever had a peculiar attraction for the criminal poisoner for we find that it was employed in twenty out of forty attempts of murder in recent years.

When arsenic is selected by the criminal it is on account of its colorless and tasteless nature and is usually administered in foods, solid or liquid, and generally in the guise of friendly solicitude.

Before white arsenic or arsenious acid was known, most of the poisons recorded by the early writers had something peculiar in regard to their taste, smell or color. White arsenic put a new instrument in the hands of the secret poisoner who sought for something powerful and tasteless for his evil designs.

In the eighth century there arose the great Arab alchemist Jabir ibn Hayyan, whose writings were known under the name of Geber. He is said to have been a native of Tarsus and believed to have been the first in Europe to obtain what is now known as white arsenic (arsenious acid) by heating realgar. His discovery was not without its disadvantages to mankind, as from this period probably dates the time when arsenic began to be used for criminal purposes. On the other hand, its medicinal properties, when properly administered, became known and recognized by physicians.

It was known to the Greeks as early as the fifth century before Christ. Hippocrates, the father of medicine, who flourished 460-377 B. C., used it as an external remedy for ulcers and similar disorders. Dioscorides knew it in its latter form and also mentions its properties when applied externally. At this period there is no allusion to its employment either as a poison or for internal treatment of disease.

The alleged practice of eating arsenic or taking it as a habit, has long been a matter of discussion, and as far back as the early part of the last century toxicologists were skeptical as to the statement that the inhabitants of Styria, and other parts of Hungary where arsenic is found, had contracted the regular habit of taking the drug until they had almost become immune to its effects.

In 1865, Maclagan of Edinburgh visited Styria for the purpose of investigating these statements, and in an account of his visit given in the Edinburgh Medical Journal, 1865, he affirms that while he was staying at the village of Legist in Middle Styria, two men were brought to him and in his presence, one took about 4½ and the other 6 grains of white arsenic. He brought back samples of what they had swallowed, and on testing it found them to be white arsenic. It was taken by one man on a piece of bread, and by the other was washed down with a draught of water. How extensively the habit existed in the district Maclagan was not able to ascertain, but he mentions that the peasants called it Hydrach or Huttereich. One of the men took a dose about twice a week, the other generally once a week, and he learned they had commenced the habit with doses of less than a grain. The effect was said to be tonic and stimulant and it was believed to aid the respiration when climbing. Once having acquired the habit, like that of other poisons, an occasional dose was much missed if omitted.

MERCURY

Mercury, one of the most fascinating of all the elements, has traditions that carry it back to an unknown period of antiquity. In the form of sulphide it is recorded in the Papyrus Ebers (1550 B. C.) as being used by the ancient Egyptians, but it is said to have been known at an even earlier date in the form of quicksilver in China and India.

The many ways in which mercury can be transformed and the numerous products which can be made from it, have had a fascination for chemists throughout the ages.

The metal was probably named after the Roman divinity Mercury on account of its volatile nature and its elusive properties when handled. It has the peculiar property of absorbing other metals and forming amalgams. As well as being found native, it was obtained by the ancients by sublimation from cinnabar, the oxide. By the alchemists it was represented by the same sign as the planet Mercury. It is alluded to by Theophrastus in the fourth century B. C., but it is to Dioscorides in the first century A. D. it owes the name of hydrargyrum or fluid silver.

The protochloride of mercury was prepared and known as far back as the time of Democritus in the fifth century B. C. In 1386 Chaucer alludes to it as "quick-silver yclept mercurie." About 1497 it was first used in the treatment of syphilis, by inunction or in the form of plasters and fumigation.

The Arabs, who doubtless derived their knowledge of the metal from the Greeks, were much attracted by it, and Geber describes perchloride of mercury, also the red oxide. Avicenna,

337

the Arab physician, was the first to doubt the poisonous properties of the metal itself, and noted that many persons swallowed it without any ill effects, as it passed through the body unchanged. Fallopius (1523-1562) records that shepherds gave quicksilver to sheep and cattle to expel worms, and Brassovola (1500-1555) says that he had given it to children in doses from two to twenty grains for the expulsion of worms.

The first to record its use internally was Peter Matthiolus, the commentator of Dioscorides (1501-1577). Paracelsus popularized its use, and since the sixteenth century the value of mercury and its salts have come to be recognized throughout the world.

Robert Boyle, who was born in 1627, and is regarded as the father of chemistry in Great Britain, made the oxide by heating mercury in a bottle fitted with a stopper provided with a narrow tube by which air was admitted. The product was known as "Boyle's Hell," on account of the belief that it caused the metal to suffer extreme agonies.

ANCIENT ANTIDOTES TO POISON

The value of the ancient remedies used as antidotes to poisons was chiefly due to the mystery surrounding their origin and the superstition connected with the source.

Apparently the ambition of the early Greek physicians was to discover a universal antidote to all poisons, and many of them devoted years, and spent a great part of their lives in endeavoring to find it. These antidotes were called by the Greeks alexipharmica or theriacs, the former word being derived from the Greek "alexipharmakos", meaning that "which keeps off poison" and the noun "antipharmakon", an antidote.

THERIAC

Theriac, which meant something pertaining to poisonous reptiles, eventually became applied to the antidote itself and

338

came to mean a treacle or confection used against poisons generally.

Theriacs have been described in a previous chapter.

BEZOAR STONE

The Bezoar Stone was regarded with great veneration as an antidote to poisons, especially in the East. It has been described in a preceding chapter (see Avenzoar).

TOADSTONE

The so-called Toadstone has from early times been reputed to possess the property of counteracting the effect of poisons. These stones were believed to be found in the heads of old toads which, when caught, were placed on a red cloth and the stone recovered through the mouth. Pomet, who wrote in the seventeenth century, threw doubt on this source of origin.

Lemery, a French writer of the same period, in describing these stones, states that when applied to the sting or bite of venomous beasts, they draw out the poison. They were usually set and worn as rings and regarded as of great value. They were generally mounted so that the back of the stone could touch the skin, and were said to notify the presence of poison by producing a sensation of heat in the finger at the point of contact.

HORN OF THE UNICORN

The so-called horn of the unicorn, which was in reality the tusk of the Narwhal, has been associated with mysterious properties since the time of Aristotle, Pliny and other ancient writers. Ctesias (about 390 B. C.) was the first to record the wonderful properties attributed to it. "Drinking vessels," he says, "were made of the horn and those who used them were protected against poisons, convulsions and epilepsy, provided that, just before or just after taking poison, they drank wine or water from the cup made from it. Other writers declared that poisoned wounds could be cured by merely holding the horn of the unicorn close to the wound."

These horns were considered of great value and in the Middle Ages are said to have been worth about ten times the price of gold. In 1553, a unicorn's horn was brought to the King of France which was valued at £20,000 sterling, and one presented to Charles I, supposed to be the largest then known, measured seven feet long and weighed 13 lbs.

Ambroise Paré doubted the value of unicorn's horn as an antidote and says: "after making a trial thereof yet could never find any good success in the use against poisons." Chapelaine, the chief physician to King Charles IX often used to say, "that he would very willingly take away that custom of dipping a piece of unicorn's horn in the King's cup, but he knew that opinion to be so deeply ingrafted in the minds of men that he feared that it would scarce be impugned by reason."

HORN OF THE INDIAN RHINOCEROS

From a time of great antiquity the horn of the Indian rhinoceros has been reputed to possess the power of absorbing poisonous substances brought into contact with it.

The traditions attached to the horn of the rhinoceros must have come to Europe at an early period, as we find that cups made from the horn, called "assay cups" were used in England as early as the fifteenth century in the time of Edward V.

TERRA SIGILLATA

Among the famous medicaments of antiquity reputed to be effective in counteracting poisons was terra sigillata or "sacred sealed earth," a peculiar clay which originally came from the Isle of Lemnos. Its reputation dates from the time of Herodotus, and it continues in use in Turkey and some parts of the East today. This red clay was formerly excavated from the side of a certain hill with great ceremony, in the presence of the principal inhabitants of the island. The ceremony was originally associated with the worship of Diana and was carried out on May 6, each year. This particular earth was not allowed to be dug by anyone on any other day of the year except that formally set apart for the operation.

According to Dioscorides, the clay was made into a paste, with goats' blood. It had a universal reputation as an antidote to all poisons, and a poisoned liquid drunk from a cup made from the clay was believed to be rendered harmless.

An analysis made some years ago showed that terra sigillata was composed of oxides of iron, aluminum, and magnesia, with a proportion of silicates. It was thus an astringent and absorbent earth.

CUPS

The Chinese, who appear to have ever been suspicious of being poisoned, made little cups of glass about 1½ in. high which they believed would crack if a poisoned liquid were poured into them.

A cup or goblet made of electrum, an alloy composed of gold and silver known to the ancients, according to Pliny, had the property of revealing any poisonous liquid which was placed in it, by exhibiting certain circles like rainbows in the liquid, which it also kept sparkling and hissing as if on fire.

NIGGER CAESER'S CURE FOR POISON

The search for antidotes to poison was not confined entirely to the Old World, for according to the Carolina Gazette of May 9, 1750, the General Assembly, the Governing Body of the Colony, authorized the publication of "Nigger Caeser's cure for poison." The General Assembly had purchased Nigger Caeser's freedom, who was apparently a slave, and granted him £100 a year for life as the price of his formula, which consisted

341

of roots of plantain and wild hore-hound, 3 oz. boiled together in 2 quarts of water down to 1 quart and strained. Of this, one-third was to be given every morning, fasting for three consecutive mornings. Certain dieting was also required, and it is stated that if in the three days' treatment no benefit had resulted, it was a sign that the patient had either not been poisoned at all or had been by such poisons as Caeser's antidote would not remedy.

CHAPTER TWENTY

Poisoners

THERE has always been an intimate connection between ancient pharmacy and poisoning. The secret poisoner who endeavored to kill his victim by the most subtle and cunning methods, unseen and mysterious, has been dreaded throughout the centuries. He was even more feared by kings, princes and nobles than the assassin with his poniard or dagger.

Poison appears to have been employed as a political agent from an early period of history, and many stories have been handed down of royal personages who used this secret and deadly method of ridding themselves of troublesome individuals and removing enemies from their path. In the same way, they themselves sometimes became the victims of jealous rivals. The greatest craft and cunning were exerted in order to introduce poison into the human body, and there are many stories concerning the curious and subtle methods said to have been employed.

Women especially seem to have had a predilection for this method of administering a lethal dose, a fact probably due to their control and direction of domestic matters, which rendered the introduction of a poisonous substance into food or drink an easy matter.

Hecate and her daughters Medea and Circe figured prominently in Greek legends as inventors and discoverers of poisons.

343

The magic arts for which they were all famous were closely associated with deadly drugs. They were supposed to live in the island of Colchis, the name of which still recalls a vegetable which for many centuries retained the reputation of possessing the most venomous properties. Colchicum was discovered by Medea, but to Hecate is attributed the earliest use of aconite.

Reginald Scot, who wrote THE DISCOVERY OF WITCH-CRAFT in 1584, quaintly states his belief that "women were the first inventors and the greatest practisers of poysoning and more materially addicted and given thereunto than men."

Of this type was Van der Linden, a Dutch woman who poisoned one hundred and two people, and Héléne Jegado, who apparently regarded poisoning as a pastime and is said to have been responsible for twenty-six deaths.

The motives actuating their crimes have generally proved to be greed of gain, jealousy or lust, while there have been others who appear to have acted from sheer love of notoriety and the power of possession.

A secret society of women was formed in Rome in 1659. Many of the members were young married women belonging to some of the best and wealthiest families of that city. They apparently met together with the chief object of plotting to destroy the lives of their husbands or members of families connected with them. They gathered at regular intervals at the house of a woman called Hieronyma Spara, who was reputed to be a sorceress. She provided the members of the Society with the poison necessary for their purposes, and planned and instructed them how to use it.

Operations had been carried on for some time before the existence of the Society was discovered, "and," says a contemporary writer, "the hardened old hag passed the ordeal of the rack without confession, but another woman divulged the secrets of the sisterhood, and La Spara, together with twelve other women implicated, were hanged. Many others were publicly whipped through the streets of the city."

Plutarch writes of the last king of Pergamus:

"And Attalus Philometor used to grow poisonous plants, not only henbane and hellebore, but also hemlock, aconite, and dorycnium, sowing and planting them himself in the royal gardens, and making it his business to know their juices and fruits, and to collect these at the proper season." Justin adds, that in in his playful moments, Attalus distributed fruits to his friends: some of these fruits were natural, and some were poisoned.

Mithridates Eupator, King of Pontus, in the second century before Christ, who was the first student of toxicology, lived in such constant fear of being poisoned that he devoted his entire time to the study of the effects of poisons, experimenting upon criminals in his realm and also taking poisons and their antidotes himself. His experiments upon himself were so successful that on the day of his defeat by Pompey he attempted to commit suicide by poison, but had developed such a high degree of immunity or tolerance that the poison failed to produce the desired effect and he called upon one of his attendants to slay him, which he did.

Livy tells the story of the earliest of the poison leagues. He is dependent on older historians for his facts, as the alleged events happened some three centuries before he wrote, about the year 330 B. C.

Down to the seventeenth century there was more exact knowledge of poison than of medicinal drugs. Theriaca, emeralds, and bezoar stones were the antidotes to all poisons recognized.

CONTROLLED POISONS

The belief that certain poisons could be so prepared that their administration controlled with such a degree of precision as to cause death at any given period, according to the will of the poisoner, has existed from ancient times. This idea was encouraged and fostered by the practitioners of alchemy and astrology, and others who professed to exercise magical powers.

They also claimed a knowledge of certain lethal bodies which could be administered to the victims that would leave no trace behind them.

The origin of the time or slow poison tradition may be found in the cunning which is usually associated with the poisoner. In order to avoid suspicion, the poison was probably first administered to the victim in minute quantities, then gradually increased, from time to time, until it was finally decided to give the lethal dose, and so the culminating time could be determined by the poisoner.

In Italy, during the Middle Ages, the highest dignitaries of the Church did not scruple to employ poisons in order to gain their ends, and statesmen used them as instruments of diplomacy. Princes and nobles became adepts in devising the most cunning methods of administering a lethal dose to those whom they wished removed from their paths. This subtle method for the destruction of human life seems to have specially appealed to the Latin races. When they desired to dispose of a dangerous enemy or an inconvenient rival, they say no distinction between using poison and the dagger. Many notable personages are said to have fallen victims to the poisoner's craft, including Pope Victor II, Christopher I, King of Denmark, and Henry VII of Germany.

On a careful investigation of the cases recorded of so-called secret and slow poisonings mentioned by writers of the Middle Ages, the substance employed in the majority of such cases was probably arsenic. La Spara's mysterious elixir, that was the cause of so many deaths in Rome in the seventeenth century, was a preparation of arsenic, and so also was the famous Aqua Toffana, which is said to have put an end to no less than six hundred persons. It is improbable that any substances of a toxic nature were used in medieval or earlier times that are unknown to science today, and most of the stories of slow and secret poisoning can be explained by the manner in which the poison was given. A common phrase used by historians of this period in closing the account of some personages of note was, "he died not without suspicion of venom."

Ambroise Paré did not altogether believe in the stories concerning the effects of the so-called slow and time poisons that were current in his time.

ENGLISH POISONERS

There are but few authenticated records of the use of poison in England for criminal purposes until the sixteenth century. According to tradition King John is said to have compassed the death of the unfortunate Maud FitzWalter by means of a poisoned egg.

According to the French Chronicles, "After the death of Gaultier Giffard, Count Buckingham, in the early part of the twelfth century, Agnes his widow became enamoured with Robert Duke of Normandy, and attached herself to him in an illicit manner, shortly after which time his wife Sibylle died of poison."

One of the earliest recorded cases of secret poisoning in England is that of Sir Walter de Scotiney, who was convicted of poisoning the Abbot of Westminster and William, brother of the Earl of Gloucester.

Robert Dudley, Earl of Leicester, Prime Minister and favorite of Queen Elizabeth, had an ambition to marry his royal mistress, who appears to have had no insight into his unscrupulous character, and was apparently the cause of his attempting by insidious methods to move every human obstacle from his path. The death of his wife, Amy Robsart, a mystery which has never been completely solved, was believed by some to be due to poison.

Leicester was also suspected of causing the death of Lord Sheffield, whose death is said to have been due to "Leicester's cold." A short time afterward, the Earl married his widow, but under pretence that the Queen would be offended at the marriage, compelled her to keep it secret. After some time, the more effectually to conceal the connexion, he required her to marry Sir Edward Stafford. This she refused to do, till under the gentle discipline of Leicester it is recorded that "her hair fell off and her nails fell out, and she did what was demanded of her to save her life." This story is certified by her own testimony on oath, and recorded by Sir William Dugdale.

The Earl of Sussex, his great rival, is also said to have been one of his victims. On his death-bed he is said to have warned his friends in the following words: "I am passing into another world and must now leave you to your good fortunes and to the Queen's grace and goodness; but beware of the gipsy's son (Leicester) for he will be too hard for you all. You know the beast as well as I do."

According to all accounts, Leicester's list of victims did not cease here. Many writers declare that he kept professional poisoners ready to do his will and carry out his designs. There seems little doubt that he had some needy physicians in his pay. His personal doctor, one Bayly, is said to have boasted of the fact that "he knew of poisons which might be so tempered that they should kill the party afterwards at what time it should be appointed."

ITALIAN POISONERS

The study of poisons for criminal purposes developed into a cult in Italy during the Middle Ages, and the Italian school of poisoners became known throughout Europe. There is an authentic record that its members were ready on receipt of certain fees to carry out murder by poison to order.

There seems little doubt that some of the Italian alchemists of the fourteenth and fifteenth centuries studied the art of combining certain poisonous substances with the object of making them more virulent; thus, Pierre le Bon of Ferrara, describes a poison he compounded, containing aconite and copper with the venom of toads.

348

From the fifteenth to the seventeenth century there were schools of poisoners both in Venice and Rome. The Venetian poisoners who first came into notoriety began their operations early in the sixteenth century. At that period the mania for poisoning had risen to such a degree that the governments of the States were formally recognizing secret assassination by poison, and considering the removal of emperors, princes and powerful nobles by this method.

On December 15th, 1543, John of Ragusa, a Franciscan brother, offered the Council a selection of poisons, and declared himself ready to remove any person out of the way whom they deemed objectionable. He openly stated his terms, which for the first successful case was to be a pension of 1,500 ducats a year, to be increased on the execution of future services. The Presidents, Guolando Duoda and Pietro Guiarini, placed this matter before the Council on January 4th, 1544, and on a division it was resolved to accept this patriotic offer, and to experiment first on the Emperor Maximilian. John, who had evidently reduced poisoning to a fine art, afterward submitted the following regular graduated tariff to the Council:

For the great Sultan, 500 ducats.

For the King of Spain, 150 ducats, including the expenses of the journey, etc.

For the Duke of Milan, 60 ducats.

For the Marquis of Mantua, 50 ducats.

For the Pope, 100 ducats.

He further adds at the foot of the document, "The farther the journey, the more eminent the man, the more it is necessary to reward the toil and hardships undertaken, and the heavier must be the payment."

What may be called the Roman school of poisoners became prominent in the early sixteenth century, and their operations continued until the early part of the eighteenth century. During this period the magnitude and daring of their crimes struck terror into the hearts of the chief nobles and rulers of the country. The books on what were termed "secrets," printed in Italy about this time, consisting of formulas of various descriptions, contain many allusions to poisons. In them stories are told of poisons supposed to be unknown, whose secrets died with their originators.

The mania for poisoning appears to have seized on all classes from the highest to the lowest, and no one who made an enemy was safe.

TOFFANA

During the early part of the seventeenth century the southern parts of Italy, including Sicily, also appear to have been infested by unscrupulous practitioners in the use of poison, and Naples became a centre for this nefarious trade. The most notorious of these criminals whose name has been left on record is the woman named Toffana, who is said to have been responsible indirectly for the deaths of hundreds of people. About 1650, when she was little more than a girl, she began her evil career in Palermo, but in 1659, during the pontificate of Alexander VII, she removed to Naples and made it the centre of her operations. Whether she herself devised the poison which is associated with her name, or whether she obtained the knowledge from a confederate, is not known. Her method was to prepare a solution and bottle it in special vials bearing the representation of some saint, generally Saint Nicholas of Bari, who was associated with a medicinal spring, the water of which had a reputation for healing. Sometimes she used other names for her poisonous solution, such as "Aquetta di Napoli," "Manna of St. Nicholas di Bari," or "Aqua Toffana."

When the manufacture and sale of the poison was at last traced to Toffana, she took refuge in a convent where, under the privileges of the place, she bade defiance for some time to the officers of justice, and continued to vend her solution from the very bosom of the Church until the scandal at length became too great to be tolerated. She was then dragged from her refuge and thrown into prison.

There was naturally much mystery at the time as to the composition of Aqua Toffana and the most extraordinary properties were attributed to it. Its alleged effects are thus described by Behrens, a contemporary writer: "a certain indescribable change is felt in the whole body, which leads the person to complain to his physician. The physician examines and reflects, but finds no symptoms either external or internal, no vomiting, no inflammation, no fever. In short, he can only advise patience, strict regimen, and laxatives. The malady, however, creeps on, and the physician is again sent for. Still he cannot detect any symptoms of note. Meanwhile the poison takes firmer hold of the system; languor, wearisomeness, and loathing of food continue; the nobler organs gradually become torpid, and the lungs in particular at length begin to suffer. In a word, the malady from the first is incurable; the unhappy victim pines away insensibly even in the hands of the physician, and thus he is brought to a miserable end through months or years, according to his enemy's desire."

Toffana had many imitators, who continued to practise for some time after her death. A similar scheme was attempted with a poisonous preparation called "Aquetta di Perugia," which was also sold for cosmetic purposes. It is said to have been prepared by killing a hog, disjointing it, and strewing the pieces with white arsenic, which was well rubbed in, and finally collecting the juices which dropped from the meat itself. This preparation was supposed to be a stronger and more powerful poison than arsenic, and more rapid in its action.

LOCUSTA

Women, who not only dealt in poisons, but also practised as poisoners for due reward were common in Rome. Among these nefarious practitioners in crime was Locusta, who appears to have been the personification of a fiendish poisoner.

She was a slave who had been condemned to death in a case which had been proved against her, but her life had been spared in order that she might be employed as a poisoner in the service of the State.

She is said to have been commissioned by Agrippina to kill the Emperor Claudius, and was instructed to prepare a poisonous dish which was to have a gradual effect. It was to be so compounded that it would destroy the Emperor's reason, lest in the course of his proposed illness he should take measures to supplant Nero by Britannicus. Locusta undertook to fulfil this commission and the dish took the form of prepared mushrooms of which the Emperor was particularly fond. He was taken ill shortly after eating them and had to be carried from the table, but as this was an incident that often occurred after his dinner, little notice was taken of it. His physician gave him an emetic and he was recovering, but when Agrippina heard of it she at once sent for Locusta and commanded her to use something stronger. She then prepared a poisoned feather and under the pretence of applying it to his throat to induce further vomiting, she introduced a lethal dose and completed her infamous work.

To Locusta also is attributed the murder of Britannicus whom Nero wished to remove from his path. It is stated that by threats and blows she was compelled to prepare a powerful poisonous draught in his presence. According to Suetonius, it was first tried on a kid but the animal survived five hours. She was then ordered to make it stronger, which she did by boiling it, until it was powerful enough to kill a pig. According to the story, the crime was committed when Britannicus was dining with his brother and the Imperial family, when, as was the custom, hot water was brought round by slaves to the table, the water being heated to varied degrees to suit the taste of the drinker. The cup handed to Britannicus was purposely made too hot and he handed it back to the slave to be made cooler. This presented the opportunity to add the fatal dose, for no sooner had he swallowed the draught than he fell back gasping for breath.

With regard to the knowledge of powerful poisons of rapid action at this period it is recorded that during the reign of Tiberius, a Roman noble accused of high treason swallowed a poison and immediately fell dead at the feet of the senators.

THE BORGIAS

Considerable mystery has ever enveloped the history of the Borgia family, whose name historians have linked with some of the most morbid stories of crime and secret poisoning of the Middle Ages. A great deal that has been written concerning their crimes is doubtless pure fiction, but there seems little doubt that some of the Borgias were guilty of terrible and sinister deeds, which were only too common in the times in which they lived.

The Borgias, who were of Spanish origin, migrated to Italy and came into notoriety about the year 1455. The first member to come into prominence was Rodrigo, who was born in 1431, and who began life as a soldier. Afterward he entered the priesthood, and finally rose to be the head of the Church under the title of Pope Alexander VI. He is said to have had five children by his mistress Vanozza de Cattanei, viz.: Pier Luigi, who died in infancy, Giovanna Duke of Gandia, Giffredo Count of Cariati, Cesare, afterward Duke of Valentinois, and Lucrezia, who eventually became Duchess of Ferrara.

Alexander is described by contemporary writers as "a handsome man of majestic and kingly bearing," and is said to have looked "more like a Caesar returned to life than a Vicar of Christ."

From father to children, who apparently put no restraint on their criminal and sensual instincts, it was not long before the most extraordinary stories were circulated about the Borgias. Cesare, in particular, appears to have been a degenerate of the worst possible type.

The following method of preparing the Borgia poison has been published:

"La Vanozza lifts the heavy red copper dish by the two handles, and on it may be noticed a mouldiness, or greenish spots caused by a settling deposit. With a hare's paw Cesare collects this powder, then with an ivory knife he carefully scrapes the copper, and mixes the residue in a marble mortar. From it he takes in small pinches some of the powder and places it in another mortar of agate, and reduces it with a pestle to an impalpable dust until it is like a morsel of polished silver.

" 'Give me the "manna," ' says Cesare. La Vanozza hands him the arsenic which he calls by that name, and he mixes some with the powder in the mortar, passing the mixture again under the pestle until thoroughly incorporated, and then, his task completed, he stands erect and exclaims: 'God said "Let there be light" and there was light. We Borgias are able to say "Let it be night," and night it shall be.' He then remarks to Vanozza, 'It is time for luncheon.' La Vanozza leaves him and retraces her way; when she is gone, the copper dish being empty, he pours urine in it in order to replace that which has evaporated, the salts of which he had just utilized. The salt which resulted, combined with the verdigris, were then mixed with arsenic and this formed the famous poison which the Borgias called 'La Cantarella.' 'That which the Borgias utilized in conjunction with arsenic without knowing it,' says Apollinaire, 'was phosphorus, a secret which had been divulged to the Borgias by a Spanish monk, who also knew the antidote for it, as well as an antidote for arsenic; one sees, therefore, that they were well armed.' "

Another account of the preparation is as follows:

"The abdominal viscera of a sow which had been poisoned with arsenic were powdered with arsenious acid; they waited until the putrefaction was complete and the liquids which flowed from it were then concentrated by evaporation and constituted a white powder which was called 'La Cantarella.' "

Several other contemporary writers claim to give the true method of its preparation, and one states that a bear was killed, then cut open and saturated with arsenic, and the liquid that dripped from it formed the poison.

This method of preparing a venom was employed by some of the Italian poisoners of the period. The combination of the animal poison contained in the products of putrefaction, together with arsenic, would no doubt furnish a poisonous substance of a very powerful nature, but there is no evidence to prove that the Borgias ever used such a preparation. Baron Corvo, in his CHRONICLES OF THE BORGIAS, denies that the family possessed any such secret, and declares that the venom never existed.

It is evident that the composition of the so-called "Cantarella," the poison said to have been employed by the Borgias, has long been a subject of dispute. According to Paolo Jovio, it was "a kind of whitish powder, that to a certain extent resembled sugar, and which has been used on a great many poor innocent people who died in a miserable state."

The probability is that when the Borgias found it necessary to use a poison for nefarious purposes they employed arsenic, which was so commonly used in Italy at that period.

Lucrezia Borgia has been accused of being guilty of the worst possible crimes, including that of poisoning, but there is said to be no historic proof of the truth of these stories. It is possible that many of the infamous crimes of her brother Cesare were erroneously attributed to her.

In justice to the Borgias one must try to visualize the condition of the people of Rome at this period. Poison may be said to have become a common weapon in this social and political life of the country. For the politician it was a weapon which procured him office, for the theologian a secret method of removing an enemy from his path, and so on throughout the whole social strata.

It seems appropriate that the earliest law to regulate the sale of poisons in mediaeval times should have been enacted in Italy. Thus as early as 1365, a statute was passed in Siena rendering it illegal to sell red arsenic or corrosive sublimate to any slave, freed or otherwise, or to any servant or person under twenty years of age. These poisons could only be sold to an adult who was well known to the apothecary.

FRENCH POISONERS

In the latter part of the sixteenth century the mania for criminal poisoning spread from Italy to France. The practice increased with great rapidity, and poisons appear to have been commonly employed by those of the highest to the lowest classes of society, to get rid of enemies and undesirable persons. The epidemic of poisoning was without precedent and L'Estoile says, in referring to the execution of a magician named La Miraille, that in Paris in 1572, the number of sorcerers and vendors of love-philtres was above thirty thousand. It is stated that the Prior of Cluny and his valet Saint-Barthélemi, with grim humour, even poisoned their physicians in order to avoid paying them. It may be said of the many stories of poison mysteries in France that have come down to us from the sixteenth century, that though their truth may be doubtful they are not without romantic interest.

Francis II, the first husband of Mary Queen of Scots, who died in 1560, was supposed to have succumbed to poison, and Beaucaire de Péguillon goes so far as to charge Ambroise Paré, the great military surgeon, with having been the cause of his death. The Duc d'Albe asserts that Mary Stuart was the cause of his death, but John Knox was nearer the mark when he wrote on hearing of it: "The potent hand of God from above sent unto us a wonderful and most joyful deliverance; for unhappy Francis, husband to our Sovereign, suddenly perisheth of a rotten ear . . . that deaf ear that never would hear the truth of God."

As a matter of fact, it was proved from an investigation by Courladon a few years ago, that Francis, who was born with an obstruction of the nose and mouth probably due to adenoids, died from chronic suppurative otitis.

A curious method of introducing poison is recorded in the story of the Cardinal of Lorraine, uncle of Mary Queen of Scots, who is said to have died after handling some gold coins on which poison had been smeared. There is, however, evidence to show that his death was due to pleurisy caused by a cold caught in walking barefooted at the head of a procession at Avignon.

Catherine de'Medici was credited with having poisoned her three sons, Charles IX, the Duc d'Anjou and Francis II, but the story has apparently no foundation.

The divorce proceedings between Henry IV and Marguerite de Valois were almost complete, when all preparations for the marriage of the King to Madame d'Estrées were brought to a sudden end in Holy Week, 1599, by her mysterious death. A post-mortem examination made by the doctors threw no light on the cause of death, and hints began to be spread abroad that she had been secretly poisoned by the Grand Duke of Tuscany. According to the story, she had arrived in Paris on Tuesday, April 6th, and stayed the night at the palace of Zametti, a wealthy Italian Jew. He presented her with an exquisite scent bottle containing a very powerful perfume. On the following Thursday, while in the Church of Saint-Antoine, she was taken ill with headache and vertigo and had to leave before the end of the service. Severe convulsive attacks followed, which increased in violence and frequency until she lost consciousness and died during the night of April 10th.

There appears little doubt that her death was due to eclampsia and her entire illness presents a true picture of this condition showing its various stages and lastly the end in coma. As the physicians were unable to account for her sudden death, rumors of poison soon gained currency.

Catherine de'Medici is said to have been instrumental in introducing the Italian methods of poisoning into France, and after her time deaths in Paris attributed to poisons increased to an alarming extent. Her Florentine perfumers were supposed to have been adepts in mixing poisons with sweetmeats and articles of food.

From the highest to the lowest all seem to have had the dread of meeting death in this way, and it is said that Henry IV, when a guest at the Louvre, ate only eggs which he cooked himself and drank only water which he drew from the Seine.

Toward the end of the seventeenth century the epidemic of poisoning appears to have again broken out and the feeling of alarm and insecurity was felt especially among people of the higher classes.

The Marquise de Brinvilliers was convicted of poisonings and shortly before her death she declared the poisonous substances she had employed, but said: "I do not know exactly what they were, I should like to know the composition of the poisons I used and which were used at my direction, but all I know about them is, there was toad's venom and that there were some that consisted of rarified arsenic."

It seems very probable that she acquired much of her knowledge of poisons from Glaser the apothecary, who states in his treatise on Chemistry that he was "an artist in his profession" and declares that he writes of "nothing he has not done and sets down as preparations but what I have made and well-experienced." Among the mineral poisons he describes are vitriol of Luna (silver), Lapis Infernalis (copper sulphate), sugar of lead, corrosive sublimate (mercury perchloride), antimony, in the form of tartar emetic and arsenic. He describes his rarified arsenic as having the same properties as antimony but more violent in action, and another powerful poison called the "corrosive liquor of arsenic." This was a combination of arsenic and corrosive sublimate made by mixing equal parts in powder and distilling them with water with slow heat. The result is a gummy liquor, "which hath the same properties as antimony but is more violent."

The following is the Marquise de Brinvilliers' recipe for making 'eye drops,' from a manuscript stated to be in her handwriting, (Translation):

"Recipe for the eyes

"Take six new laid eggs, harden them in hot ash, then shell them and afterwards remove their yolks, cutting them very neatly in half. Then re-fill the said eggs with sugar-candy and white copperas (zinc sulphate) in equal amounts well pulverized. Then join them together and tie them with thread, then attach them to a little stick so that they hang down, putting them thus hanging into the cellar, putting under them a glazed dish.

"Leave them for forty-eight hours in the cellar, then take the water which has distilled from the said eggs and put it in a phial. Then when one wishes to make use of it one must take a thimble full of it with two ounces of plaintain water. Mix together and put two or three drops of it into the eyes in the evening only, three times a week; and according as one find oneself benefitted by it, one must diminish (the amount) and only apply it twice and so on."

One of the worst of the poison-fiends in human shape was Catherine Deshayes, the wife of Antoine Monvoisin a peddling jeweler, who was popularly known as La Voisin. She practised as a fortune-teller and sorceress and although by no means beautiful she appears to have had an extraordinary influence over her dupes.

She received all kinds of secrets and confessions from her fashionable customers and had a regular trade in selling poisons to wives who wished to rid themselves of their husbands.

Madame de Montespan is said to have been one of her clients and it was La Voisin who provided her with "love-powders" to give Louis XIV which are declared to have been composed of cantharides, dried moles in powder and the blood of bats.

La Voisin's creatures claimed to know the secret of the particularly poisonous powder known as the *poudre de succession*, so-called from the real or supposed frequency with which it had been used to hasten or change the succession in the families of the rich. According to later writers, the *poudre de succession* consisted of arsenic, sometimes mixed with vegetable poisons such as aconite, belladonna and opium.

The question of the various poisons used during this period in France for criminal purposes has been investigated by Dr. Lucien Nass, who has had access to the documents relating to the various important trials that took place. He says, that according to police inventories of articles found in the domiciliary visits made by them in the course of their inquiries into these poisoning cases, many substances were employed. If one failed another was tried. The method of administration was varied with considerable ingenuity, and arsenic, opium, cantharides and lead acetate were the substances mostly used.

NAPOLEON AND POISONS

When Napoleon was driven from Leipzig in defeat and disaster, culminating in his abdication at Fontainebleau, it is said that he attempted to end his life by swallowing opium. During the retreat from Moscow, the Emperor is stated to have requested his physician to provide him with means to prevent his falling into the hands of the enemy alive, and was supplied with a drug which he carried in a small packet suspended round his neck. Either from the poison losing its properties or having become inocuous, it is stated "to have thrown Napoleon, after he took it, into a deep sleep, from which he awoke in spasms."

From these and other accounts he appears to have had a dread of being taken a prisoner alive, and Charles Louis Codet who was his personal pharmacist and accompanied him on his

Austrian campaign confirms this. Codet who died in 1821, in his biography states that after his return from Elba, Napoleon consulted him regarding the preparation of an infallible poison in as small a compass as possible, which he might use if the campaign should fail. Codet supplied him with the drug and it is said that the Emperor actually swallowed the poison after the battle of Waterloo, but quickly repenting of his act, he speedily obtained an emetic from Codet and got rid of the dose.

Spain also was not without its historic poisoning mysteries about this period. In September, 1689, Marie Louise the wife of King Carlos II of Spain was taken suddenly and seriously ill. After undergoing terrible sufferings, she died at the age of twenty-six years and it was officially announced that she had succumbed to an attack of cholera. Rumours were spread abroad that she had been poisoned and that her nails had fallen off before her death.

CHAPTER TWENTY-ONE

Love-Philters

THE EMPLOYMENT of certain substances having aphrodisiac properties in the form of charms or potions to incite the amatory passion has long been practised by both barbaric and civilized races.

The early Hebrews are said to have employed the fruits of the mandrake (not the American mandrake), which were known by the suggestive name of "love-apples," for this purpose.

The popularity of the *philtra* or *pocula amatoria* among the ancient Greeks and Romans at a later period can readily be understood in an age given to sensuality in its grossest forms. Medea was regarded as the greatest adept in the art of preparing philters, and hence the term "Medei de herbae," used by Horace and Ovid to designate the substances generally used. Next in reputation came the Thessalian women, who were supposed to have acquired the art from Medea, and who were said to be versed in all the secrets relating to poison and sorcery.

Many of the ingredients were both grotesque and filthy, such as "the hair that grew in the nether part of a wolf's tail, the penis of a wolf, the brain of a cat, the brain of a newt, the brain of a lizard, a certain fish called 'remora,' and the bones of a green frog which had been left bare by ants." Young swallows were buried in the earth and after a time disinterred.

The bodies of those that were found with open bills were believed to provoke love, while those with closed beaks were given to produce the opposite effect.

The testicles of certain animals were employed, selected doubtless for a physiological reason, and the menstrual blood, especially that of a red-haired woman, was highly esteemed and was believed to have powerful effects.

In the Anglo-Saxon Leechdoms, an ointment composed of goat's gall, incense, goat's dung and nettle seeds is recommended as an application to the genital organs to promote passion.

The mandrake root, which was a common ingredient in love-philters in ancient times, is still worn in some parts of France as a charm for that purpose, and in Germany a belief in the power of endive seed to influence the affections still exists.

In Italy, basil was used to inflame the heart of the indifferent, and a young man who accepted a sprig of this plant from the hand of a maiden was sure to be inspired with love for her. Satyrion is another herb for which amatory properties were claimed, while certain species of orchis, when eaten fresh, were believed to inspire pure love, and when dried were employed to check illicit passion.

Even at the present day belief in the efficacy of love-charms has not yet died out in some parts of England. Among the ignorant in some parts of the country "All Hallow E'en" is dedicated to the performance of certain love-charms, in which the gum-resin called dragon's blood and quicksilver play an important part.

Of other plants employed in the composition of love-philters, mention should be made of the cyclamen, carrot, purslane, cummin, maiden-hair, valerian, navel-wort, wild poppy, anemone, crocus, periwinkle, pansy and the root of the male fern, which has long had a reputation for inspiring the tender passion, although, curiously enough, its present use in medicine is as a vermifuge.

Love-philters and charms were also used by Eastern nations, and the Hindus still employ mango, champac, jasmine, lotus and asoka for this purpose. According to Albertus Magnus, the most powerful herb for promoting love is the "Provinsa," the secret of which, he says, has been handed down from the Chaldeans. The Greeks called it Vorax and it is thought to be the same plant now known to the Sicilians as "*Pizzu'ngurdu*," to which they attribute remarkable properties. They believe that if given surreptitiously it will provoke an ardent passion in the heart of the coldest and most chaste woman. The Sicilians have also great faith in the power of hemp to secure the affection of those on whom they set their hearts, and they gather the plant with certain ceremonies.

"As touching this kind of witchcraft," says a writer of the sixteenth century, "the principall part thereof consisteth in certain confections prepared by lewd people to procure love which indeed are mere poisons, bereaving some of the benefit of the braine and some of the sense and understanding of the minde."

Yet even such men as Van Helmont believed in the efficacy of the love-philter. Writing in the seventeenth century, he says: "I know a plant of common occurrence which if you rub and cherish it in the hand till it becomes warm, and take the hand of another and hold it until it becomes warm, that person will forthwith be stimulated with love for you and continue so for several days."

Reginald Scot states, wolf's penis was an ingredient in the love-philters of his time, and Frommaun mentions that human skull, coral, verbena, urine and leopard's dung were also employed in these concoctions.

Ginseng root, which has been used for centuries in China to promote longevity, was also recommended as a love-charm. It is believed by the Chinese to have the power of rejuvenating the old and stimulating the senses of the young.

Among primitive peoples the love-philter is still in vogue and is generally used among some tribes in Africa. It is a custom for a love-potion to be given by men and women to gain the hearts of those whom they desire, or to wrest affection from rivals.

The numerous wives of each chieftain are constantly employing these potions in order to secure the husband's affection and become his favorite.

That the effects of these philters were often dangerous and sometimes fatal is hardly to be wondered at, when we consider the extraordinary nature of some of the substances used in their composition. They were generally compounded with much mystery by the old or wise women, who had a reputation for sorcery, and they observed the greatest secrecy in their concoction.

Another substance highly esteemed as an ingredient in love-philters was the mysterious hippomanes, which he described as "a growth found on the forehead of a newly born foal," to which Ovid alludes in the following lines:

"Who so doth run to Haemon arts
I dub him for a dolt,
And giveth that which he doth pluck
From forehead of a colt.
Medea's herbs will not procure
That love shall lasting give,
No slibbersawces given to maids
To make them pale and wan
Will help; such slibbersawces mar the minds of
    maid and man,
And have in them a furious force of phrensie
    now and then."

Ovid, the exponent of the amatory art, judging from his verse, was evidently no believer in this method of procuring affection so much practised by his contemporaries.

CHAPTER TWENTY-TWO

Snakes in Medicine

EARLY medical men were greatly concerned about the snake. No other animal has been venerated so widely. Both in their profession and religious practices, the snake appeared to primitive doctors as a creature of great import. The present result of this long association of the doctor and the snake is that the caduceus, the wand of Hermes or Mercury, the messenger of the gods, consisting of two snakes entwined on a staff, is the symbol of the modern medical profession and may be found stamped upon the doctors' books, and military and naval uniforms, and upon the arms and crests of the medical schools and hospitals.

The mystical and medical powers of snakes were felt and acted upon in an early part of the Stone Age, and they are still worshipped and used for health charms and for healing the sick.

Snakes were found to haunt empty houses and tombs, and this characteristic led to the belief that snakes represented souls of ancestors who were revisiting the earth.

Snake worship has been common in all countries at some time in its history. This accounts for the vast lore of the serpent and associated animals. There were two aspects of snake worship: the worship of the snake as a symbol and as an actual god.

THE MYSTIC SACRED SNAKE

There were dark and hidden powers in the earth, in addition to the gods in the heavens, and these were given mysterious rituals. The Mother Earth was the most popular of the earth powers. Her followers were initiated into the mysteries of Eleusis so often mentioned by the classical writers. Dionysos and Asklepia were other earth powers. The serpent, coming out of the ground, naturally was related to the Mother Earth at an early period. In time the snake became a sacred and mystic animal, being endowed with magical powers relating to dreams, prophecies, and healing. Then it became the symbol of the underworld powers and was an associate of the physicians, who employed the tongues of serpents to cleanse ulcers and sores.

Asklepia was assigned the serpent as a ritualistic symbol, but many people often mistook the serpent or its statue as the god of medicine himself; and so we find Greek artists depicting men kneeling before the bronze model of a snake praying for relief for their ailments. The Greek Pantheon sheltered many divinities who possessed healing powers, but that of Asklepios (Aesculapius as the Romans knew him later) was the only practical healing cult developed. He was the embodiment of the earth spirit, and the serpent was his symbol and his aid. He not only possessed power to heal the sick, but also to bring the dead to life.

There was a legend relating that the secret of the healing skill of Asklepios and his followers was found, when one day, while walking in a garden, he saw a snake mourning over the dead body of another snake. After awhile, the living snake went about the garden looking at various plants. Finally, it bit off a branch of one herb, chewed the leaves, and forced the spittle into the mouth of the dead snake. Soon life revived in the dead snake, and it crawled off to its nest. Asklepios marveled at what he had seen, and noted the herb that had performed the miracle. Many cities called him the Physician.

The Athenians considered him a hero and invited him to be represented in their city, but they never made him a divinity.

Asklepia was carried to Rome in the year 291 B. C. in the form of a serpent, because the Delphic Oracle declared that was the only way to stay the plague then ravaging the city. Thereafter an Asklepieian cult was formed in Rome and the serpent became a familiar symbol everywhere.

This is a brief outline of the Chthonian associations of Asklepia and of the evolution of the serpent as a symbol of medicine and the medical profession.

Snakes performed other important duties. Sacred serpents were the locaters of shrine sites and the sites of temples and sanitariums. Snakes also chose many of the sites for the Asklepieia. One snake shipped to Cos escaped from the ship and swam ashore at Lakonia near Epidauros Limera. The site of its landing was immediately selected for an important shrine. Another serpent was sent to the sanctuary at Sikyon for healing purposes. It went in great state, drawn by a gayly caparisoned team of mules.

Temples of Asklepios were built in the eighth or early seventh century B. C. and over three hundred of them were built.

All the temples were built in elevated places amid ample grounds laid out with woods, lawns, and gardens. The site of every temple possessed a medicinal spring; because water was one great feature of the cures made by the priests. Usually a small serpent was pictured near the cypress tree of Asklepios to distinguish it from the sacred laurel of Artemis and the olive of Dionysus.

The temple snakes of the Asklepieia were large, yellow beasts caught in the Hieron Valley, tamed, and taught to lick the sleepers with their forked tongues. These snakes were perfectly harmless and easily domesticated.

Among the attributes given the snake by the ancient Greeks we find, Giver of Children, Restorer of Health and All-Wise. In one of the temples of Asklepieia a childless wife is represented as asleep and dreaming of a serpent that coils itself over her person! Should she subsequently conceive and bear a child, it will be proclaimed the son of Asklepieia.

Ancient of primative peoples throughout the world have had their snake totems, snake ancestors, snake gods and snake medicine. Theriac, from the Greek *theriakos*, pertaining to reptiles, was the result of the search for a cure-all, and was so named because it contained viper flesh.

Rattlesnake oil is considered by some in the United States to be a cure for all common ailments.

370

CHAPTER TWENTY-THREE

Folk Medicine

CHARMS, enchantments, amulets, incantations, talismans, phylacteries, and all the armoury of witchcraft and magic have been intimately mixed up with pharmacy and medicine in all countries and in all ages. If people believe that disease is caused by malign spirits, they usually assume that the way to cure it is to use some form of magic which will appease the evil spirits or frighten them away from the body they have attacked. Today, the carrying of a horse chestnut to ward off rheumatism, the wearing of a bag of camphor around the neck to avoid influenza, and superstitions in regard to horseshoes and the rabbit's foot are survivals of the ages of magic. Quackery is closely associated with magic. This appears to be because the human mind prefers delusions to truth, fallacies to realities. In the attempt to understand that part of folklore known as folk medicine, one must realize that practically nothing is known of its beginning nor of its development.

The whole of the magical rites associated with the art of healing were not based on conscious fraud. The beliefs of savage or untutored races in demons which cause diseases is natural, it may almost be said reasonable. What more natural when they see one of their tribe seized with an epileptic fit than to assume the presence of an invisible foe? Or if a contagious plague or smallpox or fever attacks their village, it is not an inevitable conclusion that angry spirits have attacked the tribe, perhaps for some unknown offence?

Medicine has grown out of and is deeply rooted in superstition. Superstition in its turn is traced back to a close allegiance with folklore or so-called folk medicine. Garrison says that it may be taken as proved that there is practical identity between folklore and primitive medicine. It would merely try the patience of the reader to enumerate even a tithe of the absurd things which have been and are being used by people, civilized and savage, as charms, talismans, and amulets.

Garrison associates the simple mind of aboriginal peoples with their inability to distinguish post from propter. This inability, he points out, is also a characteristic of the folk mind of today: Toads even today, Garrison says, are believed to cause warts, horse chestnuts to cure rheumatism, stump water to be good for freckles. In Norfolk, England, a spider tied up in a cloth bag and hung up over the mantelpiece, supposedly cures whooping cough. This same disease is treated in Donegal, by a beetle in a bottle; in Suffolk by dipping the child's head down in a meadow hole, in Lincolnshire by a meal of fried mice, in Yorkshire by owl broth.

The following tales may not be true but they are remarkable for twelfth-century recognition of healing by suggestion.

A member of the House of Buwayh suffered from the idea that he was a cow. Nothing could dispel this delusion, and the prince refused to eat, crying each day, "Kill me, so that a good stew may be prepared from my flesh." The situation grew so critical, that Avicenna was compelled to take charge of the case. He directed an assistant to shout that the butcher was on his way, and then Avicenna came with a cleaver, asking, "Where is this cow, that I may kill it?" Satisfied at last, the sick prince began to moo, and the physician ordered him thrown to the ground and bound with ropes; Avicenna felt him all over in the manner of a butcher, and announced, "This cow is too lean, and not ready for the slaughter; it must be fattened." The patient therefore ate, and with the return of strength, his mind was cured.

A young woman suffered from paralysis of the arms, and her physician asked her to stand in the presence of the assembled court; without warning, he removed her veil, causing her to blush deeply, and he added to the indignity by suddenly raising her clothes over her head; the young lady instinctively lifted her arms to pull down her garments, and was cured.

An emir was rheumatic, and could not walk, and Rhazes was summoned. Rhazes refused to cross the swollen Oxus in the boat provided for him, so the royal messengers carried him across as prisoner. His treatment was unsuccessful, and eventually he said, "Tomorrow I shall try a new treatment, but it will cost you the best horse and mule in your stable"; too ill to argue, the emir assented. Outside the city was a bath where Rhazes took his royal patient, they entered the hot room, and Rhazes carefully administered douches of hot water. Then he excused himself, and the emir was left sitting alone. When Rhazes returned he was fully dressed, and he menaced his naked patient with a knife, crying, "Thou didst order me to be bound and cast into the boat, and didst conspire against my life. If I do not destroy thee for this, my name is not Mohammed ibn Zakariyya." Consumed with fear and rage the crippled emir sprang to his feet.

He called his guards in vain, for the physician and his servant had escaped on the horse and mule that he had unwittingly provided. On the seventh day, the servant returned with the animals and this letter from Rhazes: "May the life of the King be prolonged in health and authority! Agreeably to my undertaking I treated you to the best of my ability. There was however a deficiency in the natural caloric, and this treatment would have been unduly protracted, so I abandoned it in favor of *psychotherapeusis*, and when the peccant humors had undergone sufficient coction in the bath, I deliberately provoked you in order to increase the natural caloric, which thus gained sufficient strength to dissolve the already softened humors. But henceforth it is inexpedient that we should meet." The grateful emir, rid of his rheumatism through psychotherapy, begged Rhazes to return for his fee, and despite his refusal, "rewarded him with a robe of honor, a cloak, a turban, arms, a male and female slave, and a horse fully caparisoned, and further assigned to him a yearly pension of 2000 gold dinars and 200 ass-loads of corn."

The Druids of Wales and the Celtic monks of Ireland and Scotland left an interesting lore. An example is a remedy for baldness, as follows:

"Let calcine a raven, his ashes boil in sheep's suet, and rub to the head, it cures.

With mice fill an earthen pipkin, stop the mouth with a lump of clay, and bury it beside a fire, but so as the fire's too great heat reach it not. So let it be then for a year, and at the year's end take out whatever may be found therein. But it is urgent that he who shall lift it have a glove on his hand, lest at his fingers' end the hair come sprouting forth."

An envious Druid gives Saint Patrick a cup of poisoned ale; the snake-banisher makes the sign of the cross, and recites the incantation: "Tuba fis fri ibu, fis ibu anfis; Fis bru uatha, ibu lithu," and adds the name of the Savior. At these words, the poison freezes and falls to the ground as he inverts the cup. The good ale remains, and the saint now quaffs it without harm.

"Amulets and things to be borne about I find prescribed, taxed by some, approved by others. Look for them in Mizaldus, Porta, Albertus, etc. A ring made with the hoof of an ass's right forefoot, carried about, etc. I say, with Renodeus, they are not altogether to be rejected. Piony doth help elipepsies. Pretious stones most diseases. A wolf's dung carried about helps the cholick. A spider an ague, etc. Such medicines are to be exploded that consist of words, characters, spells, and charms, which can do no good at all, but out of a strong conceit, as Pomponatious proves, or the devil's policy, that is the first founder and teacher of them."

Burton's "ANATOMY OF MELANCHOLY."

Pythagoras taught that holding dill in the left hand would prevent epilepsy. Serapion of Alexandria (B. C. 278) prescribed for epilepsy the warty excrescences on the forelegs of animals, camel's brain and gall, rennet of seal, dung of crocodile, blood of turtle, and other animal products.

ENGLISH FOLKLORE SUPERSTITIONS

Sir Kenelm Digby's method for curing a toothache: He directed that the patient should scratch his gum with an iron nail until he made it bleed, and should then drive the nail with the blood upon it into a wooden beam. He will never have toothache again, says this sage.

For warts the cures are innumerable. They are all more or less like this: "Steal a piece of meat from a butcher's stall or basket, bury it secretly at a gateway where four lanes meet. As the meat decays the warts will die away. An apple cut into slices and rubbed on the warts and buried is equally efficacious. So is a snail which after being rubbed on the warts is impaled on a thorn and left to die."

The prejudice in favour of red flannel which still exists, for tying a piece of it round sore throats is probably a remnant of the fancy that red was specially obnoxious to evil spirits.

TRANSFERRING DISEASES

It was widely believed that disease could be transferred by means of certain silly formalities. This was a very ancient notion. Pliny explains how pains in the stomach could be transferred to a duck or a puppy.

In Devonshire a child could be cured of whooping cough by putting one of its hairs between slices of bread and butter and giving these to a dog. If the dog coughed, as was probable, the whooping cough was transferred.

CONSTRICTION DEVICES

In the nineteenth and twentieth centuries constriction has been, and is still, held in great esteem. "Electric" belts are sold to credulous laymen, metallic finger rings are worn for the cure of rheumatism, and many old women wear tight garters around their legs to prevent cramp.

Pliny said: "If young twigs are made into a collar and put around a cock's neck, it will never grow."

The kings of England dispensed "cramp rings" to be used for preventing cramps and fits. Henry VIII, even after his separation from the Church, continued the practice, and there is in existence a letter from Anne Boleyn which tells of their distribution. It reads: "Mr. Stephens, I send you here cramp rings for you and Mr. Gregory and Mr. Peter, praying you to distribute them as you think best—Anne Boleyn." The practice of providing cramp rings was discontinued by Edward VI. Queen Elizabeth had a blessed ring which she wore suspended between her breasts. The ring had "the virtue of expelling infected air." It was analogous to the asafetida bags of later days.

THE ABRACADABRA MYSTERY

The abracadabra was the most famous of the ancient charms or talismans employed in medicine. Its mystic meaning has been the subject of much ingenious investigation, but even its derivation has not been agreed upon. With the passing of Galen at the end of the second century it became the distaff of the age. It is not known whether written by Serenus Sammonicus, or by his son who bore the same name, but the rubbish has survived.

Serenus Sammonicus explained that the entire word, Abracadabra, must be written out on the first line, and a letter dropped with each succeeding line, thus forcing the demon of the disease gradually to release its grip upon its victim. The sick wore this magic word and it was repeated in countless incantations.

CHAPTER TWENTY-FOUR

Is There Anything New Under The Sun?

IT IS SAID that a little part of everything in the past survives today. There is not a single development, even the most advanced of contemporary medicine, which is not to be found in embryo in the medicine of the olden time.

In very ancient times professors in luxurious medical colleges were giving lectures to students from all parts of the world. Their extensive knowledge of drugs was handed down to them from a remote antiquity.

These peoples were quite as advanced in their pathological knowledge as in their therapeutics. In dentistry, surgery, and as oculists and specialists in diseases of the eye, and in fevers, they have perhaps rarely been excelled. They were the heirs of many previous great ages, running back hundreds of thousands of years, and, when we study the records of Babylon and contemporary cities, we find that the physicians practiced under an efficient government with an excellent legal code and a good system of education.

No new basis type of disease has been shown to have occurred within geological times; but there is abundant evidence that all the common diseases of animals, plants, and insects are of the greatest antiquity. Wounded animals, plants, and insects appear in remote antiquity. They became infected with bacteria and bacilli precisely as they do today. Links in the chain of life that continue today have always been subject to the same disabilities.

Recent studies of the cave bones discovered in Europe show that fractures were well set, and that many surgical operations were carried out, by the surgeons of the Stone Age, and museum specimens show us that during the early Egyptian dynasties the physicians had a good knowledge of oral surgery and were expert operators.

The Egyptians used many animal remedies, just as we today use testicular, ovarian, liver, adrenal, thyroid and other animal extracts, therefore, the Egyptians are the forerunners of organotherapy.

The story of the medical school of Salerno illustrates very well how old is the new in education—even in medical education. There is scarcely a phase of modern interest in medical education that may not be traced very clearly at Salerno though the school began its career a thousand years ago, and ceased to attract much attention over six hundred years ago.

The Salerno treatment of goitre—the enlargement and over-action of the thyroid gland in the neck—has been improved on only in the details of technique. Medical treatment was always tried first. Today these patients are given small doses of iodine. The Four Masters achieved the same effect by giving ashes of seaweed, which has a high iodine content. If this failed, then resort was had to surgery.

Although blood transfusion was performed as early as the seventeenth century, it was not until the twentieth century that the operation became thoroughly practicable.

Some of the medical aphorisms used centuries before the Christian Era are still applicable:

"Life is short, and the medical art long; the opportunity fleeting, experiment dangerous and judgment difficult. Yet we must be prepared not to do our duty ourselves only, but also patients, attendants, and external circumstances must co-operate.

"For extreme diseases, extreme methods of cure.

"The aged endure fasting most easily; next adults; then young persons, and least of all children, and especially such as are most active and wide-awake.

"Growing bodies contain the most innate heat; they require therefore the most nourishment, and if they lack it they waste away. In the aged there is little heat, and therefore they require little food. Similarly, fevers in the aged are not so acute because they cannot be so well sustained.

"In diseased states sleep that is laborous is a deadly symptom; but when sleep relieves, the indications are good.

"Sleep that puts an end to delirium is also a favorable symptom.

"When a patient eats well, and fails to put on flesh, the symptom is bad.

"Food or drink which is a little less good but more palatable is to be preferred to such that is better but less palatable.

"Old people generally have fewer complaints than the young; but those chronic diseases which do befall them generally never leave them."

The Therapeutic Papyrus mentions many drugs that are in common use today. The ancient Egyptians had an assortment of surgical instruments and the actual cautery were in use, also steam inhalations, massage, ointments, plasters, poultices, suppositories, injections and emetics, and the importance of temperature in disease was to some extent recognized.

Chinese medical authors have been numerous from the most remote periods. Before the Christian Era volumes were written on various branches of medical practice; and the art had been reduced to a sort of system as early as the days of Solomon, or the siege of Troy.

Hippocrates enumerated the names of four hundred substances which physicians prescribed in his time. The bulk of these were handed down to the Greeks from the early Asiatic peoples, and the majority of the effective remedies came from the Near East. Pharmacists at that time were familiar with fomentations, gargles, sprays, pills, lozenges, inhalations, sulphur baths for skin diseases, suppositories, pessaries, poultices, sticking plasters, ointments, cerates, and collyria.

Avicenna, one of the later Arabian savants in medicine, introduced the gilding and silvering of pills to enhance their therapeutic values.

Moses taught two clear conceptions of sanitation—the importance of cleanliness and the possibility of controlling epidemic diseases by isolation and quarantine.

Architects of the present day go back to the hospitals of the Middle Ages in order to find the models for hospitals for the modern times. Mr. Arthur Dillon, a well-known New York architect, writing of a hospital built at Tonnerre in France, toward the end of the thirteenth century (1292), says:

"It was an admirable hospital in every way, and it is doubtful if we today surpass it. It was isolated; the ward was separated from the other buildings; it had the advantage we so often lose of being but one story high, and more space was given to each patient than we can now afford.

"The ventilation by the great windows and ventilators in the ceiling was excellent; it was cheerfully lighted; and the arrangement of the gallery shielded the patients from dazzling light and from draughts from the windows and afforded an easy means of supervision, while the division by the roofless low partitions isolated the sick and obviated the depression that comes from sight of others in pain.

"It was, moreover, in great contrast to the cheerless white wards of today. The vaulted ceiling was very beautiful; the woodwork was richly carved, and the great windows over the altars were filled with colored glass. Altogether it was one of the best examples of the best period of Gothic Architecture."

CHAPTER TWENTY-FIVE

Pharmacy

PHARMACY, or the art of selecting, extracting, preparing, and compounding medicines from vegetable, animal, and mineral substances, is an acquirement which must have been almost as ancient as man himself on the earth. The Greek word, pharmakeia, the original of our "pharmacy," had a rather mixed history in its native language. It does not seem to have exactly deteriorated, as words in all languages have a habit of doing, for from the earliest times it was used concurrently to describe the preparation of medicines, and also through its association with drugs and poisons and the production of philters as equivalent to sorcery and witchcraft.

The word "pharmakoi" in later times came to be used for the criminals who were sacrificed for the benefit of the communities, and thus it acquired its lowest stage of signification. It is remarkable and unusual for a word which has once fallen as this one did to recover its respectable position again.

Chiron, the centaur, is the originator of the pharmaceutic art, according to the mythological tale. It was he who taught Aesculapius, another mythical character commonly accepted as the patron saint of medicine. Aesculapius and Hercules are said to be the forbears of Hippocrates, who was a real character of the fifth century B. C., and from whose period the history of medicine and pharmacy may be said to begin.

The earliest records of pharmacy go back to the days before Tutankhamun, who was laid away in regal splendor in the Valley of the Kings in that country where Isis and Osiris were the dominating deities. The oldest prescriptions are found in the hieratic writing (or writing of the priesthood) of ancient Egypt.

There are several medical prescriptions in the British Museum which have never been translated nor photographed, and which are said to date from the time of Cheops, about 3700 B. C. From the ruins at Pompeii come records showing the use in the medicine and pharmacy of those days of aconite, acacia, colocynth, elaterium, garlic, anise, and mallow, and castor oil seeds have been found in the tombs of the Egyptians.

Primitive man, like every member of the animal kingdom, and like the insects, appears to have instinctly appealed to special vegetable extracts for remedies against physical ills. In the course of time certain men and women showed a special aptitude for finding such medical remedies and became herbalists. At the dawn of history we find there were herbalists everywhere who had a large store of remedies. These embryo pharmacists developed into regular drug store proprietors in Nineveh, Babylon, and in the Egyptian and Carthaginian cities, and in Athens and Rome the Pharmacies were large, finely furnished offices where medical men were wont to meet.

Several medical papyri have been discovered in Egypt, the Kahun Papyrus dating from 2000 B. C. As regards materia medica the Egyptians possessed the following drugs: lactuca, various salts of lead, such as the sulphate, with the action of which in allaying local inflammation they were well acquainted; pomegranate and acanthus pith as vermifuges; peppermint, sulphate and acetate of copper, oxide of antimony, sulphide of mercury, petroleum, nitrate of potash, castor-oil, opium, coriander, absinthe, juniper (much used as a diuretic), caraway, lotus, gentian, mustard, ox-gall, aloe, garlic, and various bitter infusions; mandragora, linseed, squills, saffron, resin, and various turpentine products; cassia, certain species of cucumis, cedar-oil, yeast, colchicum, nasturtium, myrrh, tamarisk, powdered lapis lazuli, vinegar, indigo; the oasis onion, mastic and various gums, mint, fennel, henbane or hyoscyamus, magnesia, sebeste (a tonic and a cough medicine), lime, soda, iron, and a great number of other agents, the names of which no one at present can translate.

Precious stones were employed in a finely divided condition and there were special distinctions, according to the ability of the patient to pay. Thus, emerald was used for the plutocrat and green porcelain for the proletariat; lapsis lazuli and sapphire were replaced in a similar manner by blue glass when occasion required.

The ancients used all kinds of substances as medicines— animal, vegetable and mineral. Those drawn from the animal kingdom form the most disgusting portion of the materia medica, which consisted of the flesh of lizards, crocodiles, vipers, the brains of wolves, the heads of mice, the bodies of moles, the livers, lungs, blood and organs of generation of animals, etc. This would not have been so bad, but they used the excrements of various animals, both internally and externally. The entire bodies of patients were frequently anointed with cow-manure, for numerous diseases; and poultices of mashed spiders were bound to the temples; and the heart of the hare was worn upon the back of the neck, for the cure of malarious intermittents. Newly-born puppies were boiled and eaten, for the purpose of preserving the patient from attacks of colic during the remainder of his days.

Chin-Nong, Emperor of China, who died 2699 B. C., is reckoned to have been the founder of pharmacy in the Far East. He studied plants and composed a Herbal used to this day. It is related of him that he discovered seventy poisonous plants and an equal number of antidotes to them. Other Oriental countries also have their pharmaceutical lore reaching back into forgotten ages. Japan, India, Persia—all can claim a share in the common heritage of pharmaceutical practices and traditions.

Between Hippocrates and Galen an interval of some six hundred years elapsed and, especially in the latter half of that period, pharmacy developed into enormous importance. Not that it necessarily advanced. It was during the interval between Hippocrates and Galen that the many sects of ancient medicine, the Dogmatics, the Stoics, the Empirics, the Methodics, and the Eclectics were born and flourished.

The Empirics were the boldest users of drugs. One of the most famous doctors of this sect, Heraclides, made several narcotic compounds which are commended by Galen. One of these formulae prescribed for cholera was 2 drms. of henbane seeds, 1 drm. of anise, and ½ drm. of opium, made into 30 pills, one for a dose. Another which was recommended for coughs was composed of 4 drms. each of juice of hemlock, juice of henbane, castorum, white pepper, and costus; and 1 drm. each of myrrh and opium.

There can be no question that the Empirics did a great deal to increase the medical knowledge of ancient times. During the third century before Christ, pharmacology began to take on a rapid development, and this was in great measure the fruit of the work of the Empirics. The pharmacologists of the days of the Roman Empire, Galen not excepted, borrowed freely from empirical sources.

It is generally conceded that opium, brought into general medical esteem by the empirics, is the most valuable drug in materia medica. The therapeutic reputation of opium was established by the foremost physicians. Franciscus Sylvius said he would not practise without opium; van Helmont prescribed it so frequently that he was called Doctor Opiatus.

It was the one universal medicine, the gift of the East to the West, a drug in whose traffic ignorance and corruption had combined to abuse its salutary uses. An expensive medicine, it was adulterated with dirt and inert material, and even bullets were added to increase its weight. No careful assays were required by law as they are today, and the opium purchased in the open markets of London and Edinburgh was notoriously variable in its potency and uncertain in its effects.

GREEKS IN ROME

The Greeks in Rome in pharmacy, as in medicine, were the bright lights of the period.

DIOSCORIDES, as has already been mentioned, was the greatest of the medical botanists.

MENECRATES, physician to the emperor Tiberius, labored industriously over his 155 works, including a treatise on pharmacology, but he is now remembered for his early use of escharotics, as the first who suggested that in prescriptions the capricious signs for weights be discarded in favor of actual figures, and as the inventor of the famous Diachylon Plaster.

ANTONIUS MUSA introduced into therapeutics the lettuce—of which he was an ardent champion—and chicory and endive; his brother Euphorbus was medical adviser to King Juba of Mauritania, who discovered near Mount Atlas the medical plant which he named Euphorbia in honor of his physician. Musa holds no rank among the great physicians of antiquity, but he is of historic interest because his popularity with the masters of his day acted as an antidote to the warning of Cato: "I forbid you to have anything to do with physicians."

SCRIBONIUS LARGUS, whose book on the compounding of medicines may be regarded as the earliest of pharmacopeias, was received with favor by the emperor Claudius. Scribonius acted as physician to Claudius' third wife, the loving Messallina, who was always ready to doff the purple robes of office to appear naked in the public brothel. The relationship between this medicus and the warm blooded spouse of Claudius was evidently strictly professional, in which respect the discreet Scribonius differed from his colleague Vettius Valens, who not only prescribed for his young empress, but committed adultery with her—until the day of discovery.

Scribonius Largus deserves a wreath as one of the few practitioners of his age who honored the Hippocratic Oath, as the first who presented an accurate method of obtaining opium, and as the first who suggested the repeated application of the electric ray-fish in headache and facial neuralgia, which is probably the earliest use of electricity in therapeutics.

DAMOCRATES, physician to Nero, is said to have originated a tooth powder famous in his time and for centuries thereafter, and to have also popularized many liniments, electuaries, poultices, and plasters.

PHARMACY IN ARABIA

The Arabians preserved the pharmaceutic art and carried the torch of professional and scientific knowledge from the sixth to the thirteenth centuries.

The Arabs were well skilled in pharmacy and added much valuable information about their actions. They were also responsible for the abracadabra which until recent times played such a great role as a curative agency.

The Arabians established the first pharmacies; fostered the early steps of chemistry; discovered nitric acid, aqua regia, red precipitate, corrosive sublimate; either introduced or popularized such important drugs as camphor, rhubarb, senna, cassia fistula, nux vomica, nutmeg, tamarinds, musks and clove; observed that colchicum is beneficial in gout; and gave us juleps, alkali and alembic. They certainly introduced syrups into pharmacy. They also brought the process of distillation to the attention of the world, if they did not invent it, thus giving us alcohol and the various tinctures made therefrom.

Medical historians do not allow that they contributed much original service to either anatomy, physiology, pathology, or surgery; but it is admitted by every student that their maintenance of scholarship through the half dozen centuries during which Europe was sunk in the most abject ignorance and superstition entitles them to the gratitude of all who have lived since.

It was the Arabs who raised pharmacy to its proper dignity. We do not read of any noted pharmacists among them who were not physicians, but the latter were all keen students of the materia medica, and occupied themselves largely with pharmaceutical studies. But it is evident that there was a distinct profession of pharmacy.

ALEXANDER OF TRALLES, who lived in the sixth century A. D., used rhubarb as an astringent and cantharides as a blister. He also used colchicum in gout and reintroduced that then almost forgotten combination of aloe and canella called *hiera picra* (literally sacred bitters).

ABU-MOUSSAH-DSCHAFAR-AL-SOLI, commonly called Geber, the equivalent of his middle name, is supposed to have lived in the eighth century. From him are dated the introduction into science, to be adopted later in medicine, of corrosive sublimate, of red precipitate, of nitric and nitro-muriatic acids, and of nitrate of silver. Geber is the first of the chemical authorities who describes in detail the operations of distillation, sublimation, and calcination.

AVICENNA was born at Bokhara in 980. He often prescribed camphor, and alluded to several different kinds; a solution of manna was a favorite medicine with him; he regarded corrosive sublimate as the most deadly of all poisons, but used it externally; iron he had three names for, probably different compounds; he had great faith in gold, silver, and precious stones. It has already been mentioned that it was probably he who introduced the silvering and gilding of pills to add to their medicinal effect.

389

In the tenth century in Saxon England many old documents were translated and explained, and from these the ideas of medicine in these islands a thousand years ago were made manifest. A Saxon Herbarium was written about the year 1000.

The genealogy of the modern druggist goes back to the Norman Conquest in the eleventh century, when the mercers, whose scene of operation in London was known as the Mercery, controlled the trade in drugs and spices. This business gradually passed into the hands of the pepperers and spicers of Sopers Lane and Chepe. By the time of Edward III it had been absorbed by the grocers, and Bucklersbury, its headquarters, became a famous section of old London. In fact at this time most people with minor complaints went directly to the apothecary. He prescribed for them without further ado, or if necessary secured a physician's advice, the patient himself never seeing the doctor.

In England in the twelfth century some physicians were beginning to devote themselves particularly to the compounding of medicines, and they became known as apothecaries.

RICHARD FITZNAGEL, one of the first of these apothecaries was appointed to the Court of Henry II. He became Bishop of London, and died in A. D. 1198. The prescriptions in vogue at that time were remarkable alike for the number and variety of their ingredients. Notable amongst them was theriac, a compound with a chequered history.

AVERROES OR AVERRHOES, born at Cordova in 1126, was an outstanding pharmaceutical authority in the West. He was a freethinker, who raised doubts concerning the creeds of both the Mohammedans and Christians and was accordingly hated by both. His most famous pharmaceutical work is the COLLIGET, which later appeared in many editions and translations.

There were four outstanding figures in the thirteenth century. These were Roger Bacon, Albertus Magnus, Raymond Lully, and Arnold of Villanova.

ROGER BACON did not have as close contacts with pharmacy as had the others, but he stands out as the first really great character in general science for more than thirty generations. He was born in 1210 and died in 1292. He was an English Franciscan monk, and has been aptly described as a modern scientist living centuries before methods of modern scientific thinking were known.

ALBERTUS MAGNUS was born in 1193 and died in 1280. He was a member of the Dominican Order, and was successively engaged as a teacher at the University of Paris and the University of Cologne. He did not write on medical practice, as this branch of learning was forbidden to members of his order. He wrote instead on natural history subjects and alchemy.

He was one of the first authors to intelligently describe the concentration of alcohol by distillation.

RAYMOND LULLY was born in 1235 and died in 1315. He was a native of Majorca and was a sedate family man with a wife, two sons, and a daughter at the age of 22. He then commenced to lead a wild life and became a libertine. One of the objects of his affection was a virtuous married woman of Majorca, who, in order to check his ardor, showed him her breast, which had been ravaged by cancer. This affected him so strongly that he immediately renounced not only his wild life but his family as well, and set out to study medicine with the object of discovering a cure for such a terrible disease. Later he went to Tunis and tried to convert the natives to Christianity, and was stoned to death for his zeal.

Lully is most famous in pharmaceutical history for his introduction into the profession of the alcoholic preparations of drugs known as tinctures. He had learned the art of concentrating alcohol both by distillation and by dehydration. Lully also is credited with the earliest description of the methods of preparing ammonium carbonate, nitric acid, red precipitate, and white precipitate.

Lully's SECRETA SECRETORUM is really a pharmaceutical formulary.

ARNOLD OF VILLANOVA was the last of the four great figures of the thirteenth century. He was a Spaniard and was born in 1235 and died in 1320. He was educated at Montpellier and traveled extensively, during which time he met Raymond Lully, and each seems to have influenced the other.

He had the same high regard for the physiological effect of alcoholic distillates as is attributed to Lully, and shares the honors, too, with that authority in the matter of using alcohol as a menstruum for tinctures. He came under the ban of the Church before his death as a heretic and fled to Sicily, where he died.

Pliny describes the obtaining of oil of turpentine by heating resin and collecting the liquefied vapor on wool which was suspended over the heated resin.

THOMAS AQUINAS, one of the greatest of scholastics, was a pupil of Albertus Magnus. Thomas Aquinas first used the word "amalgam" to describe the combination of mercury with another metal.

Beckmann gives much minute information concerning the establishment of apothecaries' shops in the chief cities of Germany. He mentions a conjecture that there was a pharmacy at Augsburg in the thirteenth and fourteenth centuries, but exact dates begin with the fifteenth century.

Distillation is a very ancient process. Evidence exists of its use by the Chinese in the most remote period of their history, and possibly they distilled wine. But so far as can be

392

traced spirit was not produced from wine previous to the thirteenth century.

It is worth remarking that when Henry II invaded and conquered Ireland in the twelfth century the inhabitants were making and drinking a product which they termed uisgebeatha, now abbreviated into whisky, the exact meaning of the name being water of life.

Raymond Lully, who acquired much of his chemical lore from Arnold of Villanova, was even more enthusiastic in praise of the aqua vitae than his teacher. "The taste of it exceedeth all other tastes, and the smell all other smells," he wrote. Elsewhere he describes it as "of marveylous use and commoditie a little before the joyning of battle to styre and encourage the soldiers' minds." He believed it to be the panacea so long sought, and regarded its discovery as evidence that the end of the world was near.

We are now coming to the time when pharmacy emerges more generally as a distinct and separate calling. There is quite a difference of opinion among historians as to whether the Crusades really influenced the progress of the sciences.

Whether or not the evidence is apparent as to the effect of the Crusades, we must admit that the thirteenth century is notable for the great intellectual awakening which occurred simultaneously throughout Europe.

The fifteenth century opened without any outward evidence of the marvelous changes it was to bring forth. During the centuries that had passed since the time of Geber there had grown up a new science, or rather pseudo-science, called alchemy, which had its contacts with both pharmacy and medicine.

It was in this period that there appeared the first establishments in which pharmacy was practiced as a profession separate from that of healing, although this was by no means universal.

The botanist was the physician-pharmacist who collected his own samples and subjected them to trial. The chemist was the physician-pharmacist who subjected mineral substances to various influences and observed and recorded the changes which took place. We find pharmacy, therefore, inextricably interwoven with the history of medicine and of chemistry.

The compendium of medicine of Gilbertus Anglicanus was more of a pharmaceutical than a medical work. He is the earliest author to describe minutely the method of "extinguishing" mercury to make "blue ointment." He gives details of the method of preparing a solution of potassium carbonate, which at that time was known under the title of "*oleum tartari per deliquum.*" He anticipated Minderer by several hundred years in proposing a solution of ammonium acetate for use in medicine. He gave a prescription for apoplexy for which the pharmacist had to procure ants' eggs, oil of scorpions, and lions' flesh. For calculi he employed the blood of a goat which had been fed upon diuretic herbs.

The earliest record of the exercise of authority over apothecaries in England is found in 1456, when a fine was imposed on John Ashfield "for making untrue powder of ginger, cinnamon, and saunders."

BASIL VALENTINE, at the very end of the Middle Ages, became the father of modern pharmaceutical chemistry. In chemistry the advances made during the thirteenth, fourteenth, and fifteenth centuries were, perhaps, even more noteworthy than those in any other department of science. During the fourteenth century, Arnold of Villanova, the inventor of nitric acid, and the two Hollanduses, kept up the tradition of original investigation in chemistry.

It is not surprising, then, to have a great investigating pharmacologist come along sometime about the beginning of the fifteenth century, when, according to the best authorities, Basil Valentine was born.

Basil Valentine did so much for the science of the composition of substances that he eminently deserves the designation that has been given him of the last of the alchemists and the first of the chemists. There is practically a universal recognition of the fact now that he deserves also the title of the Founder of Pharmaceutical Chemistry, not only because of the value of the observations contained in his writings, but also because of the fact that they proved so suggestive to certain scientific geniuses during the century succeeding Valentine's life.

Pharmacy seems at first glance to have made but little progress during the fifteenth century, but when we reach the next century we shall see that this period of apparent stagnation was in reality but a marking time, or a pausing for breath, for in proportion as alchemy recedes from the centre of the stage, pharmacy advances to the foreground.

The sixteenth century was the one in which the theriacs made their last stand in the original complicated form.

Early in the sixteenth century a number of Pharmacopoeias were published, beginning with "Bancke's Herbal" in 1525. This was followed by the London Pharmacopoea, work upon which was begun in 1589, and afterward many others followed.

A prominent pharmacist and physician of this period named Bulleyn, who is said to have been a cousin of Anne Boleyn, one of the King's numerous wives, laid down the following rules for the practice of pharmacy:

The apothecary must first serve God; foresee the end, be cleanly, and pity the poor. His place of dwelling and shop must be cleanly, to please the senses withal. His garden must be at hand with plenty of herbs, seeds, and roots. He must read Dioscorides. He must have his mortars, stills, pots, filters, glasses, boxes, clean and sweet. He must have two places in his shop, one most clean for physic and the base place for chirurgic stuff. He is neither to decrease nor diminish the physician's prescriptions. He is neither to buy nor sell rotten drugs. He must be able to open well a vein, for to help pleurisy. He is to meddle only in his own vocation, and to remember that his office is only to be the physician's cook.

DR. SAMUEL GARTH, a physician, politician, and litterateur of his time, wrote the following description of the seventeenth century apothecary and his shop:

> "Long has he been of that amphibious fry,
> Bold to prescribe and busie to apply,
> His shop the gazing vulgar's eyes employs
> With foreign trinkets and domestick toys.
> Here mummies lay most reverently stale,
> And there the tortoise hung her coat of mail;
> Not far from some large shark's devouring head,
> The flying fish their finny pinions spread.
> Aloft in rows large poppy heads were strung,
> And near, a scaly alligator hung,
> In this place drugs in musty heaps decayed,
> In that dried bladders and drawn teeth were laid."

The pharmaceutical and chemical progress of the seventeenth century shows remarkable advances over that of the preceding century.

The sixteenth century legislation which had united the apothecaries and grocers in Great Britain had also given the members of the Faculty of Medicine the right to practice medicine, pharmacy, and surgery. The assistants and apprentices of these medical men were called apothecaries and they performed minor surgical and medical duties, compounded their masters' prescriptions, and prepared the stock supplies of medicines.

As these assistants became skilled in the art of pharmacy they established themselves independently as apothecaries and united with the grocers in a common guild in 1606. This guild however, was subservient in some respects to the physicians, for the members were warned that when they made a dispensation of medicine (probably meaning theriac in particular) they should "expose the several ingredients to open view in their shops for six or eight days so that the physicians passing by might judge of the goodness thereof, and prevent their buying and selling any corrupt or decayed medicines."

It is natural to suppose that there would be resentment on the part of the apothecaries, both against the humiliation of being subservient to the physicians, and also against being forced to unite with the grocers, with whom they had little in common. The apothecaries soon took steps to sever their connection with the guild of grocers, and appealed to James I, who was King.

King James, in 1617, gave the apothecaries a separate charter and an independent existence as a restricted guild which has never admitted to its active membership any but actual practitioners of pharmacy. There are said to have been only 114 apothecaries in London in 1617, the year that the charter was granted to the Guild.

The Grocers' Guild resented the attainment of independence of the apothecaries, probably on account of the loss in membership which followed the withdrawal. The Grocers' Company, in 1624, petitioned the King in opposition to the new guild.

King James said to the grocers, in reply to their protest: "Grocers are but merchants; the business of the apothecary is a mystery; wherefore I think it fitting that they should be a corporation of themselves." The meaning of the word "mystery" at that time, used in such a context as that given above, was "art, craft, or profession," as opposed to merchandising.

ROBERT BOYLE, the most famous chemist of the seventeenth century, was born in 1627. He is known as the Father of Modern Chemistry. His early education was obtained at Eton College and he later traveled on horseback through Europe with a tutor. In 1654 Boyle went to Oxford.

Even the best of the scientists of that time had their weak spots. Boyle's was pharmacy and medicine. He left a book of medical recipes which in these days would excite ridicule.

The first ether made for medicinal purposes was manufactured in the laboratory directed by Robert Boyle.

JEAN BAPTISTE VAN HELMONT was born in Brussels in 1577 and died near there in 1644. He studied at Louvain, where he refused a degree because, as he said "academic distinctions ministered to pride." He studied medicine and was made professor of surgery at Louvain. He left the University and the practice of medicine because, having contracted the itch, he was nearly killed by the purging and ineffectual internal dosing of the regular physicians, while an itinerant quack quickly cured him with a preparation of sulphur applied externally. This made him a violent anti-Galenist, and a devoted disciple of the teachings of Paracelsus.

His principal chemical achievement was in connection with the discovery or rather identification of carbon dioxide. He traced this gas through many of its combinations and obtained it from various sources. He named it *gas sylvestre* or the "wild and untamed gas." He coined the word "gas," which had never before been used, in connection with this investigation.

JOHN RUDOLPH GLAUBER, who was born at Carlstadt, in Germany, in 1603, contributed largely to pharmaceutical knowledge. According to his own account he took to chemistry when as a young man he got cured of a troublesome stomach complaint by drinking some mineral waters. Eager to discover what was the essential chemical in those waters to which he owed his health he set to work on his experiments. The result was the discovery of sulphate of soda, which is called "Sal admirabile," but which all subsequent generations have known as Glauber's Salts.

Glauber was the first to distil ammoniacal liquor from bones and to synthetically prepare ammonium sulphate and ammonium chloride.

PIERRE SEIGNETTE, apothecary at Rochelle, in 1672, introduced the combination of sodium and potassium tartrate known as Rochelle salt; while in the waters of Epsom, Nehemiah Grew discovered magnesium sulphate.

Many preparations which are still in use originated during the seventeenth century. Among these are the following: Cinchona, coca, ipecac, potassium acetate (1610), milk sugar (1619), and others.

PETER ANDREW MATTHIOLUS, born at Sienna in 1500, died at Trent in 1577, the first who is known for certain to have administered mercury internally. Paracelsus, however, was without doubt the practitioner who popularized its use. He gave red precipitate, corrosive sublimate, and nitrate of mercury, and describes how each of these was made.

Calomel was introduced into practice by Sir Theodore Turquet de Mayerne about the year 1608. It has been said that he was the inventor of the product, but as it was described and, perhaps, to some extent used by other medical authorities, Crollius among these, who lived and died before Turquet was born, this was evidently impossible.

Van Swieten's solution of corrosive sublimate was introduced in the middle of the eighteenth century as a remedy for syphilis, and for a long time was highly esteemed.

Tin came into medical use in the Middle Ages, and acquired its position particularly as a vermifuge. For this purpose tin had a reputation only second to mercury.

The earliest known description of zinc as a metal is found in the treatise on minerals by Paracelsus, and it is he who first designates the metal by the name familiar to us.

A London chemist's advertisement (about 1680-1690) runs thus:

"Ambrose Godfrey Hanckwitz, chemist in London, Southampton Street, Convent Garden, continues faithfully to prepare all sorts of remedies, chemical and galenical. He hopes that his friends will continue their favours. Good cordials can be procured at his establishment, as well as Royal English drops, and other articles such as Powders of Kent, Zell, and Contrajerva, Cordial red powder, Gaskoins powder, with and without bezoar, English smelling salts, true Glaubers salt, Epsom salt, and volatile salt of ammonia, stronger than the former. Human skull and hartshorn, essence of Ambergris, volatile essence of lavender, musk and citron, essence of viper, essence for the hair, vulnerary balsam, commendeur, balsam for apoplexy, red spirit of purgative cochliaria, spirit of white cochliaria, and others. Honey water, lavender water of two kinds, Queen of Hungary water, orange flower water, arquebusade.

"For the information of the curious, he is the only one in London who makes inflammable phosphorus, which can be preserved in water. Phosphorus of Bolognian stone, flowers of phosphorus, black phosphorus, and that made with acid oil, and other varieties. All unadulterated. Every description of good drugs he sells, wholesale and retail."

The seventeenth century has been called the golden age of pharmacy, but the eighteenth century also was a great century for pharmacy, and pharmaceutists, as they were then usually called, played a very important part in the development of chemistry, which was beginning to emerge as a definite science with a worthy objective very different from that in sight at the close of the previous century.

In the eighteenth century the apothecaries became recognized medical practitioners, the Society granted medical diplomas, and a hundred years later (1815) they obtained an Act which gave them powers against other persons similar to those which the physicians thought they possessed against them.

In the course of the eighteenth century chemists and druggists had to a large extent replaced apothecaries as keepers of shops where medicines were sold and dispensed, and even when the businesses were owned by apothecaries, they usually styled themselves chemists and druggists.

400

SCHEELE, a Swedish apothecary, was perhaps the foremost investigator in the eighteenth century. Poor in purse and health, he worked with only such apparatus as he could manufacture with his own hands, and was forced to earn his livelihood as a druggist in an isolated town. Independently of Priestley, he discovered oxygen; independently of Rutherford, he discovered nitrogen; and he alone is the discoverer of chlorine and fluorine; besides his investigations of alum, ether and hydrogen sulphide, he devised methods of preparing phosphorus and calomel, discovered glycerin and barium oxide, and such acids as mucic, citric, gallic, mallic, oxalic, tartaric, and the terrible hydrocyanic, known to the public as prussic acid.

It has been said that more money has been expended upon his statute at Stockholm than the living Scheele saw during his glorious career.

ELIXIR PROPRIETATIS

"This medicine was very celebrated in all countries for several centuries, and, though not in the British Pharmacopoeia, was official under the name which Paracelsus gave it in the P.L. 1724, as Elixir of Aloes in the P.L. 1746, and later as Tinct. Aloes Co. In the Ph. Ed. it was called Tinct. Aloes et Myrrhae, and this was the most usual name for it until quite recent times, and probably is still. Paracelsus wrote about it and extolled it as a compound which would prolong life to its utmost limits. That he used the same ingredients mainly as his successors is certain, but he never gave any clear formula. His disciple, Oswald Crollius, however, deduced from his writings that it was a tincture of aloes, myrrh, and saffron, with sulphuric acid. Boerhaave substituted vinegar for the sulphuric acid and left most of that behind by distillation. Van Helmont had previously made an Elixir Proprietatis without any acid; and in many continental pharmacopoeias the elixir was made alkaline by the addition of carbonate of potash. This also originated with Boerhaave. Other authors added a few spices."

The first medicine to be actually patented in Great Britain was "Goddard's Drops."

The history of nineteenth century pharmacy is more difficult to write than that of any other period that has been considered. One reason is that we are closer to it and the task of selecting the salient features is increased in direct proportion to the wealth of material available.

JOSEPH PELLETIER (1788-1842) was the son of a Paris pharmacist, and was one of the most brilliant workers in pharmacy known to us. He is best known for his isolation of quinine. Either alone, or in association with others, he investigated the nature of ipecac, nux vomica, colchicum, cevadilla, hellebore, pepper, opium, and other drugs, and a long series of alkaloids is credited to him. He also contributed valuable researches on cochineal, santal, turmeric, and other coloring materials.

The advance in every section of chemistry during the nineteenth century, and especially during the latter half of it, has literally been by leaps and bounds. Although practically a creation of our own time, no branch has been more fruitful in result, in suggestion, or in possibility, than that of organic analysis.

Three great achievements characterize the pharmacy of the nineteenth century, namely, the discovery of alkaloids in its early years, of anesthetics in the middle period, and of synthetic organic products in its later years.

Iodine was discovered by Bernard Courtois in 1811. Iodoform was first prepared by Serullas about 1828. Lithium, the oxide of which was discovered in 1807 by Arfwedson, was first suggested as a remedy for gout by Dr. Ure in 1843.

The inauguration of synthetic chemistry is understood to date from the year 1828 when Wohler, then a professor of chemistry at Berlin, produced a supposed cyanate of ammonium by the action of ammonium chloride on silver cyanate.

402

A factor of outstanding importance in the nineteenth century, and which affected both pharmacy and medicine, was the appearance of synthetic remedial agents, the "products of the tar barrel," as they have been called. From the unsuccessful search for synthetic quinine which was conducted by Perkin in 1856, and which led to the discovery of the first coal tar dye called "mauve" or "Perkin's purple," came unexpected developments in the way of scientific research.

Many factors combined in the nineteenth century to bring about great changes in the practice of pharmacy. One of the earliest factors to appear was the introduction of machinery in the manufacture of drugs and the introduction of many elegant pharmaceutical products to supersede many of those whose chief virtue was often their vile smell and taste. The newer forms of medication that have become popular are pills, tablets, filled capsules and ampuls.

During the twentieth century legislation affecting pharmacy has been particularly rife. Many new drugs have been discovered that appear to be of lasting value. The manufacture of ready-to-use drugs in large laboratories has increased enormously. The isolation and preparation of vitamin and gland products has become an important field of pharmacy.

We are constantly in the midst of history in the making. With our perspective distorted by too close proximity we are usually unable to differentiate between what is historically important and what is not.

CHAPTER TWENTY-SIX

Pharmacy in America

THE ABORIGINES of America, the Aztecs, and the Incas, all had their combination of priest-prophet-physician-pharmacist.

In 1620 the Mayflower at Plymouth included among its passengers an apothecary, Giles Firmin.

The London Company sent two apothecaries to the Virginia Colony before 1624. After that we hear nothing of apothecaries in Virginia until the eighteenth century. Every bit of evidence points to the entire control by physicians of the drug business in the colony.

In the earliest years of the seventeenth century there were several apothecaries in the colony. Thomas Field and Thomas Harford came over with the first settlers, and Fitch and Townshend were apothecaries to John Pott. But by 1621 there was a great scarcity, as the following will show: "It was signified unto the Court that an Apothecary offered to transport himself and his wife at his own charge to Virginia if the Company would please to give them their transport of two children, the one being under the age of eight and the other a youth of good years: which offer the Court did very well like of in respect of the great want of men of his profession, and being put to the question did agree hereunto; provided that the Apothecary at his coming over did exercise his skill and practice in that profession."

In 1646 the first store devoted distinctly to pharmacy in Boston was opened by William Davies.

The first intimation of prescription writing in Virginia in the eighteenth century was William Stark's announcement in Petersburg in 1771 that prescriptions would be made in his shop "in the most elegant and accurate manner." The practice had probably become more general, at least in the cities, when J. K. Read advertised his new "medicinal store" in Norfolk in 1800, assuring the public that "prescriptions elegantly prepared under his own inspection" would be an important part of the business.

An item in the Virginia Gazette in 1737 gives us our earliest glimpse of the colonial Virginia drug business: "Just imported from London, A Parcel of Choice Medicines; which are to be sold at reasonable Rates, by Wholesale or Retail, at Mrs. Sullivan's in Williamsburg, by Thomas Goodwin, Chymist." A few weeks later another advertisement appeared: "All Sorts of Chymical and Galenical Medicines, faithfully prepared and Sold by Robert Davidson and Thomas Goodwin, chymists, at Williamsburg."

The first physician to make a practice of writing prescriptions in America was Abraham Chauvet, who came to Philadelphia in 1770. He was followed in that city by John Jones.

A PHARMACIST'S HANDBILL OF 1784

The brothers Whiting sold dry goods, groceries, and pharmaceutical supplies. The final note on the handbill is a commentary on the finance of the period. Cash payment only was accepted, but wood ashes served as tender, as did also many other marketable commodities. The ashes were used in the preparation of soft soap, the alkali being leached out of them.

Benjamin Franklin, born early in the eighteenth century, taking all fields of human endeavor into account, was the most richly endowed of all Americans. Without either wealth or influence, by sheer force of native ability, Franklin became one of the broadest and most versatile characters the world has ever seen.

Franklin had several interesting contacts with pharmacy. He is said to have sold drugs himself for a few years; it is known that as a printer he published a number of articles upon medical and other scientific subjects, and, as will be seen presently when we come to discuss American pharmacy in particular, he had a profound influence upon the development of both pharmacy and medicine by the aid and encouragement he gave to a young man named John Morgan, who later became prominent in both medicine and pharmacy.

However, Franklin made a mistake when at the age of sixteen he editorialized opposing the inoculation against smallpox.

Pharmacy as an independent profession did not receive the support of American physicians until after the Revolutionary War. At the Pennsylvania Hospital in 1754 were written the first prescriptions to be filled by an apothecary in the United States. John Morgan, who as a student in Europe had learned the advantages of the separation of the two professions, wrote: "I am now preparing for America, to see whether after fourteen years' devotion to medicine, I can get my living without turning apothecary or practitioner of surgery."

John Morgan (1735-1789), was born in Philadelphia. When the Pennsylvania Hospital opened its apothecary shop in 1755 Benjamin Franklin appointed Morgan as chief dispenser. Two years later he was graduated with the first class from the College of Philadelphia. After two years' study in Edinburg and Paris he returned to found America's first medical school in Philadelphia College, which later became the University of Pennsylvania. In 1821 the Philadelphia College organized the first college of pharmacy in the new world.

Dr. Morgan is said to have been the first man in Philadelphia to carry a silk umbrella. Dr. Morgan served with George

Washington in the French and Indian Wars as lieutenant and surgeon and was Physician-in-Chief of the Revolutionary Army. He had professional enemies and became the victim of false charges and political abuse. When the war ended and George Washington had time to review the charges, he exonerated Morgan of neglect or wrongdoing. Congress declared he had conducted himself ably and honestly. But the mischief was done. Morgan retired to private life, a heart-broken, grief-stricken man. He would sit for hours looking at a book without turning a leaf. When his wife died he lost all interest in life.

On October 15, 1789, he was found dead in a squalid house, on an untidy bed littered with books and papers.

* * *

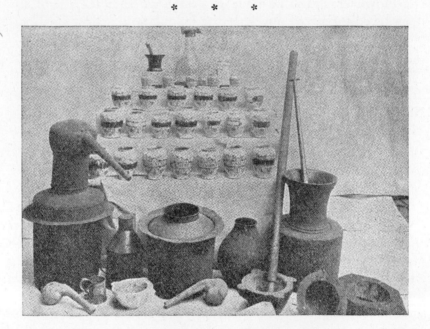

"AMERICA'S OLDEST PHARMACY"

The oldest pharmacy in America which has been in continuous operation was established in 1743 in the Moravian settlement at Bethlehem, Pennsylvania. "Die Apotheke," as it was early known, was seventh in order of founding, but is the sole survivor of those earlier shops. It was founded by Dr. J. F. Otto and has been operated by various owners up to the present time, now being owned by the R. A. Smith estate.

There is no picture extant of the original building. The picture on page 408 represents some of the original apparati.

*   *   *

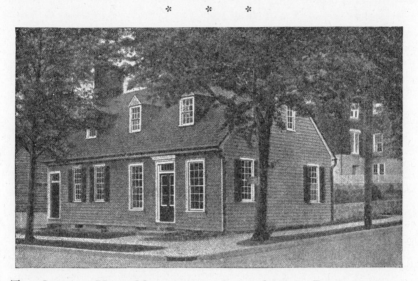

THE GENERAL HUGH MERCER APOTHECARY SHOP AT FREDERICKSBURG, VIRGINIA, ERECTED BEFORE 1771

This is not a restoration, but the original building that was used as an apothecary shop, office and dwelling, therefore, it is the oldest pharmacy building in America. The left door opens into the office which was used jointly by George Washington and Dr. Mercer. Washington's boyhood home was at Fredericksburg and he retained a large landed interest there. The building is now used as a museum.

Hugh Mercer (1725-1777), a young surgeon one year out of medical school, was among the Scots who fought in the battle of Culloden in 1745. After this disastrous battle Mercer came to America and settled at Greencastle, Pennsylvania. He served as an officer in the French and Indian Wars. At the age of thirty-five he put aside the profession of arms and moved to Fredericksburg, Virginia, where he set up an apothecary shop in a portion of his house and soon became the leading physician of the community. Mercer's fifteen years' residence in Fredericksburg terminated with the outbreak of the Revolution. He again took up the profession of arms. He became a brigadier-general and died Jan. 12, 1777, of wounds received on the 2nd of the same month near Princeton, New Jersey.

The deed to the historic apothecary shop of Hugh Mercer passed into the hands of the AMERICAN PHARMACEUTICAL ASSOCIATION, on February 28, 1941, and was formerly dedicated on April 30, 1941.

The Association acquired title to the property through the Friends of Historical Pharmacy, Inc., an organization created for the purpose of perpetuating this and other shrines of the profession. Officers of the organization: President, Wortley F. Rudd, Dean of the School of Pharmacy, Medical College of Virginia, Richmond; vice-president, Dr. Richard A. Deno, of the Rutgers University College of Pharmacy, Newark, N. J.; secretary and treasurer, Dr. E. F. Kelly, secretary of the American Pharmaceutical Association, Washington; members of the board of managers: W. B. F. Cole, Commonwealth's Attorney, Fredericksburg; Roger Clarke, of Fredericksburg; Charles H. Lewis, Fredericksburg pharmacist; and Robert W. Rodman, Editor of the Practical Pharmacy Edition of the Journal of the American Pharmaceutical Association, Washington. Every member of the American Pharmaceutical Association becomes a member of the Friends of Historical Pharmacy, Inc., automatically, and can feel that he has a part in the restoration and preservation of this and other pharmaceutical shrines.

Dr. Deno was made chairman of a committee to arrange details of the transfer of ownership. This involved the raising of sufficient funds to make necessary repairs and to provide for the maintenance of the shop on a self-sustaining basis.

Among the friends of the Association who responded to Dr. Deno's appeal for the necessary funds were Elmer H. Bobst, Bodeker Drug Co., Bristol-Myers Co., Turner F. Currens, Dr. H. A. B. Dunning, Emerson Drug Co., Henry B. Gilpin Co., Dr. J. Leon Lascoff, Eli Lilly, Dr. S. E. Massengill, National Association of Retail Druggists, Dr. E. L. Newcomb, Owens and Minor Drug Co., Parke, Davis & Co., S. B. Penick, G. A. Pfeiffer, Standard Drug Co., and the Virginia State Pharmaceutical Association.

* * *

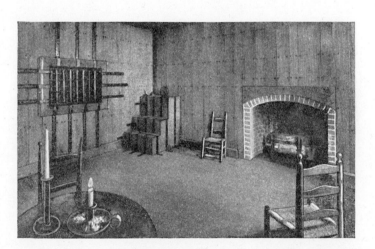

A RESTORATION OF THE GENERAL COURT PRISON
FOR DEBTORS AT WILLIAMSBURG, VIRGINIA

The Gaol was built about 1701 and about ten years later an addition was made containing cells such as these. The commode in the far corner, operated by water, was the first attempt at sanitation in America.

411

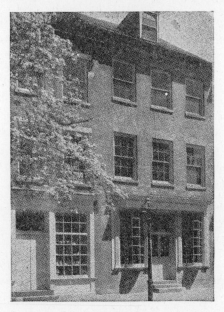

THE STABLER-LEADBETTER APOTHECARY SHOP,
ALEXANDRIA, VIRGINIA

The Stabler-Leadbetter Apothecary Shop founded in 1792, by Edward Stabler, before being converted into a museum, was the third oldest in America in continuous operation. It was owned and operated by the same family for 141 years. This unique drug shop is almost exactly as it appeared when George Washington, Robert E. Lee and other leading figures of Alexandria and Northern Virginia were regular patrons of this firm.

The documentary records retained here are extraordinary. One is from Mount Vernon, April 22, 1802:

"Mrs. Washington desires Mr. Stabler will send by the bearer A quart bottle of his best Castor Oil and the bill for it."

Daniel Webster, Henry Clay, John Calhoun and other early patriots are known to have engaged in the "drug store conversations" in this historic building.

412

Robert E. Lee was here to get his mail and chat with his friend, Mr. Leadbetter, when J. E. B. Stuart, later chief of cavalry under Lee, handed him the order from the War Department to proceed at once to Harper's Ferry to end the John Brown insurrection. The spot is marked where Lee stood at the time.

This Apothecary Shop, now conducted as a museum, is replete with a stock of ancient wares used by early Americans, including three items of the original order of 1792.

* * *

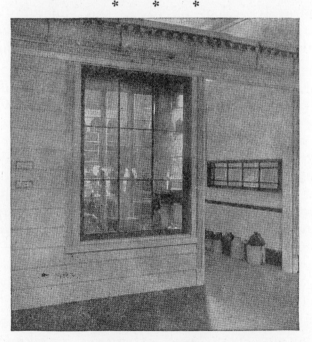

EXTERIOR OF APOTHECARIES' HALL AS INSTALLED
IN THE CHARLESTON, S. C., MUSEUM IN 1921

The museum presents the original room's proportions (17 x 17 ft.), which was the corner room of a private house in 1780. Nothing remains certainly identified as from the founder's time beyond the bits of antique chairboard and cor-

413

nice. Otherwise the interior woodwork goes back to 1816. The golden mortar and pestle (called by some, "De Big Yalluh Bucket"), which was raised in 1838, still hangs over the door of "Schwettmann's."

Apothecaries' Hall was founded in 1780 by Dr. Andrew Turnbull and has been in continuous operation since that time, being the second oldest drug store in America.

Dr. Turnbull was born and educated in Scotland, settled in Asia Minor, and became a distinguished medical practitioner. He married a wealthy Greek merchant's daughter, and with others planted a colony of Greeks and Minorcans at New Smyrna, Florida. There was an insurrection and armed strife among the Minorcans at the outbreak of the Revolution. Dr. Turnbull lost everything.

In May, 1781, during the British occupation, he came from St. Augustine to Charleston with his family, which was large, and a few servants, in great distress. But by his attainments and talent he soon rose to the front of his profession, and engaged in the business of a dispensing physician, prescribing, preparing, and dispensing medicines. Having taken no part on either side but to heal the sick, and having, during the early imprisonment of the Charleston exiles in St. Augustine, been enabled to show much kindness to their distress, he remained, unquestioned, a citizen at the close of the Revolution. He was one of the founders and charter-members of the Medical Society of South Carolina, was esteemed and respected by all who knew him, a kindly, friendly, courteous gentleman.

Apothecaries' Hall has been owned by a continuous line of prominent druggists. Much of interest in regard to this notable drug store may be found in the Charleston Museum.

BOND'S DRUG STORE, FREDERICKSBURG, VA.
(No Picture)

A drug store was opened at this location in 1791 by Dr. Elisha Hall with equipment which he had secured from the

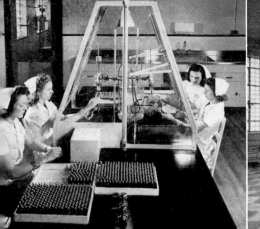
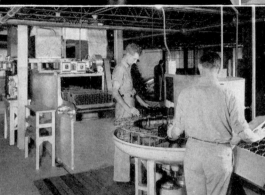
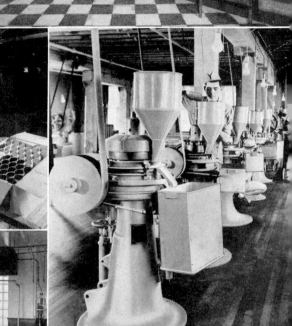
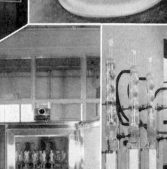
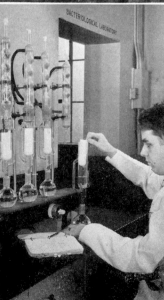

Actual scenes which show the manufacture of pharmaceutical products in the S. E. Massengill Company laboratories.

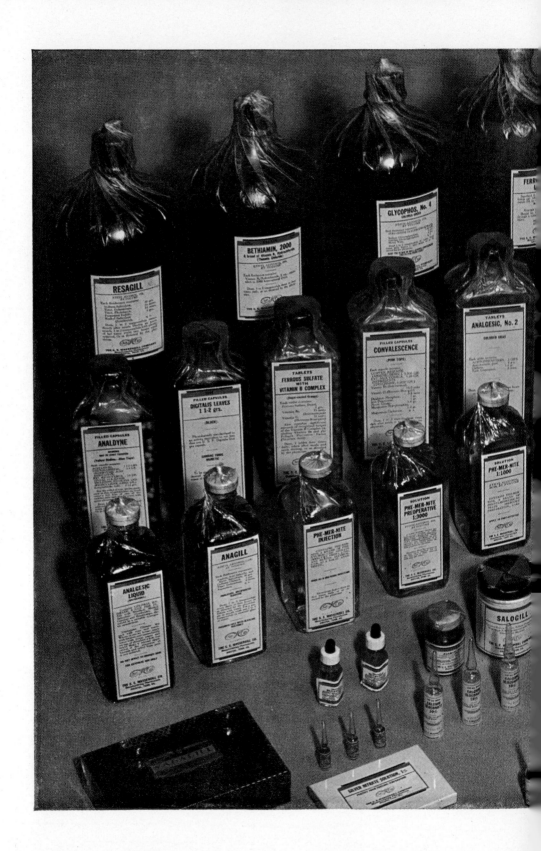

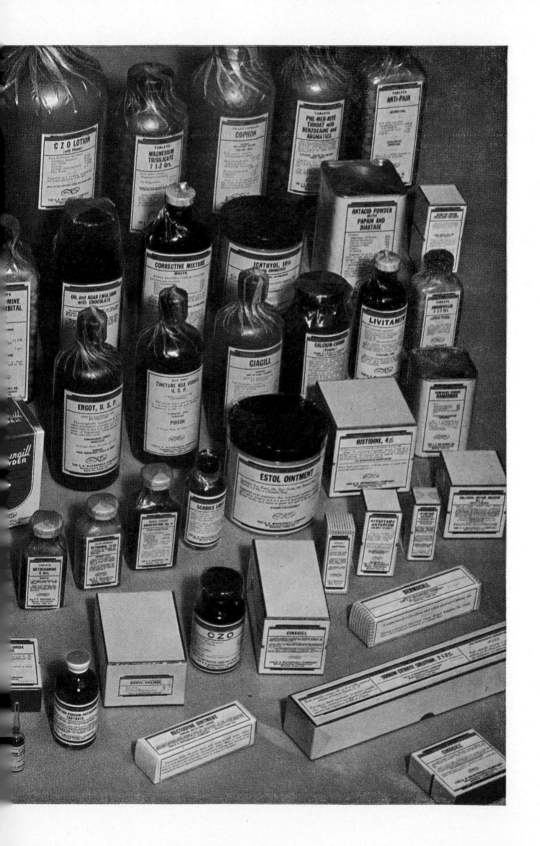

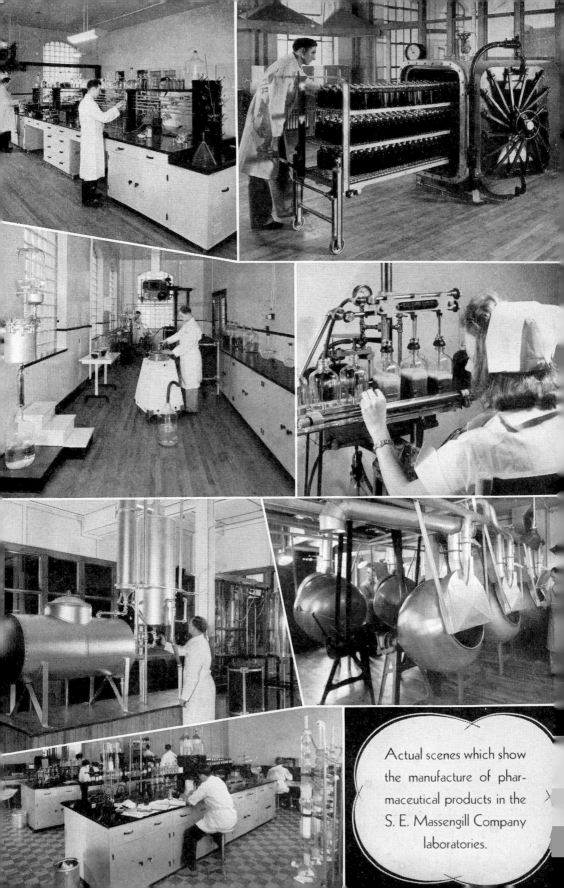

Actual scenes which show the manufacture of pharmaceutical products in the S. E. Massengill Company laboratories.

widow of Dr. Hugh Mercer. It is located a block away from the Mercer Apothecary Shop, which is now preserved as a national shrine. The original store remains the same, though an annex was later erected.

The second proprietor was John Byrd Hall and, following his death in 1862, the store was operated under the name of J. B. Hall's Sons. In 1907 the store passed from the founder's family to William L. Bond.

*   *   *

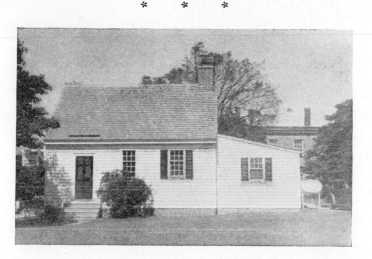

A RESTORATION OF THE 1769 APOTHECARY SHOP OF DR. CORBIN GRIFFIN, YORKTOWN, VIRGINIA

Dr. Griffin, a physician, had studied at the University of Edinburg in 1765 and was a man of culture and learning, not confining his lore, as was the custom of the day, to "blood-letting, calomel and cathartics." Dr. Griffin was an ardent patriot during the Revolution and served as a surgeon in the Virginia line.

The addition to the building was added recently and the building is now used as the post-office at Yorktown.

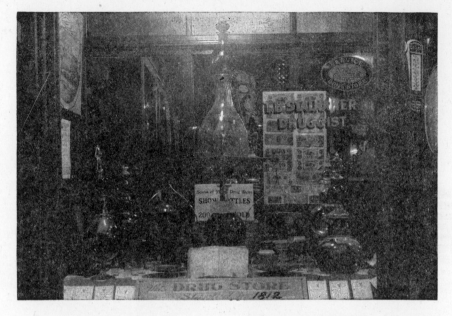

A VIEW OF THE SHOW BOTTLES AND SCALES THAT HAVE BEEN USED IN THE STALNAKER DRUG STORE, CHARLESTON, W. VA., FOR 120 YEARS.

When founded by Dr. Henry Rogers in 1812 it was the first store in Charleston. When Dr. Rogers died in 1837, ownership passed to his son, J. H. Rogers, and later to his grandson, J. A. Rogers.

T. B. Stalnaker purchased the business in 1909 and it is now operated as Stalnaker Drug Co., Inc.

The owners began a collection of historical documents and articles, which are now on display in the store. Visitors may also see a collection of rare show bottles, some of which Dr. Rogers brought from Williamsburg, Va., and some of which were purchased from Dr. Blair, the early proprietor of Blair's Drug Store, Richmond, Va.

Among the collection of old medical and pharmacy books is "The Anatomy of Humane Bodies," 1703.

Among the collection of old prescription bottles is found an early nursing bottle which sold for $1.50.

Henry Clay, Sam Houston and other notables were served in this store. * * *

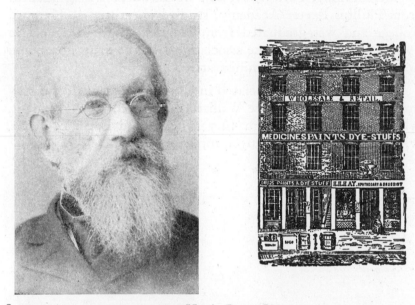

SHOWN AT RIGHT IS A CUT OF HAY'S DRUG STORE AS IT LOOKED WHEN 21-YEAR-OLD HENRY H. HAY FOUNDED IT IN 1841 AT PORTLAND, MAINE. AT THE LEFT IS A PORTRAIT OF THE FOUNDER.

Henry H. Hay, the founder, was the great-grandson of Dr. William Hay, a Scotch doctor who came to America in 1683. His father and grandfather also were physicians.

Edward Hay, youngest son of Henry, entered the business in 1885, and upon returning from the College of Pharmacy of Columbia University in 1887, soon after became a partner. In 1905 the business was incorporated and in 1907 Edward Hay became President and Treasurer, continuing as directing head of the organization ever since. He is one of the oldest Life Members of the American Pharmaceutical Association, and of the Alumni Association of the Class of '87, Columbia College of Pharmacy.

417

Hay's Drug Stores have occupied several locations and now consist of two stores that have been entirely modernized and streamlined in keeping with the times.

Merrill Hay, born 1901, son of Edward, was graduated from Phillips Exeter Academy, studied chemistry at Harvard College and was graduated from Harvard Business School in 1926. In 1930 he became associated with the drug stores, and now is active in their administration.

The other officers associated in the management of the Hay Stores for many years, are William A. Lowell, Vice-President, who started with the firm 40 years ago, and Isaiah E. Davis, who has been principal buyer for many years.

* * *

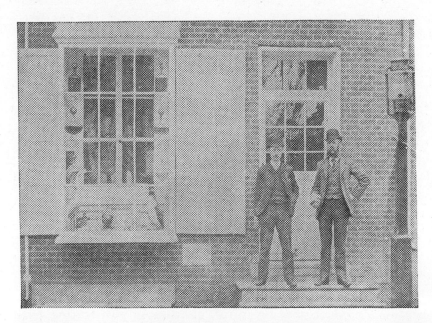

CARL'S DRUG STORE, GREENCASTLE, PENNSYLVANIA, AS IT APPEARED ABOUT 1880, THIS BEING THE EARLIEST PICTURE AVAILABLE. FOUNDED IN 1825 BY DR. ADAM CARL, AND OPERATED SINCE THAT TIME BY HIS DESCENDENTS. THE OLDEST CONTINUOUSLY-OPERATED DRUG STORE IN PENNSYLVANIA.

Dr. Adam Carl, the founder, was born at Hanover, Pennsylvania, December 16, 1800, and received his M.D. degree from the Washington Medical College, Baltimore, Maryland.

His medical practice covered a radius of thirty miles. Most calls had to be made on horse-back. Following the retreat from the battle of Gettysburg, Dr. Carl treated hundreds of the wounded soldiers. His office and store became a hospital for some time. He continued in active practice until one week before his death in April, 1891, at the age of 91 years.

William Carl, son of Dr. Adam Carl, took over the management about 1850, and Charles B. Carl, grandson of the founder, after having graduated from the Philadelphia College of Pharmacy in 1880, succeeded to the management.

Dr. Adam Carl continued to own the store until 1889, when it was purchased by his grandson, Charles B. Carl. The present owners are, John J. Carl and Edward R. Carl, sons of the late Chas. B. Carl, and great-grandsons of the founder.

The drug store "day book" for the year 1825 is still preserved. It contains many interesting items. It indicates that much material for the making of paints, dye-stuffs and many other now obsolete items were then staple drug store merchandise. In that year quinine was selling at 12 1-2 cents per grain.

Dr. Adam Carl's saddle-bags, medicine kits, etc., are preserved. Also many of the old iron mortars, show-globes and other drug store utensils of another day.

EXTRACTS FROM THE MASSENGILL MEMORIAL ERECTED BY SAMUEL EVANS MASSENGILL

Erected to the memory of Henry Massengill and his Pioneer Family.

Came from North Carolina to the Watauga settlement in 1769. His plantation near the mouth of Boone's Creek adjoined William Bean's, who was the first permanent white settler west of the Alleghany Mountains.

In 1775 was appointed to an office in the Watauga Association which adopted the first written constitution for the government of American-born freemen.

Built the Massengill House of Worship, 1777. Served two years as sheriff of Washington District. In 1778 was chairman of the committee of safety.

Served on the staff of Captain William Edmiston in General Shelby's Expedition against the Chickamauga Indians in 1779.

Furnished three sons to the Revolutionary Army.

THE MASSENGILL HOUSE OF WORSHIP

From the memoir of Henry Massengill:

"In April, 1777, Rev. Charles Cummings, a Presbyterian minister from Wolf Hills Settlement, came to Watauga and preached three days. We hailed his coming among us with great joy, for our souls were hungering and thirsting for spiritual nourishment. He urged the settlers to build a House of Worship, which we decided to do. I was to furnish logs, boards and all timbers needed to build a large house, with a section of benches in the back side for the Massengill and Cobb negroes, numbering at this time 151 souls. So these slaves can come out and be refreshed in body and soul. This house was completed by July, 1777, and was known as the Massengill

420

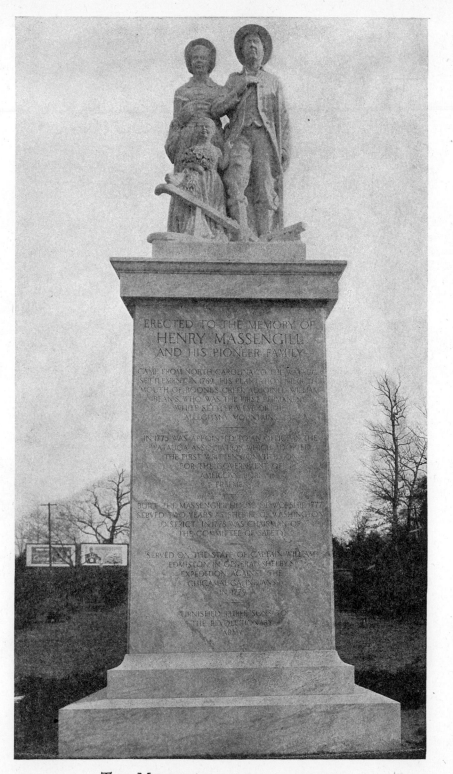

ERECTED TO THE MEMORY OF
HENRY MASSENGILL
AND HIS PIONEER FAMILY

CAME FROM NORTH CAROLINA TO THE WATAUGA
SETTLEMENT IN 1769. HIS PLANTATION NEAR THE
MOUTH OF BOONE'S CREEK ADJOINED WILLIAM
BEAN'S, WHO WAS THE FIRST PERMANENT
WHITE SETTLER WEST OF THE
ALLEGHANY MOUNTAINS

IN 1775 WAS APPOINTED TO AN OFFICE IN THE
WATAUGA ASSOCIATION WHICH ADOPTED
THE FIRST WRITTEN CONSTITUTION
FOR THE GOVERNMENT OF
AMERICAN-BORN
FREEMEN

BUILT THE MASSENGILL HOUSE OF WORSHIP 1777
SERVED TWO YEARS AS SHERIFF OF WASHINGTON
DISTRICT. IN 1785 WAS CHAIRMAN OF
THE COMMITTEE OF SAFETY

SERVED ON THE STAFF OF CAPTAIN WILLIAM
EDMISTON IN GENERAL SHELBY'S
EXPEDITION AGAINST THE
CHICAMAUGA INDIANS
IN 1779

FURNISHED THREE SONS TO
THE REVOLUTIONARY
ARMY

THE MASSENGILL FAMILY MEMORIAL

421

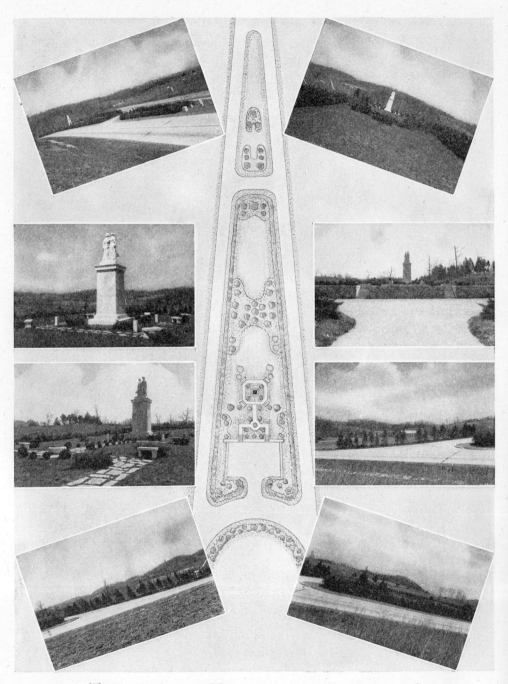

THE SITE OF THE MASSENGILL FAMILY MEMORIAL

House of Worship. Revs. Cummings and Mulkey preached several times to the settlers. I marched with Shelby against the Indians in 1779. While I was away Tories came, abused my family, destroyed my property, burnt the Massengill House of Worship to the ground."

* * *

William Cobb, a brother-in-law of Henry Massengill, closely followed him to the Watauga settlement. His residence, in connection with the surrounding forest, was used by Governor Blount in 1790, as the first capitol of a recognized government west of the Alleghany mountains.

From Ramsey's Annals of Tennessee:

"Mr. Cobb was a wealthy farmer, an emigrant from North Carolina. No stranger to comfort and taste nor unaccustomed to what for the day was style. Like the old Virginia and Carolina gentlemen he entertained elegantly with profusion rather than with plenty, without ceremony and without grudging. Like theirs, his house was plain, convenient without show. His equipage was simple and unpretending. He kept his horses, his dogs, his rifles, and even traps for the use, convenience and comfort of his guests. His servants, his rooms, his grounds were all at their bidding. They felt themselves at home and never said adieu to him or his family without the parting regret and the tenderness of an old friendship."

* * *

"Andrew Jackson, 7th President of the United States, was related to William Cobb's wife, and in 1788, while awaiting his license to practice law in Washington County, stayed at the William Cobb residence for six weeks and spent the time hunting and fishing."

423

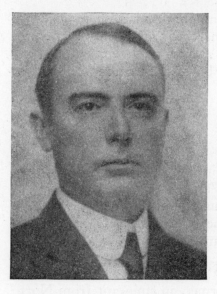
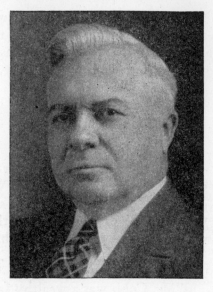

NORMAN HOOD MASSENGILL
(1869-1926)

SAMUEL EVANS MASSENGILL,
M. D.

FOUNDERS OF THE S. E. MASSENGILL COMPANY

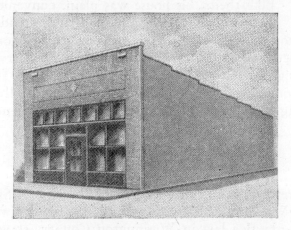

THE FIRST LABORATORY OF THE S. E. MASSENGILL
COMPANY, BRISTOL, VIRGINIA, 1899

424

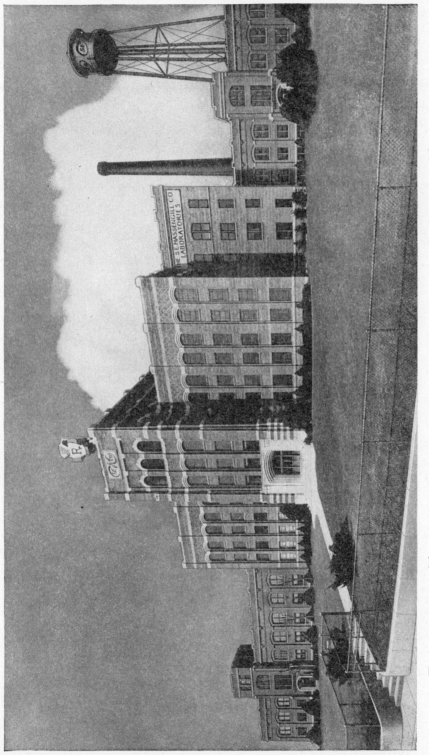

FRONT VIEW OF THE S. E. MASSENGILL COMPANY'S LABORATORIES, BRISTOL, TENNESSEE

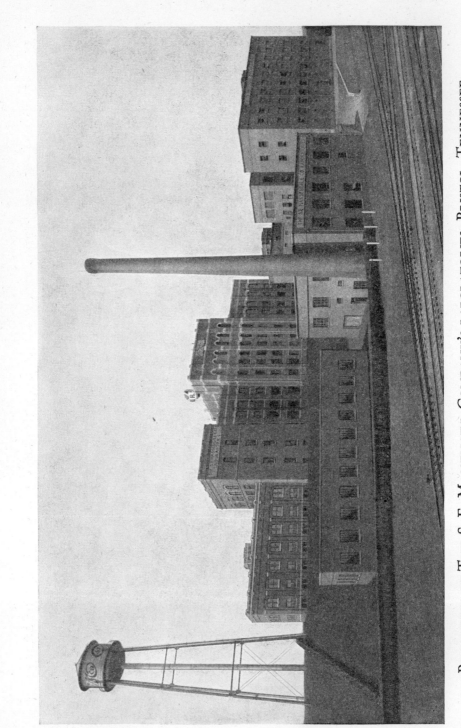

Rear view of The S. E. Massengill Company's Laboratories, Bristol, Tennessee

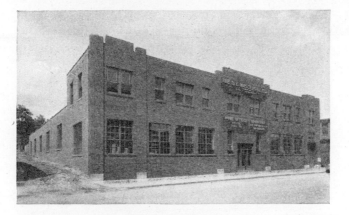

The S. E. Massengill Company, 208-214
W. Nineteenth Street, Kansas City, Mo.

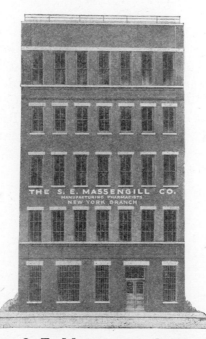

The S. E. Massengill Company,
59-61 Barrow Street, New York, N. Y.

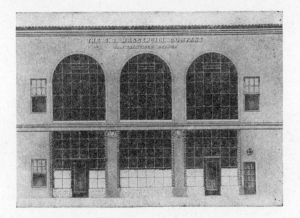

The S. E. Massengill Company, 240-244
Fourth Street, San Francisco, Calif.

Warehouses and offices of The S. E. Massengill Company are strategically located and carry over a million dollars worth of pharmaceutical products for immediate distribution to doctors and druggists in the United States. Agencies provide distribution in the following foreign countries: Cuba, Dominican Republic, Mexico, Nicaragua, Peru, Costa Rica, Guatemala, Panama, Colombia, Venezuela, Uruguay, Argentina, and Ecuador. Special representatives are located in Hawaii, T. H., Puerto Rico, and Alexandria, Egypt.

INDEX OF NAMES AND SUBJECTS